T0140630

Internet of Things Use Cases for the Healthcare Industry

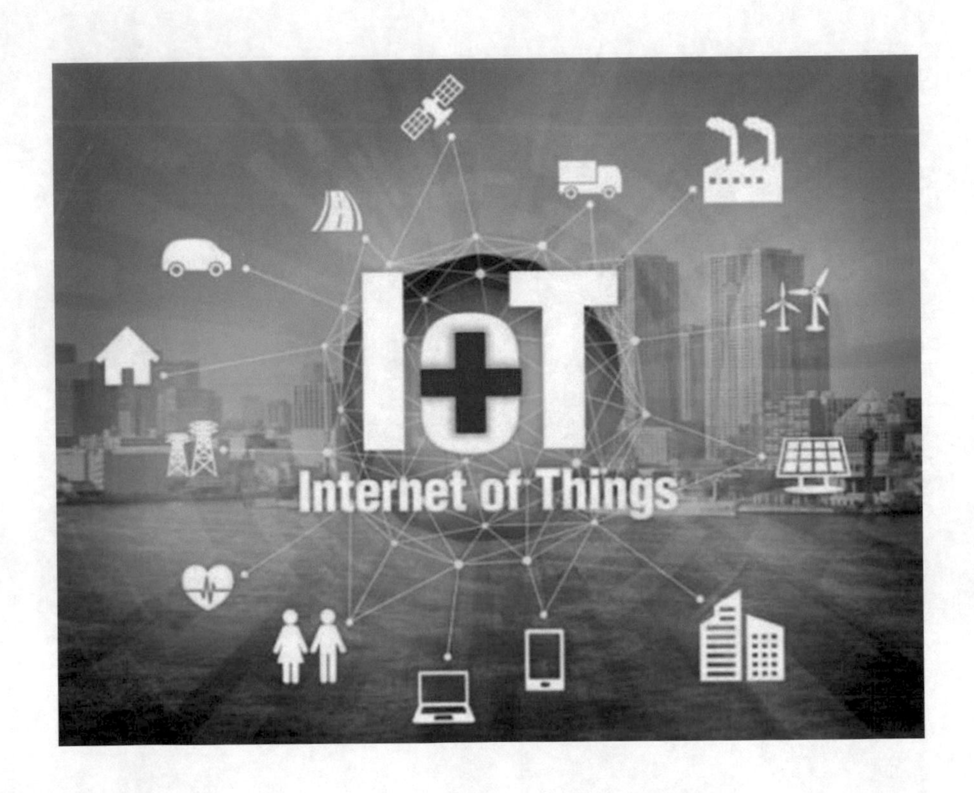
IoT
Internet of Things

Pethuru Raj · Jyotir Moy Chatterjee ·
Abhishek Kumar · B. Balamurugan
Editors

Internet of Things Use Cases for the Healthcare Industry

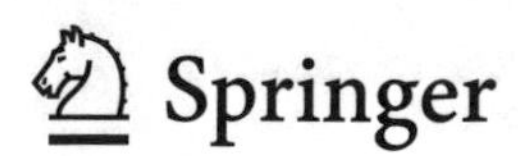

Editors
Pethuru Raj
Site Reliability Engineering (SRE) Division
Reliance Jio Infocomm Ltd. (RJIL)
Bangalore, India

Jyotir Moy Chatterjee
Lord Buddha Education Foundation
Kathmandu, Nepal

Abhishek Kumar
Computer Science & Engineering
Department
Chitkara University Institute of Engineering
and Technology
Chandigarh, Punjab, India

B. Balamurugan
School of Computer Science & Engineering
Galgotias University
Greater Noida, Uttar Pradesh, India

ISBN 978-3-030-37528-7 ISBN 978-3-030-37526-3 (eBook)
https://doi.org/10.1007/978-3-030-37526-3

This Springer imprint is published by the registered company Springer Nature Switzerland AG
The registered company address is: Gewerbestrasse 11, 6330 Cham, Switzerland

Preface

The utilization of the IoT in health care (the industry, personal health care, and healthcare installment applications) has forcefully expanded crosswise over different explicit Internet of Things use cases. Simultaneously we perceive how other healthcare IoT use cases are getting speed and the associated healthcare reality is quickening, regardless of whether obstacles remain. Up to this point, most IoT activities in health care rotated around the improvement of care all things considered with remote observing and telemonitoring as fundamental applications in the more extensive extent of telemedicine. A second region where numerous activities exist is following, checking and support of advantages, utilizing IoT and RFID. This is done on the degree of medical gadgets and healthcare resources, the individual's level and the nonmedical resource level (for example, medical clinic building resources). Be that as it may, these arrangements and use cases are only the start and, simultaneously, are a long way from inescapable. Further developed and incorporated methodologies inside the extent of the computerized change of health care are beginning to be utilized concerning health information angles where IoT assumes an expanding job, as it does in explicit applications, for example, smart pills, smart home care, personal health care, robotics, and Real-Time Health Systems (RTHS).

Inside the large associated health care and eHealth picture, increasingly coordinated methodologies and advantages are looked for with a job for the supposed Internet of Healthcare Things (IoHT) or Internet of Medical Things (IoMT). The period from 2017 until 2022 will be significant in this progress, with a few changes before 2020. From 2017 until 2022, development in IoT healthcare applications is to be sure ready to quicken as the Internet of Things is a key part in the advanced change of the healthcare business and different partners are increasing their determination.

The delectable advancements in the IoT space result in a staggering number of connected and embedded devices (resource-constrained as well as intensive). On other hand, the IoT paradigm leads to the realization of billions of digitized entities. Precisely speaking, our everyday environments are being stuffed with digitized systems and connected devices in order to produce self-, surroundings, and situation-aware applications. With flourishing of data analytics platforms, all kinds of IoT data are being consciously collected, cleansed, and crunched in order to extricate actionable insights in time. Thus, capturing data-driven insights and enabling insights-driven decisions, deals and deeds are seeing the grandiose reality with the bevy of improvisations and innovations in the Information and Communication Technologies (ICT) space.

Now, the healthcare sector is being blessed with a variety of devices, instruments, equipment, appliances, machineries, wares, toolsets, utensils, robots, highly integrated software solutions, data sources, etc. With extreme connectivity between the physical and the cyber worlds, hitherto unheard applications can be conceived and concretized. All kinds of healthcare data can be subjected to a variety of investigations in order to extract highly useful and usable intelligence in order to automate several manual tasks. Also, next-generation healthcare applications can become greatly intelligent through the integration with various knowledge discovery and dissemination tools. Thus, with the growing ecosystem of healthcare sensors and actuators, the ready formation of ad hoc and application-specific sensor and actuator networks, data capture, processing, storage and mining, the pioneering machine and deep learning algorithms, and other noteworthy advancements in the Artificial Intelligence (AI) and Ambient Intelligence (AmI) domains, the breakthroughs in the Internet of Things (IoT) and Cyber-Physical Systems (CPS) fields, the faster stability and maturity of mobile, social and edge computing models, etc. are to bring forth a litany of smarter and sophisticated applications in the healthcare domain. This book is being specially prepared with the aim of telling all about the forthcoming healthcare-specific use cases that are going to get realized through the disruptions and transformations happening in the IoT landscape.

Now, the healthcare sector is being blessed with a variety of devices, instruments, equipment, appliances, machineries, wares, toolsets, utensils, robots, highly integrated software solutions, data sources, etc. With extreme connectivity between the physical and the cyber worlds, hitherto unheard applications can be conceived and concretized. All kinds of healthcare data can be subjected to a variety of investigations in order to extract highly useful and usable intelligence in order to automate several manual tasks. Also, next-generation healthcare applications can become greatly intelligent through the integration with various knowledge discovery and dissemination tools. Thus, with the growing ecosystem of healthcare sensors and actuators, the ready formation of ad hoc and application-specific sensor and actuator networks, data capture, processing, storage, and mining, the pioneering machine and deep learning algorithms, and other noteworthy advancements in the Artificial Intelligence (AI) and Ambient Intelligence (AmI) domains, the breakthroughs in the Internet of Things (IoT) and Cyber-Physical Systems (CPS) fields, the faster stability and maturity of mobile, social and edge computing models, etc. are to bring forth a litany of smarter and sophisticated applications in the healthcare domain. This book is being specially prepared with the aim of telling all about the forthcoming healthcare-specific use cases that are going to get realized through the disruptions and transformations happening in the IoT landscape.

Bangalore, India	Pethuru Raj
Kathmandu, Nepal	Jyotir Moy Chatterjee
Punjab, India	Abhishek Kumar
Noida, India	B. Balamurugan

Contents

Contributors

A. Aymond University of North Dakota (UND), Grand Forks, ND, USA

F. Badrouchi University of North Dakota (UND), Grand Forks, ND, USA

S. Badrouchi University of Tunis EL Manar (UTM), Tunis, Tunisia

Heena Farooq Bhat Department of Computer Science, University of Kashmir, Srinagar, India

A. R. Charulatha Department of Computer Science, Stella Maris College, University of Madras, Chennai, India

Jyotir Moy Chatterjee Lord Buddha Education Foundation, Kathmandu, Nepal

Maitreyee Dutta Computer Science and Engineering Department, NITTTR-Chandigarh, Panjab University, Chandigarh, India

Sumathy Eswaran MGR Educational and Research Institute, Chennai, India

Shahnaz Fatima Amity University, Lucknow, Uttar Pradesh, India

E. GangaDevi Loyola College, Chennai, Tamil Nadu, India

M. Haerinia University of North Dakota (UND), Grand Forks, ND, USA

G. Jeya shree Department of Information Technology, Thiagarajar College of Engineering, Madurai, India

Deepa V. Jose Department of Computer Science, CHRIST (Deemed to be University), Bangalore, India

Latika Kharb Jagan Institute of Management Studies, Rohini, Delhi, India

M. Lawanya Shri School of Information Technology and Engineering, Vellore Institute of Technology, Vellore, India

S. Nathiya School of Information Technology & Engineering, Vellore Institute of Technology, Vellore, India

S. Padmavathi Department of Information Technology, Thiagarajar College of Engineering, Madurai, India

G. Priya School of Computer Science and Engineering, Vellore Institute of Technology, Vellore, India

P. Ranganathan University of North Dakota (UND), Grand Forks, ND, USA

Sudipendra Nath Roy Management Science, Ivey Business School, Western University, London, Canada

Jagriti Saini Electronics and Communication Engineering Department, NITTTR-Chandigarh, Panjab University, Chandigarh, India

D. F. Selvaraj University of North Dakota (UND), Grand Forks, ND, USA

Tuhin Sengupta Department of Information Technology and Operations Management, Goa Institute of Management, Goa, India;
Indian Institute of Management Indore, Indore, Madhya Pradesh, India

Junaid Latief Shah Department of Information Technology, Sri Pratap College, Cluster University Srinagar, Srinagar, India

Prateek Singh Jagan Institute of Management Studies, Rohini, Delhi, India

Rashbir Singh Department of Information Technology, Amity University, Noida, Uttar Pradesh, India

Sonia Singla University of Leicester, Leicester, UK

R. Sujatha School of Information Technology & Engineering, Vellore Institute of Technology, Vellore, India

K. Tavakolian University of North Dakota (UND), Grand Forks, ND, USA

Parul Verma Amity University, Lucknow, Uttar Pradesh, India

A. Vijayalakshmi Department of Computer Science, CHRIST (Deemed to be University), Bangalore, India

AI and IoT in Healthcare

Sonia Singla

Abstract The web of things has various applications in therapeutic organizations, from remote checking to sharp sensors and medicinal gadget blend. It can keep patients verified and sound, in any case, to improve how pros pass on thought also. Human organizations Internet of Things (IoT) can in like way help getting obligation and fulfilment by engaging patients to contribute greater imperativeness collaborating with their specialists. In any case, remedial organizations IoT is not without its impediments. The measure of related gadgets and the huge extent of information they collect can be a test for remedial focus IT to coordinate. Diabetes is an essential unending illness that effects in excess of 30 million individuals in the United States. The illness results from high blood (glucose) because of a fragility to appropriately get importance from sustenance, in a general sense as glucose. Insulin is a hormone that normally helps to process glucose in the body. Regardless, by ethicalness of diabetes, insulin is inadequate (Type 2 diabetes) or obsolete (Type 1 diabetes).

Keywords Diabetes mellitus · Cardiovascular disease · Mental illness · Artificial intelligence · Parkinson's diseases

1 Introduction

Man-made intelligence and the improvements above will alleviate many migraines of tasks and techniques in the medicinal field today. Medicinal experts have been battling with electronic well-being records (EHRs)—capacity techniques, safety efforts and access. Enormous information and AI will give an answer for each of the three of these issues.

Besides, AI can help with the analysis and treatment of patients, distinguishing ailment quicker and with better precision through the historical backdrop of a patient's EHRs. Through prescient examination, AI can glance back at a patient's past medicinal records and discovers designs that could recommend that the patient is made a beeline for a specific disease—like the recently referenced malignancy. Specialists can take this data and get them back on the correct way, keeping them

S. Singla (✉)
University of Leicester, Leicester, UK

P. Raj et al. (eds.), *Internet of Things Use Cases for the Healthcare Industry*,
https://doi.org/10.1007/978-3-030-37526-3_1

from the beginning of more things like a heart assault, diabetes and other hazardous diseases [1].

2 Role of AI in Diabetes

An expected 425 million individuals all around have diabetes, representing 12% of the world's well-being uses, but then 1 out of 2 people stay undiscovered and untreated. Utilizations of man-made consciousness (AI) and subjective registering offer guarantee in diabetes care. The motivation behind this chapter is to more readily comprehend what AI advances might be significant today to People With Diabetes (PWDs), their clinicians, family and guardians. The writers directed a predefined, online PubMed search of freely accessible wellsprings of data from 2009 forward utilizing the pursuit terms 'diabetes' and 'man-made reasoning'. The investigation included clinically significant, high-sway articles, and rejected articles whose design was specialized in nature. An aggregate of 450 distributed diabetes and AI articles met the consideration criteria. The investigations speak to various and complex arrangements of imaginative methodologies that intend to change diabetes care in four fundamental territories: mechanized retinal screening, clinical choice help, prescient populace chance stratification and patient self-administration apparatuses. Many of these new AI-controlled retinal imaging frameworks, prescient displaying programmes, glucose sensors, insulin siphons, cell phone applications and other choice helps are available today with additional in transit. Simulated intelligence applications can possibly change diabetes care and help a great many PWDs to accomplish better blood glucose control, diminish hypoglycaemics scenes, and decrease diabetes comorbidities and confusions. Artificial intelligence applications offer more noteworthy exactness, effectiveness, convenience and fulfilments for PWDs, their clinicians, family and guardians [2].

A key finding was the fruitful upgrades found in the inconstancy of individual postprandial and post-action glucose results, proposing that Sugar.IQ with AI learning may give a powerful, minimal effort technique for streamlining singular patient administration through customized experiences and commitment prompts, as per Dr. Neemuchwala.

Highlights of the Sugar-IQ application include the following:

Customized bits of knowledge that uncover time and day of practices identified with glucose levels connected to bolus requests, quick change in glucose levels, for example, post-insulin highs and lows, time-sensitive activities and supper substance designs.

- Inspirational signals to empower continued positive activities.
- Glucose prompts are made dependent on examples and sent to the showcase board.
- Brilliant sustenance log to make section of suppers and snacks simple and consistent.
- Stores past glucose measurements to educate future practices.

As indicated by patient criticism, while 80–85% of members enjoyed the prompts, full acknowledgment expanded after some time and introduction to the gadget input, achieving 100% by day 18.

The specialists showed that the key finding was less inconstancy in individual postprandial and post-action glucose results, recommending that the enhancements discovered after the utilization of the Sugar.IQ aide gave a viable technique to improving individual patient administration thought customized bits of knowledge and commitment prompts.

The application right now can keep running on iOS cell phones; applications for other cell phone stages are being developed. Furthermore, the Sugar.IQ application additionally will be incorporated into the Guardian Connect CGM framework (Medtronic) when it is propelled in towards the finish of the late spring 2018 [3].

Diabetes mellitus, for the most part known as diabetes, is a metabolic infection that causes high glucose. The hormone insulin moves sugar from the blood into your cells to be secured or used for essentialness. With diabetes, your body either does not make enough insulin or cannot satisfactorily use the insulin it makes.

Diabetes is the main source of death around the world. Absence of mindfulness and learning among urban and provincial zones is the fundamental driver of diabetes in India. Like in urban region, in rustic region, additionally, diabetes is expanding, i.e. two men and ladies are at high hazard for diabetes. Corpulence cases are expanding in men and subsequently sugar level is expanding and hazard to diabetes. It tends to be averted by doing work out, staying away from fat nourishment and desserts. Besides being limited to the standards of diabetes care in India, there is a specific prerequisite for a broad diabetes care programme which must be even more wide going. Essential diabetic thought should be all around accessible, regarding advancement and ability, to the comprehensive network and qualified to them at a sensible cost. To reduce repulsiveness and mortality on account of diabetes, conscious undertakings of experts practicing diabetes care, family specialists, individuals with diabetes, the comprehensive network, material affiliations and those blessed with general prosperity in India are a flat-out need. In context on the openings between the guidelines and real practice thus as to improve diabetes control in India, a reasonable method to manage and improve care about diabetes and its control both among patients and the remedial club is the desperate need vital. For the Indian subcontinent in like manner, the best-fit pertinence of thing and organization structure for patient-centred diabetes care might be overviewed and care levels among the diabetic patients might be extended to incorporate them in their treatment plans [3, 4].

Untreated high glucose from diabetes can hurt your nerves, eyes, kidneys and various organs.

There are two or three different sorts of diabetes:

Type 1 diabetes is an invulnerable framework illness. The safe structure attacks and pulverizes cells in the pancreas, where insulin is made. It is murky what causes this ambush. Around 10% of people with diabetes have this sort.

Type 2 diabetes happens when your body ends up impenetrable to insulin, and sugar is produced in your blood.

Prediabetes happens when your glucose is higher than commonplace, anyway it is not adequately high for an assurance of sort 2 diabetes.

Gestational diabetes is the presence of high amount of glucose during pregnancy. Insulin-blocking hormones made by the placenta cause this sort of diabetes [5].

The diabetes crisis in the United States cannot be overstated. The numbers are horrible: beginning at 2012, 29.1 million Americans, or 9.3% of the masses, had diabetes, and 86 million more were prediabetic.

All things considered, diabetes prompts in any occasion 243,000 passing's yearly, and type 1 and 2 diabetes record for a totalled yearly direct therapeutic cost of $176 billion in the United States, as it were, in view of diabetic perplexities and related crisis centre affirmations.

Crucial in turning away these affirmations and weakening bothers is control of blood glucose levels, evasion of unsafe lows (routinely implied as hypoglycaemic events).

While various relationships over all organizations are using AI to help comprehend the heavy slide of data made by the multitudinous number of devices accessible for use, the social protection division has a momentous opportunity to use AI for the most significant of causes: improving patient outcomes for people who experience the evil impacts of diabetes, and finally saving lives.

For an instance of how AI has been displayed to improve diabetes patients' outcomes, look not any more remote than a continuous observational starter held at the Diabetes Clinic in the Netherlands, one of Europe's driving diabetes offices.

The Diabetes Clinic's continuous observational starter used a system based over a self-streamlining AI organize. The structure, called Rhythm, gauges and regulates blood glucose measurements of people with diabetes, in perspective on non-prominent biometric sensors and AI.

By using modified blood glucose desire models that acclimated to all of the eight patients who checked out the observational starter, the experts controlling the primer found that in seven of the eight patients, the Rhythm system alone cultivated a 20% development in time in range and a 9% decline in unsafe lows—both key estimations for diabetes patients—appeared differently in relation to diabetes' starting at now suitable, high-contact approach.

The observational starter of Rhythm exhibited that the Diabetes Clinic had the alternative to not simply coordinate the blood glucose control results it as of late achieved through standard human checking, yet truly improve them. Thusly, expecting a motorized, AI-fuelled structure can improve—than the Diabetes Clinic's masters at controlling blood glucose levels, we should have the choice to achieve the office's low diabetes hospitalization rates inside the general open of diabetics.

Despite diminishing the amount of possibly fatal extreme scenes related to diabetes, this would result in $67 billion in yearly cost speculation reserves. Finally, extrapolating the results achieved by Rhythm over the general U.S. masses would astoundingly influence our overall population's prosperity [6, 7].

This starter not simply centres a way ahead for watching out for the stunning size of diabetes in the United States, it similarly plots how much the therapeutic administrations division—and patients in all cases—stay to get from man-made intellectual competence.

Believe it or not, the certification that AI advancement shows up in human administrations is provoking an impact of endeavour: plans to social protection related AI associations have been extending year over year since 2011, and financing jumped from $64 million out of 2013 to a colossal $358 million of each 2014 [8, 9].

There is an essential work to be done to improve the consequences of diabetes patients in the United States; anyway, AI has, in any occasion, huge potential to help with a noteworthy piece of the diligent work.

Everything considered, that is, the certifiable assurance of AI: to take the world-changing contemplations that the human character is prepared for envisioning and apply those musings at a scale that nobody, yet machines can reach [10].

Diabetes mellitus is a vital unending affliction, impacting up to 3% of the masses in the industrialized countries. Insulin-Dependent Diabetes Mellitus (IDDM) patients need exogenous insulin mixtures to oversee blood glucose assimilation, to turn away ketoacidosis and stupor-like state, and to lessen the peril of later life disproving bothers. It has been exhibited [11] that Intensive Insulin Therapy (IIT), including 3 to 4 mixtures reliably or the usage of subcutaneous insulin siphons, is the best strategy to adjust blood glucose, and along these lines to lessen or delay IDDM troubles; the extension in treatment organizing flightiness and in costs is the unquestionable drawback. IDDM the administrators consistently contain in visiting patients every 2/4 months; during these visits, the data beginning from home-checking are dismembered, to review the metabolic control achieved by the patients [12]. It has been maintained that the use of current advances of information developments and decision sincerely strong systems may improve cost-feasibility of IIT, by diminishing the amount of periodical control visits, while growing the patient/specialist correspondence rate. A couple of gadgets and cautioning systems for helpful game plan assessment are right now available, both on a well ordered and on a visit-by-visit premise [13], and for some of them the capacity of giving real decisions has been shown probably [11]. The exponential advancement in the availability and in the use of media transmission organizations pushes towards the blend of such instruments in a framework's organization condition, to give long-expel help to seeing, similarly as long-separate checking ability to the specialist [14]. The usage of fitting Artificial Intelligence (AI) techniques, for instance, data-based systems, intelligent data analysis and case-based reasoning, may overhaul the structure of the general organization: it ought to be possible to allow the customers abusing an insightful work territory for infrequent treatment evaluation and update [15].

By virtue of an appropriated structure, the nearness of an around the world, shared cosmology is fundamental to ensure the probability of correspondence between the building portions: the way of thinking goes about as the ordinary expressing to which all of the modules suggest while exchanging information, and is used to choose the direct of the whole system. The T-IDDM theory is secured in a learning base fabricated using an edge system [11] that reinforces diverse heritage and made spaces.

It is dealt with into logical orders, which depict substances (for instance, patients explore office regards), events (for instance, checking data estimations), reflections (for instance, hyperglycaemia), drugs, accommodating shows and so forth. Since spaces are created, we in like manner expected to define a chain of significance of classes addressing types (for instance, the class of numerical characteristics and the one of fixed-length-string regards). Types are theoretical classes: no events are produced using them; anyway, they are used to store information required by the case openings. The database was used essentially as a conclusive instrument, to depict the space theory, while we misuse a social database to manage the certifiable data. The structure of the database tables, similarly as the bearings to store and recuperate the data, is created normally dependent on the cosmology information. A SQL interface, prepared to get the request steered to the database, besides, to re-establish the ensuing data, ensures the correspondence between the customer and the data file [15].

The data accumulated by patients during home-watching and sent through the PU-MU affiliation are time-ventured and acquired a couple of times (from three to four) multi-day. To allow a suitable comprehension of the data, we have subdivided the 24 h ordinary length into a great deal of successive non-covering time cuts, concentrated on the period of dinners or insulin implantations; each datum is from this time forward identified with a given time cut. The MU mishandles the home-checking information through a great deal of mechanical assemblies to picture and to separate accumulated data. Data examination ranges from a great deal of real systems, for instance, the extraction of the step-by-step ordinary estimation of Blood Glucose Level (BGL), the step-by-step insulin need and the amount [16, 17].

Way of life and Daily-Life Support in Diabetes Management Lifestyle the executives is a crucial part of diabetes care. Inactive living, stress, non-adherence to drug, absence of customary medical examinations and negative behaviour patterns can prompt cessation of treatment for patients with diabetes. From the season of determination, patients are required to advance their lifestyles to manage complications and other comorbid conditions, with the general objective of improving their own care. Current advancements and information distribution centres enable solutions that model information and settle on quality choices dependent on them. Choice emotionally supportive networks (DSSs) comprise of tools concentrated on helping patients or specialists to oversee diabetes treatments. These frameworks for the most part have checking highlights that encourage precise account of data about eating routine, PA, prescription, glucose estimations and so on, and join it with instruments to help the two patients and clinicians, with the general objective of upgrading remedial results. Multiple investigations went for creating DSSs to oversee diabetes have been proposed since 2010. One of the most productive approaches is the METABO venture. This task involves monitoring and advanced highlights including devices to counteract future journeys, progressively enhance care pathways, remove designs via knowledge discovery and guide health improvement plans. The creators directed a few pilot trials, including usability tests in 36 T1D patients. The MOSAIC project, another significant project, is concentrated on the improvement of a DSS for T2D the executives, with a unique spotlight on the hazard evaluation of related intricacies utilizing information mining techniques. Another everyday life emotionally supportive network has progressed tools, such as a recommender framework that utilizes CBR and an integrated BG forecast apparatus dependent on developmental calculation. As of late, Everett et al. presented a DSS utilizing AI to elevate adherence to physical activity and weight decrease. Creators approved the framework with 55 patients with prediabetes. Previously, Yom-Tov et al. proposed a DSS dependent on an RL algorithm that consequently sends messages to patients who are following a customized arrangement for physical exercise. The methodology was approved in stationary T2D patients. Daily-life emotionally supportive networks using AI devices for GDM were additionally examined. A weight the executive's proposal was introduced in the MediClass system. The system, which depends on the use of a characteristic language preparing (NLP) algorithm, was approved during the postpartum visits of 600 GDM patients. Rigla et al. also explored devices for GDM patients. They proposed a versatile application dependent on an AI-enlarged telemedicine DSS as a device for aiding GDM patients. Later, they introduced a platform to remotely assess patients utilizing a classifier dependent on a grouping calculation and a DT learning calculation. The system was evaluated in 90 GDM patients. The results showed a decrease in the time devoted by clinicians to patients and in face-to-confront visits per patient. Six different investigations have proposed options in contrast to the manual formation of patient care work processes. The studies offer support for the structure and sending of diabetes the board conventions, just as approaches to consistently improve patient tracking all through the whole procedure. Cleveringa et al. presented a framework for diminishing cardiovascular danger of T2D patients by optimizing patient care work processes. The creators approved their framework by administering polls to 3391 T2D patients. Mill operator et al. used an AI way to deal with concentrate data from drug medicines from electronic well-being record (EHR) information and distinguish elements related with patient consideration stream deviations. Another DSS with consideration stream apparatuses was displayed in the work of Al-Otaibi et al. This system focuses on the administration of T2D patients utilizing progressed features, such as modernized cautions and updates. It was tried in 20 T2D patients for a half-year, and resulted in diminished HbA1c levels and improved diabetes mindfulness. Fernandez-Llatas et al. proposed utilizing information mining techniques to empower the dynamic plan of consideration conventions, however, featured the requirement for instruments to decrease the Spaghetti Effect and make DSSs usable by specialists. Contreras et al. developed a diabetes management system to coordinate a progression of AI models and devices with a motor to oversee diabetes patient care streams. At last, Suh et al. proposed a dynamic consideration stream framework that connected information grouping together with rule mining methods to organize required client tasks. Other devices have been proposed for improving daily-life support for diabetes treatments. Four different instruments have been intended to investigate online dialogue discussions and social systems to remove pertinent information. First, grieves et al. compared various AI methods (DT, SVM, bagging, and Bayes) to analyse patients' online comments with the point of predicting patient assessment of hospital execution. Second, Valdez et al. propose a k-implies clustering analysis to distinguish correspondence designs both on and off

Facebook. They validated their device in a cohort of 700 T2D patients. Third, Chen et al. proposed bunching dependent on continued bisecting k-means with the objective of obtaining patient experience data, including enthusiastic and transient parts of diabetes the board. At long last, Hamon et al. proposed utilizing NLP strategies to extricate data about patients' expertise in overseeing diabetes [18].

3 AI in Cardiovascular

The impact of high peril leads by diabetes, hypertension, smoking between the age of 35 and 70 and nonappearance of treatment is critical explanation behind death in India [19, 20].

Within the near future, man-made mental aptitude (AI) frameworks, for instance, AI, significant learning and abstract enrolling, may accept a fundamental occupation in the improvement of cardiovascular (CV) medicine to support exact CV solution. CV clinical thought starting at now faces down to earth challenges identifying with cost diminishes in shirking and treatment, insignificant exertion sufficiency, overutilization, lacking patient thought, and high readmission and passing rates. Productive associations among specialists and data analysts are relied upon to engage clinically significant modernized and judicious data assessment. Until this point in time, colossal data, for instance, 'omics' data, human gut microbiome sequencing, online life and cardiovascular imaging, are exorbitantly enormous and heterogeneous, and change too quickly, to be secured, analysed and used. Re-enacted insight can mishandle huge data and be used in front line relentless thought. For sure, Cardiovascular Disorders (CVDs) are unusual and heterogeneous in nature, as they are realized by various genetic, biological (e.g. air pollution) and lead factors (e.g. diet and gut microbiome). At present, much more movements ought to be made to envision results definitely and feasibly, instead of looking over a direct score structure or standard CV chance components [13, 21].

Man-caused insight frameworks have been associated with cardiovascular medication to explore novel genotypes and phenotypes in existing afflictions, improve the idea of patient thought, enable cost-practicality, and decline readmission and passing rates. Over the earlier decade, a couple of AI strategies have been used for cardiovascular contamination examination and gauge. Each issue requires some degree of appreciation of the issue, the extent that cardiovascular medicine and estimations, to apply the perfect AI count. Within the near future, AI will bring about an adjustment in context towards precision cardiovascular prescription. The ability of AI in cardiovascular medicine is tremendous; regardless, negligence of the challenges may overshadow its potential clinical effect [22].

The presentation of such computerized innovations as automated inserts, home-checking gadgets, wearable sensors and portable applications in social insurance has created critical measures of information, which should be deciphered and operationalised by doctors and human services frameworks crosswise over different fields.

Most frequently, such advances are executed at the patient level, with patients turning into their own makers and customers of individual information, something which prompts them requesting progressively customized care.

This computerized change has prompted a move away from a 'top-down' information of the board technique, 'which involved either manual section of information with its characteristic impediments of exactness and fulfilment, trailed by information investigation with moderately essential measurable instruments... and frequently without authoritative responses to the clinical inquiries posited'. We are currently in a period of a 'base up' information of the executives methodology that includes constant information extraction from different sources (counting applications, wearables, emergency clinic frameworks and so on.), change of that information into a uniform configuration and stacking of the information into a logical framework for last analysis.

Each one of this information, be that as it may, represents a genuine test for doctors: the test of boundless decision. As indicated by a white paper by Stanford Medicine, 'the sheer volume of social insurance information is developing at a galactic rate: 153 exabytes (one exabyte = one billion gigabytes) were created in 2013 and an expected 2,314 exabytes will be delivered in 2020, meaning a general rate of increment at any rate 48% every year'. With such a great amount of information on the day-by-day choices of a large number of patients about their physical action, dietary admission, drug adherence and self-checking (for example, circulatory strain, weight), to give some examples, doctors are at a misfortune with respect to which information to concentrate on, to scan for what and for which wanted result?

Expanded information stockpiling, high registering force and exponential learning abilities together empower PCs to adapt a lot quicker than people and address the test of boundless decision. Man-made consciousness (AI) is the advancement of wise frameworks, equipped for taking 'the most ideal activity in an offered situation' To grow such savvy frameworks, AI calculations are required to empower dynamic learning abilities in connection to evolving conditions. AI takes various structures and is related with a wide range of ways of thinking, including reasoning, brain research and rationale (with learning calculations dependent on reverse finding), neuroscience and material science (with learning calculations dependent on backpropagation), hereditary qualities and developmental science (with learning calculations dependent on hereditary programming), insights (with learning calculations dependent on Bayesian surmising) and scientific advancement (with learning calculations dependent on help vector machine). Each of these ways of thinking can apply their learning calculations for various issues. Be that as it may, none of these calculations are flawless in tackling every single imaginable issue and none have achieved a degree of 'superintelligence' that will almost certainly anticipate, analyse and give suggestions for treating complex ailments. In any case, when capability joined—and gave they are encouraged the suitable information to gain from—these calculations can produce what has been known as an 'ace calculation', which could possibly tackle substantially more mind-boggling issues than people can.

AI can decidedly affect cardiovascular sickness forecast and finding by creating calculations that can demonstrate portrayals of information, a lot quicker and more effectively than doctors can. For instance, at present, a doctor who wishes to foresee the readmission of a patient with congestive heart disappointment needs to screen a huge, however, unstructured electronic well-being record (EHR) dataset, which incorporates factors, for example, the International Classification of Diseases (ICD) charging codes, drug remedies, research centre qualities, physiological estimations, imaging studies and experience notes. Such a dataset makes it very hard to choose from the earlier which factors ought to be incorporated into a prescient model and what sort of strategies ought to be connected in the model itself.

Such prescient models can be delivered with 'managed learning' calculations that require a dataset with indicator factors and named outcomes. For instance, an ongoing report examined the prescient estimation of an AI calculation that 'consolidates spot following echocardiographic information for computerized separation of Hypertrophic Cardiomyopathy (HCM) from physiological hypertrophy seen in athletes'. The investigation's outcomes demonstrated a positive effect of AI calculations in aiding 'the segregation of physiological versus neurotic examples of hypertrophic renovating… for robotized translation of echocardiographic pictures, which may help beginner perusers with constrained experience'.

A different arrangement of calculations utilized in cardiology is called 'solo learning' calculations, which spotlight on finding shrouded structures in a dataset by investigating connections between various variables. For instance, one examination researched the utilization of such learning calculations to recognize worldly relations among occasions in EHR; these fleeting relations were then inspected to survey whether they improved model execution in anticipating beginning conclusion of heart failure. Thus, results from unaided learning calculations can nourish into regulated learning calculations for prescient demonstrating.

A third arrangement of calculations is support learning calculations, which 'learn conduct through experimentation given just information and a result to optimize'. Designing unique treatment regimens, for example, dealing with the rates of re-intubation and directing physiological soundness in escalated care units, is one territory where the utilization of fortification learning calculations may hold extraordinary potential. For what reason Does Cardiology Need Artificial Intelligence? [21]

Man-made intelligence developed because progressively commonplace calculations can regularly be enhanced for certifiable assignments. Think about the instance of strategic relapse. To empower measurable deduction, for example, estimation of coefficients and, this model requires various solid suspicions (e.g. autonomy of perceptions and no multicollinearity among factors). At the point when calculated relapse is utilized for different purposes, the presumptions that empower measurable derivation might be random to the objective and can prevent the model's presentation. Conversely, AI calculations are commonly utilized without making the same number of suppositions of the hidden information. Although this methodology prevents the likelihood for customary factual surmising, it brings about calculations that by and large are increasingly exact for expectation and grouping. In this manner, cardiovascular medication can profit by the consolidation of AI and AI [13].

3.1 Profound Learning in Cardiology

As opposed to other innovative fields, profound learning in social insurance is as yet creating, and its applications hitherto to cardiology are fairly constrained. The most punctual business utilizations of profound learning were for PC vision or the computational investigation of pictures. Also, many of the underlying biomedical utilizations of AI have been in the space of picture handling. For instance, Gulshan et al. bridled a CNN to identify diabetic retinopathy from a database of 128,00 retinal pictures. These examiners got an affectability of 97.5% and explicitness of 96.1% when contrasted and a best quality level arrangement by 7 to 8 ophthalmologists. Esteva et al. utilized a CNN on 129,000 of dermatological injuries to order whether the injury was a kind of seborrheic keratosis versus a keratinocyte carcinoma or a kind-hearted nevus versus a threatening melanoma. This gathering found that their CNN performed about just as a board of 21 board-guaranteed dermatologists. Critically, these two papers show a significant downside of profound learning: it takes a gigantic measure of information to prepare a profound learning model due to the tremendous number of parameters that must be assessed. The cost and trouble of procuring biomedical information contrasted and different fields are restricting components for the use of AI in certain conditions.

Regardless of its beginning, profound learning connected to the area of cardiology indicates extraordinary potential. For instance, in 2016, resident researchers took part in the Second Annual Kaggle Data Science Bowl, 'Changing How We Diagnose Heart Disease'. The bowl moved researchers to make a strategy to quantify end-systolic and end-diastolic volumes in cardiovascular attractive reverberation pictures from excess of 1,000 patients consequently. The top-performing group had no earlier foundation in drug. They were information researchers who worked for a money-related foundation. What's more, towards the start of 2016, the principal paper was distributed applying CNNs for electrocardiographic inconsistency location [23]. The strategy comprised of a two-arrange learning process, first, finding a suitable element portrayal for every patient and afterwards utilizing the main educated highlights for peculiarity identification at later time focuses for a similar patient.

Abdolmanafi et al. [24] utilized a CNN called AlexNet to arrange coronary vein optical soundness tomography pictures in Kawasaki infection consequently. In a case of noncomputer vision-based neural system, Choi et al. [19] utilized an RNN to anticipate heart disappointment analysis from EHRs. Their RNN possibly humbly beaten other AI calculations when utilizing a year of EHR information. At the point when these specialists extended their dataset to incorporate an additional half-year of information, their model beats other AI calculations. Quite, as a feature of this work, Choi et al. [19] built up a creative technique to incorporate fleeting sequencing as a major aspect of the neural system [13].

4 AI in Mental Well-Being

Schizophrenia is an authentic and profound established neurodevelopmental issue that impacts how an individual considers, feels and continues.

'Negative' signs insinuate social withdrawal, inconvenience showing up or inconvenience working consistently. People with contrary reactions may require help with standard errands. Negative appearances include

- Talking in a dull voice.
- Appearing outward appearance, for instance, a smile or glare.
- Having inconvenience experiencing fulfilment.
- Having inconvenience organizing and remaining with a development, for instance, looking for sustenance.
- Talking by no to different people, despite when it is huge.

These signs are more truly to see as a component of schizophrenia and can be mistaken for wretchedness or various conditions [11, 14].

4.1 Emotional Symptoms

Emotional symptoms are hard to see; be that as it may, they can make it hard for people to have a work or manage themselves. The element of mental limit is a champion among the best markers of a person's ability to improve how they work. Much of the time, these reactions are perceived exactly when unequivocal tests are performed. Emotional reactions incorporate the following [25]:

- Trouble planning information to choose.
- Issues using information following learning it.
- Inconvenience centring.

The utilization of significant learning with solo features for enormous data examination holds important potential for perceiving novel genotypes and phenotypes in heterogeneous CV infirmities, for instance, Brugada issue, HFpEF, Takotsubo cardiomyopathy, white-coat hypertension, HTN, pneumonic hypertension, familial AF and metabolic issue. Additionally, the improvement of AI application and precision drug stages will energize precision CV solution. Afterwards, abstract PCs, for instance, IBM Watson, will be standard in social protection workplaces and help specialists with their essential administration and desire for patient outcomes. Various development associations, for instance, IBM, Apple and Google, are placing strongly in human administration assessments to energize precision medicate. We believe that AI will not supersede specialists; be that as it may, it is noteworthy that specialists acknowledge how to use AI satisfactorily to deliver their hypotheses, perform colossal data examination and streamline AI applications in clinical practice to assist the time of exactness CV tranquilize. Regardless, carelessness of the challenges of AI may rule the impact of AI on CV prescription. Artificial intelligence, significant learning and mental preparing are promising and can change how medication is penetrated, yet specialists ought to be set up for the best in class AI period [26].

Diminish Trainor is the kindred advocate of US AI, an item architect having some ability in man-made awareness. Trainor and his gathering have made SU, which he calls an 'add-on bot' that could continue running in existing talk applications, for instance, Facebook Messenger and Twitter Direct Messages. 'Various mental prosperity philanthropies or social occasions starting at now have a kind of assistance instrument on their destinations', Trainor explains. 'SU can be snared onto these instruments to help recognize "trigger" words or articulations, which can alert the master on the furthest edge and after that triage a reaction or offer up substance and associations. SU has been set up to see "desire", and it utilizes AI to organize language against different conditions or conditions'.

SU, due to dispatch 1 year from now, is being made using direction from the Campaign Against Living Miserably (CALM). 'Specifically', Trainor says, 'SU scans for lost reason; that could be a business mishap or a partition, for example. Troublesome tongue is furthermore hailed, for example when someone feels that their family would be in a perfect circumstance without them'.

SU, Trainor says, is being made considering the 'shocking' inescapability of male suicide. 'Suicide is the best foe of men developed under 45. Suicide can happen so quickly, so the idea is to use AI to recognize those crises demonstrates and stall out in a shocking circumstance essentially quicker. Reckless ideation may make over some unclear time allotment, anyway when someone contacts a consideration gathering like CALM, the showing itself can happen in only minutes, so driving someone up in a line of calls could be a life saver'.

Similarly, as seeing emergency conditions, SU can in like manner be used to go-to individuals towards master help. 'SU jumps on watchwords, so if the program on a charity's visit mechanical assembly, for example, made sense of how to perceive that an individual was ex-military and encountering PTSD, by then it could control them to an ace magnanimity that dealt with that, like Help for Heroes'.

Dr. Paul Tiffin and Dr. Lewis Paton, both division of prosperity sciences at the University of York, starting late drove an assessment into the odds and troubles related with using automated thinking to treat mental prosperity issues. Paton says development can 'increase access to mental assistance', and that 'guided personal growth is an earlier framework for treating mental prosperity issues'. Where this as of late included using books and exercises, Paton perceives that applications made responsive by AI 'may be better than tolerating no treatment in any way shape or form'. He raises, regardless, that 'motorized and online medications do will when all is said in done have higher dropout rates diverged from those that incorporate a human'.

What precisely degree can a machine's bits of learning into mental health genuinely be trusted? Tiffin says that since clinicians 'much of the time need to override a computerized decision', machines are 'saw even more unfavourably for submitting mistakes' than individuals are. The precision of a machine's encounters, he says, depends upon the points of reference the system has been set up to get it. 'There are well-seen conditions where counts have wound up being uneven as a result of the general population that gave the arrangement data'.

Given the wide range and complexities of mental prosperity conditions, the openness of good getting ready data could be an important issue for any fashioner of this development. 'Medications subject to social measures, those that urge people to put more vitality in activities they find pleasurable just as satisfying', Tiffin says, 'advance themselves to robotization. That is because they are commonly unsophisticated and rely upon "right here and now"'. However, medications that 'incorporate delving into the patient's past in order to fathom their present inconveniences would be generously harder for an erroneously keen system to ever duplicate'.

Paton believes the whole deal occupation of AI in treating mental well-being issues should incorporate a 'blend of both real and phony consultants' time'. While there is apparently an understanding over the passionate well-being system that distinctive issues snappier would be useful, there remain inquiries over the advancement's ability to isolate between signs, to break down and to copy the compassion that patients regard in human educators. Holly says her experience of Woebot and proposes it could be a useful transient fix, yet Sally Brown alerts that such advancement, in any case huge in its own particular way, should not be viewed as an answer.

As Artificial Intelligence (AI) turns out to be progressively able and refined, so does the potential for abuse of the innovation. In the field of drug, groundbreaking professionals, scientists and policymakers are perceiving (and quickly grasping) AI—both for its unmistakable current advantages and for the progressive abilities these advances guarantee for the not really removed future. Leaders in AI are additionally perceiving the requirement for creating moral prescribed procedures when applying these advances in social insurance.

In a 'major information' medicinal condition, savvy machines are vital parts. Why? Since AI exceeds expectations in the tedious accumulation and examination of complex information—the centre capacities of cutting-edge therapeutic practice. Also, as medicinal information develops (both in amount and quality), human services experts just need to depend on shrewd machines to open the mysteries of these profitable information resources.

4.2 *Mental Disorders Are the Costliest Condition in the US*

As per the National Institute of Mental Health (NIMH), one out of five grown-ups in the United States (17.9%) encounters some sort of psychological well-being issue. Psychological instability diminishes a person's personal satisfaction, yet it likewise interfaces with expanded well-being spending.

Charles Roehrig, Establishing Executive of the Center for Sustainable Health Spending at Altarum Institute in Ann Arbor, Michigan, takes note of that psychological issue, including dementia, presently top the rundown of ailments with the most noteworthy evaluated spending.

Truth be told, psychological wellness is currently the costliest piece of our medicinal services framework, overwhelming heart conditions, which used to be the costliest.

Roughly $201 billion is spent on emotional wellness yearly. As more individuals achieve maturity, expanding the predominance of certain well-being conditions, for example, dementia is relied upon to push this figure higher, with going with calls for new administration techniques.

As a result of the expenses related with treatment, numerous people who experience emotional well-being issues do not get auspicious expert info. Cost is not the main contributing component; different reasons incorporate a lack of specialists and the shame related with psychological instability (www.verywellmind.com).

The twenty-first century has made fake human knowledge (AI) trying to artificially reproduce the human personality. Science is creating calculations that could figure out how to improve critical thinking over numerous fields. With ongoing years seeing a noteworthy ascent in wretchedness, tension and suicide, there is space for AI's application in psychological sickness.

Suicide rates in the United States have expanded 24% in the previous 20 years. Although ordinarily thought of disarranges like real burdensome issue can put a person in danger for suicide, others like schizophrenia, bipolar turmoil and significantly malignant growth can lead a person to mull over suicide. Because of this differing populace of patients with different issues who might experience the ill effects of self-destructive musings or activities, pinpointing symptomology to recognize an in-danger individual is amazingly troublesome and conflicting. As of late, science has started to apply AI and AI innovation towards mental research to enable clinicians to address this issue [27, 28].

Woebot is an AI-sponsored chatbot that enables individuals to examine their tension and wretchedness. It leads individuals in discussion, recollects what they state and follows-up after some time. The best part about it is that it utilizes instant messages, emoticon and short recordings to connect with clients. On the off chance that you approach Facebook Messenger, you approach Woebot.

It is not intended to supplant human-to-human treatment, obviously, however rather expands on the way that simply discussing your state of mind every day is demonstrated to help battle nervousness and sorrow. Alison Darcy, CEO and author of Woebot, had this to state about the job machines can play in tending to the psychological social insurance emergency [29, 30].

5 Role of AI in Parkinson's Disease

Parkinson's ailment is a confusion where synapses continuously kick the bucket, prompting tremors, inflexibility, lopsidedness and outrageous gradualness, among different indications, which can take a very long time to create. More explicitly, Parkinson's disease causes the loss of nerve cells that ordinarily discharge the synapse dopamine, a concoction utilized by neurons to send sign to other nerve cells. It is one of various neurodegenerative illnesses—a wide term that alludes to conditions that influence the neurons in the mind—that incorporates Lou Gehrig's infection and Alzheimer's ailment.

5.1 Pervasiveness and Costs of Parkinson's Disease

In excess of 10 million individuals worldwide live with Parkinson's ailment, and almost one million individuals in the United States will be harassed with the condition by 2020, as indicated by the Parkinson's Foundation. That is more than the joined number of individuals determined to have different sclerosis, strong dystrophy and Lou Gehrig's illness. Men are 1.5 occasions bound to have Parkinson's sickness than ladies.

Parkinson's ailment is a turmoil of the sensory system causing tremor, solidness and gradualness of development. The principle issue for clinicians is that it is difficult to analyse Parkinson's initial enough to offer patients gainful treatment. When they appear in facility, the illness is progressing and it is just the side effects which can be overseen, instead of the reason tended to [31].

The Oxford Parkinson's Disease Center, driven by Consultant Neurologist Professor Michele Hu close by Professor Richard Wade-Martins, is making incredible walks forward on numerous fronts in the battle to comprehend this condition. Most as of late, they have been granted a 5-year award from the NIHR Oxford Biomedical Research Center to investigate the connection among Parkinson's disease and a rest condition known as Rapid Eye Movement Sleep Behaviour Disorder (or RBD for short). In RBD, the turn that regularly turns off development during rest is broken, making individuals move or yell while sleeping.

Rest issues are fascinating for nervous system specialists since they can be an early pointer of issues with the sensory system. Michele and her associates are especially concentrating on the connection among RBD and Parkinson's disease on the grounds that numerous individuals with Parkinson's disease are thought to experience the ill effects of RBD too. An individual who proceeds to build up Parkinson's disease may have RBD for a long time before the issues start with their development when they are wakeful. So, may it be conceivable to utilize RBD as a kind of 'biomarker' for Parkinson's disease? [32].

6 Role of AI in Chronic Kidney Disease

Chronic Kidney Disease (CKD) influences around 1 of every 7 grown-ups or an expected 30 million Americans. CKD is portrayed by kidney harm which hinders legitimate filtration of the blood. Therefore, other medical issues may happen because of overabundance liquid and waste in the body. As per the American Society of

Nephrology, yearly human services expenses related with treating kidney (renal) disappointment are evaluated at more than 32 billion [33, 34].

With an end goal to improve personal satisfaction for people living with perpetual kidney infection and thus decrease the monetary effect of this ailment, scientists are trying the conceivable outcomes of AI applications.

A portion of the inquiries that need offering an explanation to all the more likely comprehend the job of man-made brainpower in endeavours to treat unending kidney ailment.

- What kinds of AI applications are being developed to help treat kidney malady?
- How is the social insurance market reacting to these AI applications?

6.1 *Kidney Disease AI Applications Overview*

Most of AI use cases and rising applications for treating kidney ailment seem to fall into two noteworthy classes:

Patient Monitoring and Prediction Models: Companies are utilizing AI to screen patients and to anticipate and avert the beginning of kidney disappointment.

Medicinal Image Analysis: Researchers are creating programming utilizing AI to break down kidney biopsy pictures to help counteract ailment [35].

A ceaseless infection is a condition you can control with treatment for quite a long time. Asthma, diabetes and sadness are normal models. Frequently, they do not have a fix, yet you can live with them and deal with their side effects. With an end goal to improve personal satisfaction for people living with constant malady and thus decrease the monetary effect of this ailment, specialists are trying the conceivable outcomes of AI applications.

Most of AI use cases and developing applications for treating ailment seem to fall into two noteworthy classifications:

Patient Monitoring and Prediction Models: Companies are utilizing AI to screen patients and to foresee and anticipate the malady. This forecast is finished by the detailed examination on the information of patients who had perpetual sicknesses as of now. By cross-checking the new patient's information with more established information, we can foresee. On the off chance that the new information is generally like the information of past patients, the model will anticipate the ailment as indicated by it [34].

Therapeutic Image Analysis: Researchers are creating programming utilizing AI to dissect biopsy pictures to help forestall illness. The model will break down pictures and will foresee is it like biopsy of a past patient or not.

6.2 Utilizing AI to Reveal Patients with the Most Noteworthy Hazard

There has been a tonne of discussion about AI in human services, and it is not preposterous to reason that quite a bit of it is publicity. In any case, there have been immense unmistakable favourable circumstances in a subset of methods called profound discovering that can create superhuman outcomes in exceptionally cantered errands, for example, picture acknowledgment or language interpretation. These systems are more A than I: they are approximately impacted by how the mind functions, are executed with PCs and exploit gigantic measures of information and computational power.

However, notwithstanding these advances—and what mainstream culture may let us know—there's no motivation to expect that aware robots will supplant clinicians as a group at any point soon. Rather, the convergence between these AI procedures and advanced well-being, the board exhibits an interesting and groundbreaking chance to intensify crafted by clinicians.

At the point when associations convey advanced well-being, the executives answers for patients, for example, portable applications, they can produce a totally new dataset on patient action, tolerant detailed results and more bits of knowledge. It can likewise be joined with information from the well-being framework, for example, claims information and electronic restorative record information. Through AI, associations would then be able to tackle that information to organize individuals dependent on continuous needs, create intercession cautions and suggest line-up activities with their suppliers.

This innovation eventually makes a constructive criticism circle: since patients get auspicious, customized support, they draw in with clinicians more regularly. This produces more information, which thusly gives care groups the bits of knowledge they must give the privilege clinical intercession to the correct patient at the opportune time. In addition, this methodology enables the association, in general, to realize which intercessions are best and where clinical assets can be most successfully conveyed [36].

7 Role of AI in Dementia

Dementia (an extreme decrease in mental capacity) is positioned as the sixth driving reason for death in the United States and affects an expected 5 million Americans. As per the Alzheimer's Association, social insurance expenses related with dementia totalled $259 billion out of 2017 and are anticipated to reach $1.1 trillion by 2050.

With an end goal to improve personal satisfaction for people living with dementia and thus decrease the monetary effect of this ailment, scientists are trying the conceivable outcomes of AI applications.

A portion of the inquiries that need offering an explanation to more readily comprehend the job of man-made reasoning in endeavours to analyse and treat dementia:

What kinds of AI applications are at present being used to analyse dementia?

How has the social insurance market reacted to these AI applications?

Are there any normal patterns?

7.1 Dementia AI Applications Overview

Most of AI use cases for anticipating dementia seem to fall into four noteworthy classes:

Discourse Monitoring: Companies are utilizing AI to break down discourse examples to recognize and screen dementia movement.

Restorative Image Analysis: Companies are creating programming utilizing AI to break down mind disintegration from outputs to help anticipate the beginning of dementia.

Visual Indicators: Companies are preparing calculations to evaluate eye development examples to track and connect intellectual capacity and cerebrum action.

Hereditary Analysis: Companies are utilizing AI to dissect hereditary information to anticipate the beginning of dementia [33].

Utilizing a typical sort of mind filter, scientists modified an AI calculation to analyse beginning period Alzheimer's ailment around 6 years before a clinical analysis is made—conceivably allowing specialists to intercede with treatment.

No fix exists for Alzheimer's infection; however, encouraging medications have risen as of late that can help stem the condition's movement. Be that as it may, these medicines must be controlled from the get-go throughout the illness so as to do any great. This race with time as the opponent has enlivened researchers to look for approaches to analyse the condition prior.

'One of the troubles with Alzheimer's infection is that when all the clinical indications show and we can make a complete finding, such a large number of neurons have kicked the bucket, making it basically irreversible', says Jae Ho Sohn, MD, MS, an occupant in the Department of Radiology and Biomedical Imaging at UC San Francisco.

In an ongoing report, distributed in Radiology, Sohn consolidated neuroimaging with AI to attempt to foresee whether a patient would build up Alzheimer's sickness when they originally gave a memory hindrance—the best time to mediate.

Positron Discharge Tomography (PET) checks, which measure the degrees of explicit particles, similar to glucose, in the mind, have been researched as one instrument to help analyse Alzheimer's infection before the manifestations become serious.

Different sorts of PET outputs search for proteins explicitly identified with Alzheimer's ailment, yet glucose PET sweeps are substantially more typical and less expensive, particularly in social insurance offices and creating nations, since they are likewise utilized for malignant growth arranging.

Radiologists have utilized these outputs to attempt to identify Alzheimer's disease by searching for diminished glucose levels over the mind, particularly in the frontal and parietal projections of the cerebrum. In any case, in light of the fact that the infection is a moderate dynamic issue, the adjustments in glucose are exceptionally unpretentious and thus hard to spot with the unaided eye.

To tackle this issue, Sohn connected an AI calculation to PET outputs to help analyse beginning time Alzheimer's infection more dependably.

'This is a perfect use of profound learning since it is especially solid at finding unobtrusive however diffuse procedures. Human radiologists are extremely solid at distinguishing minor central discovering like a mind tumour; however, we battle at identifying all the more moderate, worldwide changes', says Sohn. 'Given the quality of profound learning in this kind of utilization, particularly contrasted with people, it appeared to be a characteristic application'.

To prepare the calculation, Sohn sustained its pictures from the Alzheimer's Disease Neuroimaging Initiative (ADNI), a huge open dataset of PET sweeps from patients who were in the long run determined to have either Alzheimer's illness, mellow psychological debilitation or no confusion. In the end, the calculation started to learn without anyone else in which highlights are significant for foreseeing the determination of Alzheimer's sickness and which are not. Once the calculation was prepared on 1,921 sweeps, the researchers tried it on two novel datasets to assess its presentation. The first were 188 pictures that originated from the equivalent ADNI database yet had not been exhibited to the calculation yet. The second was a totally novel arrangement of outputs from 40 patients who had introduced to the UCSF Memory and Aging Centre with conceivable subjective weakness.

The calculation performed without a hitch. It effectively recognized 92% of patients who built up Alzheimer's sickness in the principal test set and 98% in the subsequent test set. Furthermore, it made these right expectations overall 75.8 months—somewhat more than 6 years—before the patient got their last finding.

Sohn says the following stage is to test and adjust the calculation on bigger, increasingly various datasets from various medical clinics and nations.

'I accept this calculation has the solid potential to be clinically applicable', he says. 'In any case, before we can do that, we have to approve and adjust the calculation in a bigger and progressively assorted patient partner, in a perfect world from various mainlands and different various kinds of settings'.

On the off chance that the calculation can withstand these tests, Sohn supposes it could be utilized when a nervous system specialist sees a patient at a memory canter as a prescient and demonstrative device for Alzheimer's illness, getting the patient the medicines they need sooner [36].

7.2 *Mental and Physical Health Screening*

Another part of social insurance that is prepared for assistive AI—now and again, officially observing the utilization of AI—is the demonstrative screening process. This is normally performed by a patient talking with a specialist or other medicinal services proficient and responding to a progression of inquiries concerning their restorative history and portraying side effects, which the human services supplier uses to make an analysis or prescribe a game plan for the patient.

8 Conclusion

As AI frameworks worked around common language acknowledgment and preparing become progressively capable at collaborating with human clients, scientists are creating AI instruments that can play out these underlying analytic evaluations—regularly as chatbots over a cell phone or PC interface.

This is basically the idea of telemedicine, which as of now exists and is accessible in numerous pieces of the world. Patients have remote access to a social insurance supplier and the capacity to cooperate, pose inquiries and get medicinal services counsel. Most present telemedicine frameworks utilize connective advances including live talk, video calling or normal telephone utility to interface patients with specialists or attendants. There are a few frameworks working in the U.S. offering telemedicine administrations; however, these frameworks are particularly essential to third world and creating countries where there is almost no formal medicinal services foundation and no standard nearby social insurance suppliers [37].

References

1. "What is Artificial Intelligence (AI)?—Definition from Techopedia." (n.d.). Accessed June 1, 2019, from https://www.techopedia.com/definition/190/artificial-intelligence-ai
2. Dankwa-Mullan I, Rivo M, Sepulveda M, Park Y, Snowdon J, Rhee K (2019) Transforming diabetes care through artificial intelligence: the future is here. Popul Health Manag 22(3):229–242
3. Diabetes Care Gets a Boost with Artificial Intelligence Technology
4. https://www.ijitee.org/wp-content/uploads/papers/v8i9/I8403078919.pdf
5. "Diabetes: Symptoms, Causes, Treatment, Prevention, and More." (n.d.). Accessed June 1, 2019, from https://www.healthline.com/health/diabetes#symptoms
6. The Diabetes Control and Complication Trial Research Group (1993) The effect of intensive treatment of diabetes on the development and progression of long-term complications in insulin-dependent diabetes mellitus. N Engl J Med 329:977–986
7. Lasker RD (1993) The diabetes control and complication trial: implications for policy and practice. N Engl J Med 329:1035–1036
8. Lehmann ED, Deutsch T (1995) Application of computers in diabetes care - a review (I and II). Med Inform 20:281–329

9. Gomez EJ et al (1992) A Telemedicine distributed decision-support system for diabetes management, 1238–1239. In: IEEE 14th annual international engineering in medicine and biology conference 1992-CH3207-8
10. "How AI can improve patient outcomes for type 1 and 2 diabetes." (n.d.). Retrieved June 1, 2019, from https://www.information-age.com/ai-can-improve-patient-outcomes-type-1-2diabetes-123467505/
11. Using AI for Mental Health Effectively
12. Andreassen S et al (1994) A probabilistic approach to glucose prediction and insulin dose adjustment: description of metabolic model and pilot evaluation study. Comput Methods Programs Biomed 41:153–165
13. Johnson KW, Torres Soto J, Glicksberg BS, Shameer K, Miotto R, Ali M, Ashley E, Dudley JT (2018) Artificial intelligence in cardiology. J Am Coll Cardiol 71(23):2668–2679
14. Alexa, Will You Be My Therapist?: The Role of AI and Machine Learning in Mental Health
15. Montani S (2019) Artificial intelligence techniques for diabetes management: the TIDDM project. In: Proceedings of the 14th European conference on artificial intelligence, Berlin, Germany, August 20–25, 2000 presented at the ECAI 2000, Berlin, Germany: ECAI
16. Fang KY, Bjering H, Ginige A (2018) Adherence, avatars and where to from here. Stud Health Technol Inform 252:45–50
17. Fulmer R, Joerin A, Gentile B, Lakerink L, Rauws M (2018) Using psychological artificial intelligence (tess) to relieve symptoms of depression and anxiety: randomized controlled trial. JMIR Mental Health 5(4):e64. https://doi.org/10.2196/mental.9782
18. Contreras I, Vehi J (2018) Artificial intelligence for diabetes management and decision support: literature review. J Med Internet Res 20(5):e10775
19. Hoermann S, McCabe KL, Milne DN, Calvo RA (2017) Application of synchronous text-based dialogue systems in mental health interventions: systematic review. J Med Internet Res 19(8):e267. https://doi.org/10.2196/jmir.7023
20. Ramesh AN, Kambhampati C, Monson JRT, Drew PJ (2004) Artificial intelligence in medicine. Ann R Coll Surg Engl 86(5):334–338. https://doi.org/10.1308/147870804290
21. Artificial intelligence in cardiology: applications, benefits and challenges (2018) Br J Cardiol
22. Baranowski T, Lytle L (2015) Should the IDEFICS outcomes have been expected? Obes Rev 16(Suppl 2):162–172. https://doi.org/10.1111/obr.12359
23. Stephens TN, Joerin A, Rauws M, Werk LN (2019) Feasibility of pediatric obesity and prediabetes treatment support through Tess, the AI behavioral coaching chatbot. Transl Behav Med 9(3):443–450
24. Kramer J-N, Künzler F, Mishra V, Presset B, Kotz D, Smith S, Kowatsch T (2019) Investigating intervention components and exploring states of receptivity for a smartphone app to promote physical activity: protocol of a microrandomized trial. JMIR Res Protoc 8(1):e11540. https://doi.org/10.2196/11540
25. Van den Eijnden R, Koning I, Doornwaard S, van Gurp F, Ter Bogt T (2018) The impact of heavy and disordered use of games and social media on adolescents' psychological, social, and school functioning. J Behav Addict 7(3):697–706. https://doi.org/10.1556/2006.7.2018.65
26. Ferrara P, Corsello G, Ianniello F, Sbordone A, Ehrich J, Giardino I, Pettoello-Mantovani M (2017) Internet addiction: starting the debate on health and well-being of children overexposed to digital media. J Pediatr 191:280–281.e1. https://doi.org/10.1016/j.jpeds.2017.09.054
27. Brand L, Beltran A, Hughes S, O'Connor T, Baranowski J, Nicklas T, Baranowski T (2016) Assessing feedback in a mobile videogame. Games Health J 5(3):203–208. https://doi.org/10.1089/g4h.2015.0056
28. Bardus M, van Beurden SB, Smith JR, Abraham C (2016) A review and content analysis of engagement, functionality, aesthetics, information quality, and change techniques in the most popular commercial apps for weight management. Int J Behav Nutr Phys Activity 13:35. https://doi.org/10.1186/s12966-016-03599
29. Rivera J, McPherson A, Hamilton J, Birken C, Coons M, Iyer S, Stinson J (2016) Mobile apps for weight management: a scoping review. JMIR mHealth uHealth 4(3):e87. https://doi.org/10.2196/mhealth.5115

30. Quelly SB, Norris AE, DiPietro JL (2016) Impact of mobile apps to combat obesity in children and adolescents: a systematic literature review. J SpecIsts Pediatr Nurs JSPN 21(1):5–17. https://doi.org/10.1111/jspn.12134
31. When Will There Be a Cure for Parkinson's Disease?—Nanalyze
32. The role of artificial intelligence in spotting the onset of Parkinson's disease—Nuffield Department of Clinical Neurosciences
33. AI Applications for Managing Chronic Kidney Disease | Emerj
34. Using AI to Amplify Care for Patients with Chronic Disease
35. Artificial Intelligence for Dementia Diagnosis—Genetic Analysis, Speech Analysis, and More | Emerj
36. Artificial Intelligence Can Detect Alzheimer's Disease in Brain Scans Six Years Before a Diagnosis | UC San Francisco
37. A Healthy Future for Artificial Intelligence in Healthcare | ENGINEERING.com
38. AI is a powerful tool in the fight against anxiety and depression

Sonia Singla Currently Advisory editorial Board Member at IJPBS https://ijpbs.net/editorial-board.php. Have done B.Sc from St. Bede's college affiliated to Himachal Pradesh University, MSc in Biotechnology from Bangalore University, India and MSc in Bioinformatics from University of Leicester, U.K. Have worked as research trainee in IARI, New Delhi for two years, apart from it have done many online courses related to Data Science from that of Coursera, is interested in Data Science, Artificial intelligence, health sector. Have done few projects in CSIR-CDRI related to Data Science.

Proposing Real-Time Smart Healthcare Model Using IoT

Rashbir Singh, Prateek Singh and Latika Kharb

Abstract In this chapter, author will discuss our proposed model for real-time management of smart health care that can be utilized both by hospitals, ambulance, and even at normal day-to-day activity tracker and requires no technical or medical knowledge to start with. As per the survey, about 40% of world's total deaths due to any disease can be prevented if an earlier diagnosis is made. People tend to avoid health and healthcare practices now either it is due to the busy schedule or lack of money. So, the research work focuses on incorporating technology into people life without disturbing their daily routine and does not require separate time to use. This technology is powered by IoT and uses many biosensors to give real-time solutions, prescribe medication, earlier detection of diseases, give a better understanding of patients current health and past health and significantly reduces medical expenses, and by having more information about patient health doctors can operate and treat the patient with a better approach. This technology works when the user sleeps and learns when the user performs day-to-day task with the help of machine learning.

Keywords Internet of Things (IoT) · Arduino software · Microcontroller · Android software · Ultrasonic sensor · EEG · ECG · EMG · Temperature sensor · Capnography · Antimony electrode sensor · Piezoelectric sensor

1 Introduction

Due to the widespread diseases around, there is a radical increase in demand for health care and healthcare support facilities. Health system has considered different levels of the healthcare services such as central-level health care, state/provincial-level health care, regional/zonal/district-level health care, and local-level health care [1]. Health is wealth and people nowadays are ready to spend an enormous amount of money without even giving a second thought but the need is not to spend in

R. Singh
Department of Information Technology, Amity University, Noida, Uttar Pradesh, India

P. Singh · L. Kharb (✉)
Jagan Institute of Management Studies, Sector-5, Rohini, Delhi, India
e-mail: latika.kharb@jimsindia.org

P. Raj et al. (eds.), *Internet of Things Use Cases for the Healthcare Industry*,
https://doi.org/10.1007/978-3-030-37526-3_2

millions but to develop smart solutions to health-related problems. The widespread use of Internet of Things (IoT), especially smart wearables, will play an important role in improving the quality of medical care, bringing convenience for patients and improving the management level of hospitals [2]. This can be achieved with the help of the combination of IoT with our day-to-day objects like beds and clothing. This research work proposes a model for smart healthcare system for personal, hospital, and general use which is easy to operate and implement and can be utilized by people of urban and rural backgrounds. The motive of this research work is to convert a regular bed into a smart self-managing health bed and a smart healthcare clothing system to monitor your body and help one with a better understanding of one's own body. The proposed solution will provide health support and will reduce one's expenses over health and help hospitals with a better understanding of patient's data which is collected daily 24 × 7. This can potentially reduce initial delay due to various tests the doctor has to perform on patient before operating on the patient, and hence the patient can be admitted for treatment which less to no delay and doctors can start operating as soon as possible and can also be used as a daily body checker which can be used to create your health database and to inform the nearest hospital and relatives in case of an emergency. Since there are some areas in India that do not have access to [3] hospitals, about 80% of Indian population still do not have proper access to health-related facilities and healthcare treatment; so the proposed model could help them to manage health at their home or office in a cost-effective manner and utilize it when so ever they feel. It can be used as a smart hospital beds, smart house beds, or even smart ambulance bed with a health monitoring clothes which can save many life with technologies like EEG (electroencephalogram), ECG (electrocardiogram), EKG (Electrocardiogram), temperature sensor, skin quality sensor pressure sensor, and many other biomedical sensors powered by the advance technology of IoT (Internet of Things), hence connecting a regular bed to the Internet and detecting several health-related issues and reducing overall cost of health and time of treatment of health which can make health treatments approachable for all.

2 Literature Survey

The literature survey consists of the analysis of deaths due to delayed disease detection and multiple reasons regarding death in humans. Survival rates were considerably low in developing countries [4], as compared to developed ones. Of the 57 million deaths worldwide in the year 2016, more than half (54%) were due to the top ten reasons. Ischaemic heart disease and stroke have become greatest top reason behind the death worldwide, considering as a combined 15 million deaths in the year 2016. These conditions have persisted to be of death worldwide in the last 15 years. The chronic obstructive pulmonary disease took nearly three million lives in the year 2016, while lung carcinoma (along with trachea and bronchus cancers) caused two million deaths. Diabetes alone took two million human lives in the year 2016, up from less than one million in the year 2000. Losses due to dementias have been doubled in the year between 2000 and 2016, and hence is the fifth leading cause of deaths in the year 2016 compared to fourteenth in 2000 all around the world.

Lower respiratory diseases and infections continued to be the most deadly contagious condition, creating three million losses around the world in the year 2016 alone. The death rate due to diarrhoeal conditions reduced over nearly one million between the year 2000 and 2016 but still managed to affect two million lives in the year 2016. Likewise, the deaths due to tuberculosis declined around the same time still are among one of the top ten reasons for the death of two million. As of now, HIV/AIDS is no longer reason for deaths and is not in the world's list of top ten agents of death, causing deaths of one million humans in the year 2016 as related to 1.5 million in the year 2000.

Road injuries took almost 1.4 million human lives in the year 2016 and from that nearly three-quarters, i.e., 74% of what remained men and boys (Fig. 1).

Similarly, late determination of diseases remains one of the usual medical failures. It might occur if the doctor fails in the diagnoses of the patient correctly and it involves long duration of time than expected for making a reliable diagnosis. When determination of disease is delayed, the valuable medication time is wasted. In some circumstances, this can create added difficulties for the patient, prolonged healing period, with additional medical debts and even can result in loss of life.

The late determination of diseases can happen due to several reasons: doctor negligence, complicated medical history, incomplete patient information, or simply due to testing errors all can contribute to late determination of diseases. The failure to determine the cause of disease quickly, and also treat it immediately, may have serious outcomes such as heart attack or paralysis. Some illnesses or conditions could or could not be analyzed because their symptoms and signs may be similar to that of other medical conditions. Ill health symptoms, viz., cough, pain in chest, and respiration problems may be related to symptom of other problems of health and if

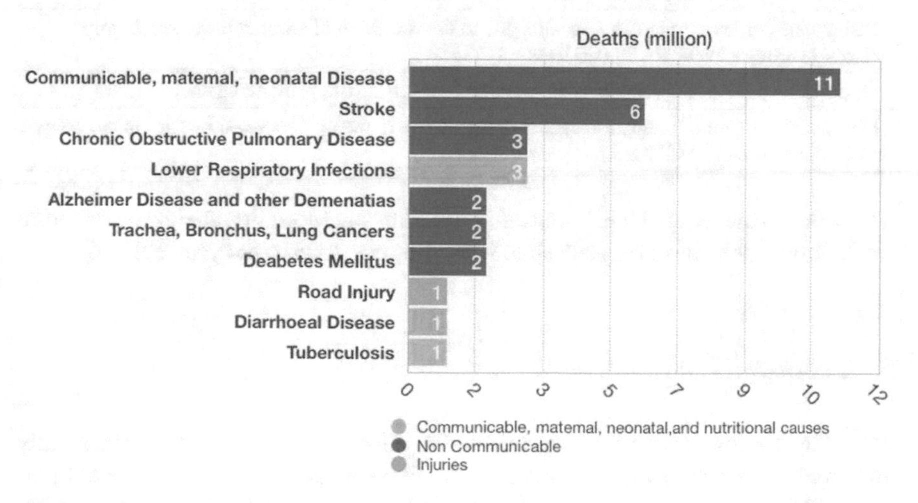

Fig. 1 Ranking of top 10 reasons for deaths (in millions) in year 2016 around the world

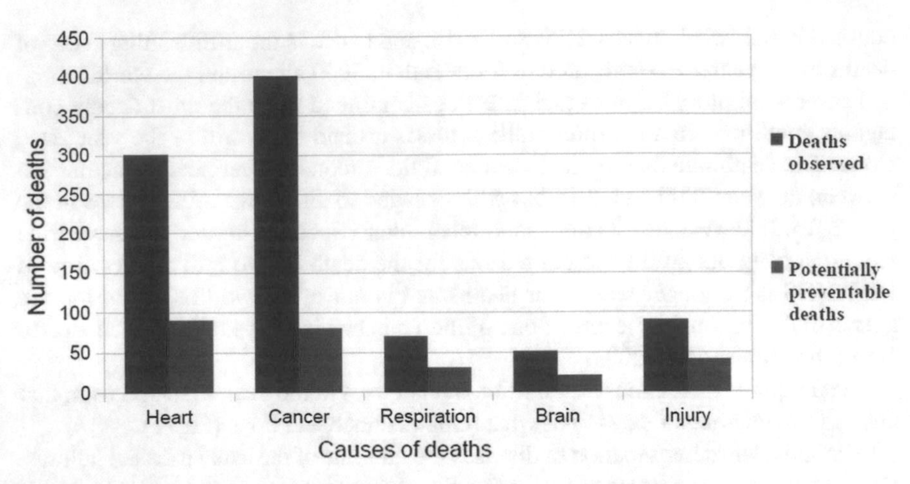

Fig. 2 Potentially preventable deaths from the five leading causes of death

delayed, it may lead to a problem. There are many other types of conditions that can lead to an unwarranted disease or progression if not properly diagnosed in a timely manner [5] (Fig. 2).

Some of the top causes of death worldwide include cancer, respiratory diseases, heart diseases, and stroke. Collectively, they represent 62% of all the deaths in the year 2010 only.

Thirty-four percent of premature deaths caused due to heart diseases, prolonging about 92,000 lives
Twenty-one percent of premature deaths caused due to cancer, prolonging about 84,500 lives
Thirty-nine percent of premature deaths due to the condition of chronic lower respiratory diseases, prolonging about 29,000 lives
Thirty-three percent of premature deaths caused due to stroke, prolonging about 17,000 lives
Thirty-nine percent of premature deaths occurred due to the unintentional injuries in the body, prolonging about 37,000 lives

According to the report, CDC's journal, Morbidity and Mortality, analyzed premature deaths from each cause for each state from the year 2008 to the year 2010 [6].

3 Proposed System

With the improvement of living standards, people's quality of life has greatly improved. Meanwhile, due to unreasonable diet, excess energy, environmental pollution, and other factors, the development of chronic diseases becomes more quickly which kills more and more people [7]. All of these lead to a shortage of qualified healthcare professionals and equipment to treat sick persons [8]. Keeping all these things in mind, author has proposed a system that can help people well in advance and it consists of the following modules.

- **EEG (electroencephalogram) sensor**

An electroencephalogram (EEG) is used to discover inconveniences related to an electric movement of the brain.

An EEG tracks and insights mind wave fashion. Little metallic plates (electrodes) with small electric wires are placed above the head of the user, the amplifier amplifies the electromagnetic brain waves and captures and plots a real-time graph of the electric movements inside the brain. The graph is shown which depicts the events and impacts happened inside the brain. A person's day-to-day activity and his interest create electric brainwaves into a recognizable pattern. Through an EEG, therapeutic specialists can scan and anticipate the seizures and different issues and can give the recommendation changes in lifestyle/medication to help the person.

- **ECG (electrocardiogram) sensor**

An ECG sensor with electrodes is attached at the top chest area to count the heartbeat. Their electrodes convert every count of heartbeat into a raw electric signal. ECG sensors are very less in weight and slim while having the capability to accurately measure continuous heartbeat produced by the heart and generates rate data of the heartbeat. This device is being used for the cardiovascular health analysis by the medical assistant and trained doctors.

Electrodes of an ECG sensor consist of three pins which are connected by a 30-inch-long cable which makes it easy for ECG sensor to connect and communicate with the microcontroller placed at the waist, pocket, or different location on the body. The sensor collects values through arm and leg pulse and every sensory electrode of the ECG has methods to be assembled on the body.

This research work uses the AD8232 module which has nine connections that are being used to solder wires, pins, and other connectors as well. The pins are, namely, GND, LO+, OUTPUT, LO−, 3.3 V, SDN which provides required pins for operating and monitoring with the microcontroller board. It also provides three pins, namely, RA: Right Arm, LA: Left Arm, and RL: Right Leg and pins to connect sensors. Moreover, there is an indicator light that will blink according to the heartbeat.

- **EMG (Electromyography) sensor**

The EMG sensor measures the muscle activation on to the concept of electric potential and is called as electromyography (EMG) and is traditionally been used in the field of research in the medical profession and for the analysis of neuromuscular dysfunctions. Through the development of ever smaller and smaller yet powerful integrated circuits and microcontrollers, it has become possible for the EMG circuits and sensors to find their usage in the field of prosthetics, robotics, and other control systems.

This research work uses Myoware Muscle sensor (AT-04-001), which is an appropriate sensor to be used to produce raw electric EMG signal which is analog output signal and can be analyzed with the microcontroller-based application, the Myoware Muscle sensor is designed for a reliable output. It operates with the single power supply ranging from (+2.9 V) to (+5.7 V) with security for polarity reversal and provides a supplementary feature with this sensor so that user can easily regulate the sensitivity gain of the electrodes. These sensors are suitable for the purpose of the wearable device and are the compact ones, and hence it is easy to handle and measure the muscle activation signal.

- **Antimony electrode sensor**

Antimony anodes are medicinally valuable since they are low in expense and have a basic development as there is no glass part to break. There is only a resistance which is of couple of hundred ohms between an antimony pH anode and the reference cathode, so if the voltage is generated it would be easy to record it with the straightforward low-impedance recorder which is associated with the microcontroller.

Antimony is an exceptional metal with the normal for an immediate connection among pH and its deliberate potential. The electric potential difference developed between that in antimony and a copper electrode is due to variations in the pH.

- **Temperature Sensor**

A temperature sensor IC works for the nominal IC temperature of −55 to +150 °C. This sensor comprises a material that plays out the task as per temperature to adjust the resistance and compute temperature.

This research work is using LM35 as the body temperature monitoring sensor which will be connected to the microcontroller. The LM35 temperature sensors operate amid the range of −55 to +120 °C. LM35 Temperature sensor has the following features:

- Calibrates in degree Celsius,
- Appropriate for application demanding remote access,
- Lower cost,
- Operates in volts between the range of 4–30 V, and
- Lower Self-heating.

The LM35 can be attached easily like any other temperature sensors. This expects the surrounding air temperature around it is just about equivalent to that of surface temperature and if the air temperature is much lower or higher than that of the surface temperature, then the real temperature of the LM35 would be at a mean temperature between the surface temperature and that of the air temperature (Fig. 3).

- **Capnography**

Waveform capnography addresses the proportion of carbon dioxide (CO_2) in inhaled out air, which assesses ventilation. It contains a number and an outline. The number is capnometry, which is deficient load of CO_2 recognized close to the completion of exhalation. This is end-tidal CO_2 ($ETCO_2$) which is routinely 35–45 mm Hg. The capnography is the waveform that shows the measure of CO_2 is accessible at every time of respiratory cycle, and it normally has a rectangular shape. Capnography

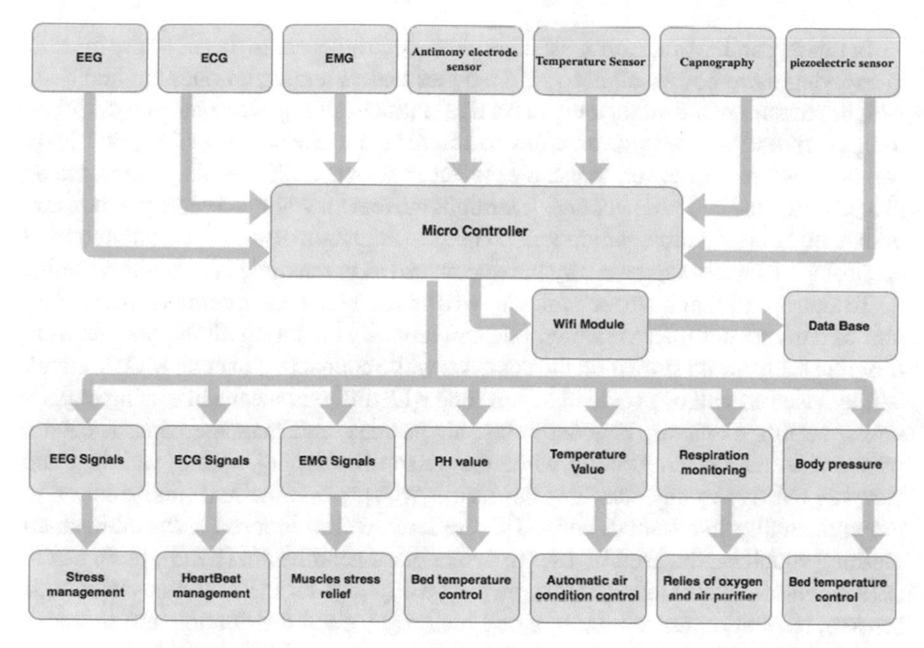

Fig. 3 Proposed model architecture

furthermore measures and shows respiratory rate. Changes in respiratory rate and tidal volume appear as changes in the waveform and $ETCO_2$. In people with solid lungs, the cerebrum responds to changes in CO_2 levels in the circulatory framework to control ventilation. Author overviews this by watching chest rise and fall, assessing respiratory effort, including respiratory rate and checking out breathing sounds. $ETCO_2$ adds an objective estimation to those revelations. The patient's respiratory rate should increase as CO_2 rises and decrease as CO_2 falls. In the event that a patient has moderate or shallow breaths, and a high $ETCO_2$ perusing, this reveals to us that ventilation is not successfully taking out CO_2 (hypercarbia) and that the mind is not reacting legitimately to CO_2 changes. This may be achieved by an overdose, head damage, or seizure by estimating the end-tidal CO_2 ($ETCO_2$, the dimension of carbon dioxide discharged toward the finish of lapse) through a sealed mask, and EMS professionals can get an "early warning" of a patients intensifying condition.

With precise and instantaneous CO_2 estimations required for capnography, the COZIR high-speed wide-range CO_2 sensor appeared the ideal answer for the issue.

- **Piezoelectric sensor**

The piezoelectric impact will be utilized by the piezoelectric sensor that estimates the adjustment in power, body temperature, increasing speed, weight, and strain and is consequently utilized through its transformation into an electrical charge. The piezoelectric sensor demonstrates three elementary activities, namely, transverse powerful, transducer impact, and shear impact.

In this research work, author used the piezoelectric sensor to detect where the user is applying more body weight to give a better understanding on ones applied body weight pressure while doing daily tasks like walking, sitting, sleeping, and detecting the pattern and suggesting remedies to improve the one's sense of applied body weight pressure. Moreover, to use piezoelectric sensor while sleeping which can be placed inside the bed to detect ones overnight movement while sleeping, posture, and body weight distribution, which will be used to adjust the bed temperature required according to what is suggested by the doctors, so as to maximize the health benefits.

To sum up, all the above technologies will be combined into a common processing unit of a microcontroller which will be continuously capturing all the outputs from different sensors and store it on the database while connecting over an MQTT client. While remedies will be provided in real time with different means like using oxygen tanks, heating elements, air conditions, air purifies, and massage pads, it cannot only collect data of one's body while the person is sleeping, sitting, walking, and carrying out day-to-day activities but also it will provide the real-time solution to the abnormality in a human body. This research work proposed a wearable smart clothing which can be used by user to detect one's heart health (EKG), brain health (EEG), muscle conditions (EMG), sweat quality and its PH (antimony electrode sensor), respiration (capnography), and his body weight distribution and center of gravity shift (piezoelectric) which will be placed in both clothing and bed.

The bed will be equipped with heating elements to control the temperature of the bed only in the area where the user is sleeping which will be sensed with the help of piezoelectric. A small oxygen tank will be placed over the headrest area of user and CO_2 exhaled during respiration is detected to be abnormal in order to provide the required amount of oxygen supply, while the user behaving choices either to use oxygen tanks, air purifier, or both. If stress is detected with the help of EEG then various remedies like playing meditation sound like alpha music will be taken with the help of speakers attached to the bed. Small massaging motors inside the bed will help in muscle relief. The wearable clothing with the heating element will help in managing healthy body temperature which is required for the body to function properly and will maximize physical and mental output.

As being powered with technology of IoT (Internet of Things), it will not only be providing remedies in physical world in real time but also the data collected will be user specific and will be used by doctors for better understanding of patients health as the data is collected every day and stored which can be used in early disease detecting like cancer, high or low blood pressure, distress, respiratory diseases, low Na+ ions level in body fluid, fever, etc.

4 Methodology

In this research work, main seven components are being used, i.e.,

- EEG,
- EKG,

- EMG,
- Antimony electrode sensor,
- Temperature sensor,
- Capnography, and
- Piezoelectric sensor.

Various components of the proposed model monitor different parts of human body and the output from different components when analyzed in combination provides detailed information about the human user as given below:

- One's sleep pattern,
- One's body natural center of gravity,
- Variation of body temperature with time,
- One's lung capacity,
- Amount of oxygen absorption capability of bodies and immunity and resistance to diseases,
- Cardiovascular health,
- Muscular health,
- Quality of one's sweat,
- Acidity and basicity of fluids,
- Mental health, and
- Stress and hypertension.

Doctors cannot gain much information with the short-term test to know all the physical and mental health issues before operating on the patient. But the model proposed by this research work can help doctors with a better understanding of patient's health and his medical background and can provide the best suitable treatment to the patient. Hence, resulting in elongation of one's life and disease-free healthy life.

This proposed model can even reduce medical expenses by using a machine learning model based on the K-NN algorithm to suggest user with best remedies for small health-related issues like cold, headache, cough, etc. and can judge the acuteness of the fever which can help the user to know the severity of the disease. The model is based on a single controller and multiple sensor methods where several sensors are connected to a single microcontroller and are dependent on the microcontroller to supply sensors with power, process the output from sensor's use decision tree to provide real-time solutions, and collect and upload the received data onto the database. The microcontroller is powered by 5 V supply and various other sensors are connected to the different I/O pins of the microcontroller and ground of each sensor is connected to the common microcontroller ground. As being so low in power consumption, it requires a low input electric supply and can be attached to various objects as desired by the user. In this model, the IoT-based mechanism is attached to two day-to-day objects making them smart, i.e.,

- Wearable clothing (thin and comfortable vest and pants) and
- Beds (room beds, ambulance beds, or hospital beds).

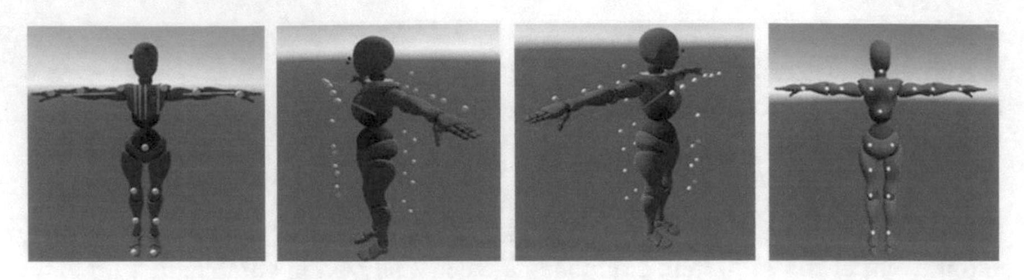

Fig. 4 Wearable smart health management clothing with sensors at various positions

A wearable smart full body cloth will be having different components placed at various locations in order to monitor different parts.

Figure 4 shows the wearable smart health management clothing which is displaying where different sensors will be placed and their significance in those positions. Figure 4 shows four views from different angles, i.e.,

- Depiction of placement of sensors and heating element from front.
- Depiction of placement of sensors and heating element from left.
- Depiction of placement of sensors and heating element from right.
- Depiction of placement of sensors and heating element from back.

Figure 4 shows green straight line above chest and stomach area and above arm which represents the placement of insulated Teflon wire or heating pad to heat the coating when the temperature detected is too low. The temperature sensor along with CO_2 can be seen around the sky blue portion of the neck.

Whereas two black dot/spheres can be seen on the forehead area and ear lobe area, which are EEG sensors containing two small electrodes connected to the brain region to detect brain's different alpha, beta, gamma, theta, and delta brain waves generated from the brain and amplify them to record user's brain activities.

A blue color object can be seen around the area above where there is the heart, and it is an ECG sensor to monitor cardiovascular health. Then, white spears can be seen in Fig. 4 which are nothing but combination of EMG and piezoelectric material sensor around the body to provide the detailed information about person's muscles and pressure applied to carry out day-to-day activities (Fig. 5).

All the above sensors and temperature management system is fully controlled with the help of an Android application and data is received with the help of the microcontroller. The heating pad will be connected to the ground for the ground wire and digital input pin of the microcontroller, so the functionality can be controlled over Android application and can be automated with a click. Following the similar mechanism, all the sensors ground will be connected to the common ground of the microcontroller and for the sensors.

ECG consists of three electrode—RA, i.e., right arm, LA, i.e., Left arm, and RL, i.e., right leg microcontroller 3.3 V—which will be used as a power supply for the ECG module, whereas L0+ and L0− pins are connected to microcontroller digital pin and output of ECG module will be connected to the analog. For EEG, this research work uses NeuroSky MindWave with two electrodes and connects the ground of

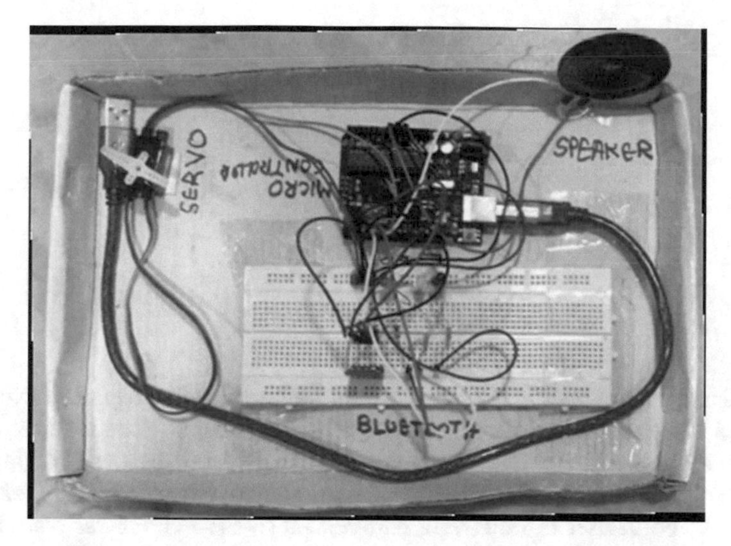

Fig. 5 EEG-based stress management and detection with alpha music to calm the mind

EEG with the ground of microcontroller while using digital pins as transmission and receiving pins, and the piezoelectric material is used to judge the amount of pressure according to the electricity generated when the piezoelectric material is under pressure. EMG sensors are placed above main muscle groups like biceps, triceps, shoulder, chest, abdomen, thighs, calves, etc.

All the collected data is then transmitted over MQTT broker where the microcontroller acts as an MQTT publisher, publishing the data to the MQTT broker and MQTT receiver is Android application and online cloud database.

5 Capability

A practical implementation of EEG was taken with the help of NeuroSky MindWave to measure patient's mental state. EEG detects different alpha, beta, theta, and gamma brain waves along with user's concentration and meditation level. The headgear has one electrode for frontal lobe and one electrode for an ear. As soon as the electrodes are at their desired places, the EEG begins sensing brain data and then that data is used to make the prediction in K-NN-based classification model.
Five classifications are being made, i.e.,

- Eyes open,
- Eyes close,
- Relaxed,
- Excited, and
- Not excited.

- **Data acquiring**

$$\int_a^b f(x)\,dx \tag{1}$$

$$\int_a^b f(x)\,dx \approx (b-a)\big((f(a)+f(b))/2\big) \tag{2}$$

The training dataset is from reference [9]. The dataset has five sections divided into dataset A discussed as Z, dataset B discussed as O, dataset C discussed as N, dataset D discussed as F, and dataset E discussed as S each containing set of EEG fragments with the recording of the electromagnetic movement of a healthy person for 23.6 s. Dataset A and dataset B are having data related to EEG chronicles from healthy volunteers with categorization as eyes open and eyes close, individually.

The second dataset characterized in reference [10] include healthy people who volunteered and analyzed under EEG to collect the data as playing particular PC computer games with a class as excited, not excited, and relaxed on the basis of the various different values of the alpha, beta, theta, and gamma.

- **Data extraction**

Ambiguous data are removed and polished/refined to get more refined information for unique groups differently. The element utilized here is categorized underneath the graph. The trapezoidal rule can be used to find the area under the graph which is formed in the dataset from the first source which is in raw graphical form. On numerical examination, the trapezoidal governs (likewise alluded to as the trapezoid control or trapezium run) is a strategy for approximating the particular imperative.

Equation 1 shows the differentiation with the upper bound as (b) and lowers bound as (a). The working of the trapezoidal rule can be understood as by approximating the region underneath the diagram of the element f(x) as a trapezoid and computing its locale.

With this, author can derive different values for different waves. It takes after that the district of the recurrence groups (delta, theta, alpha, and beta) is ascertained for every EEG section.

- **Training data and Test Data**

The acquired data is then divided into two parts, i.e.,

- Training dataset and
- Test dataset.

Training dataset is used for teaching purposes of the system while the test dataset is used for the purpose of testing the prediction accuracy of the model. Training dataset consists of 800 classified data as eyes open, eyes close, relaxed, excited, and not

(a)

S.No	Gamma	Theta	Alpha	Beta	Classification
1	1.609	0.0968	0.0697	2.0751	Eyes open
2	2.1102	0.1515	0.1014	2.6351	Eyes open
3	1.6851	0.1152	0.079	2.2138	Eyes open
4	2.1054	0.268	0.165	3.7274	Eyes open
5	1.6558	0.1632	0.109	2.1241	Eyes open
6	1.8004	0.1133	0.0711	2.3644	Eyes open
7	2.0154	0.1357	0.0989	3.496	Eyes open
8	1.3267	0.0781	0.0499	1.9388	Eyes open
9	1.0111	0.1119	0.0765	1.4273	Eyes open
10	1.2582	0.0911	0.064	1.6643	Eyes open
11	1.6092	0.0958	0.0617	2.0651	Eyes open
12	2.1002	0.1505	0.1012	2.6341	Eyes open
13	1.685	0.1122	0.0796	2.2118	Eyes open
14	2.1052	0.267	0.166	3.7284	Eyes open
15	1.6458	0.1732	0.1092	2.124	Eyes open
16	1.8	0.1137	0.0721	2.364	Eyes open
17	2.0152	0.1359	0.098	3.4969	Eyes open
18	1.3367	0.0881	0.049	1.9398	Eyes open
19	1.0211	0.1019	0.0755	1.4283	Eyes open
20	1.2581	0.0912	0.062	1.6663	Eyes open

(b)

S.No	Gamma	Theta	Alpha	Beta	Classification
1	69.4383	45.8321	49.4259	221.6474	
2	69.6446	46.5568	57.7681	102.4994	
3	91.8594	42.6131	51.5499	103.0682	
4	67.4971	40.4624	59.9489	174.7884	
5	84.6949	36.1484	72.1629	134.2374	
6	67.0467	62.3433	60.2728	189.6933	
7	79.9600	51.1087	37.0466	129.3347	
8	86.5892	42.7766	49.2190	147.3661	
9	88.7903	36.4910	34.4092	197.5100	
10	66.3496	42.6570	42.2607	220.0897	
11	76.9733	59.2717	47.9967	160.7117	
12	95.7824	48.1827	85.6501	219.9220	
13	93.5209	35.8558	50.6149	98.5616	
14	70.8636	42.8352	77.9335	183.5369	
15	74.8070	45.6797	50.9562	198.5286	
16	87.6967	42.4205	38.7483	139.3835	
17	82.0244	44.9508	80.3661	190.7009	
18	93.7250	58.3833	58.0030	128.3926	
19	80.1814	38.4987	65.4532	101.0202	
20	87.5264	43.1170	41.0551	159.5389	

Fig. 6 **a** Training dataset. **b** Test dataset

excited. Figure 6a shows the snap of training dataset and Fig. 6b shows the snap of test dataset. Attributes that were used for making prediction were

- Gamma,
- Theta,
- Alpha, and
- Beta.

Test dataset consists of 100 datasets which are unclassified and prediction is made for those 100 datasets.

- **Accuracy and prediction of model**

Figure 7 shows the prediction made by the K-NN model using five nearest neighbors, i.e., K = 5. Figure 8 shows the accuracy level which is 97.50% for the particular model and on the basis of prediction, a pie chart and a bar graph are obtained (Fig. 9a, b) viewing the mental state of the user during real-time testing, where

- Red is for not excited,
- Blue is for excited,
- Yellow is for relax,
- Green is for eyes closed, and
- Sea blue is for eyes open.

ExampleSet (100 examples, 7 special attributes, 4 regular attributes) Filte

Row No.	Classif...	predict...	confide...	confide...	confide...	confide...	confide...	Gamma	Theta	Alpha	Beta
1	?	Excited	0	0	0	0	1	69.438	45.832	49.426	221.647
2	?	Excited	0	0	0	0	1	69.645	46.557	57.768	102.499
3	?	Excited	0	0	0	0	1	91.859	42.613	51.550	103.068
4	?	Excited	0	0	0	0	1	67.497	40.462	59.949	174.788
5	?	Excited	0	0	0	0	1	84.695	36.148	72.163	134.237
6	?	Excited	0	0	0	0	1	67.047	62.343	60.273	189.693
7	?	Excited	0	0	0	0	1	79.960	51.109	37.047	129.335
8	?	Excited	0	0	0	0	1	86.589	42.777	49.219	147.366
9	?	Excited	0	0	0	0	1	88.790	36.491	34.409	197.510
10	?	Excited	0	0	0	0	1	66.350	42.657	42.261	220.090
11	?	Excited	0	0	0	0	1	76.973	59.272	47.997	160.712
12	?	Excited	0	0	0	0	1	95.782	48.183	85.650	219.922
13	?	Excited	0	0	0	0	1	93.521	35.856	50.615	98.562
14	?	Excited	0	0	0	0	1	70.864	42.835	77.933	183.537
15	?	Excited	0	0	0	0	1	74.807	45.680	50.956	198.529
16	?	Excited	0	0	0	0	1	87.697	42.420	38.748	139.383
17	?	Excited	0	0	0	0	1	82.024	44.951	80.366	190.701
18	?	Excited	0	0	0	0	1	93.725	58.383	58.003	128.393
19	?	Excited	0	0	0	0	1	80.181	38.499	65.453	101.020
20	?	Excited	0	0	0	0	1	87.526	43.117	41.055	159.539
21	?	Eyes open	1	0	0	0	0	1.982	0.242	0.053	3.423

Fig. 7 Prediction made using K-NN

Table View Plot View

accuracy: 97.50%

	true Eyes open	true Eyes close	true Relax	true Not Excited	true Excited	class precision
pred. Eyes open	15	2	0	0	0	88.24%
pred. Eyes close	0	13	0	0	0	100.00%
pred. Relax	0	0	15	0	0	100.00%
pred. Not Excit...	0	0	0	15	0	100.00%
pred. Excited	0	0	0	0	20	100.00%
class recall	100.00%	86.67%	100.00%	100.00%	100.00%	

Fig. 8 K-NN prediction model with 97.50% accuracy

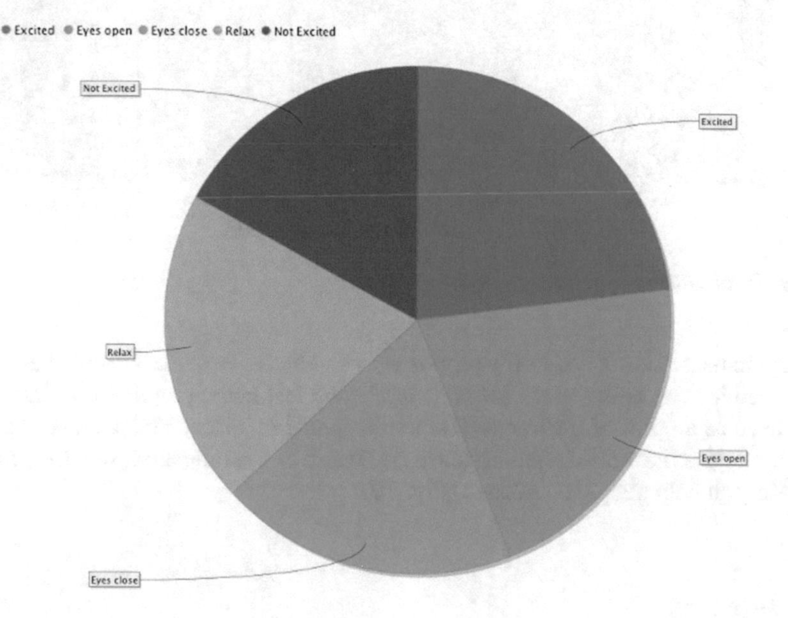

Fig. 9 Pie chart

6 Conclusion and Future Work

The process of building applications has been a journey and it varies depending on one's application requirements and purpose [11]. The proposed system will prove to be triumphant in providing automated health benefits at home with high accuracy and reducing the expenses on overall health care, generating data of person's mental and physical health at each moment and successful in early detecting of diseases and can save many people from injury or even deaths. It is easy to use and provide healthcare support even when the user is sleeping. With accuracy as high as 97.50%, the proposed model can completely revolutionize people's idea about health care and

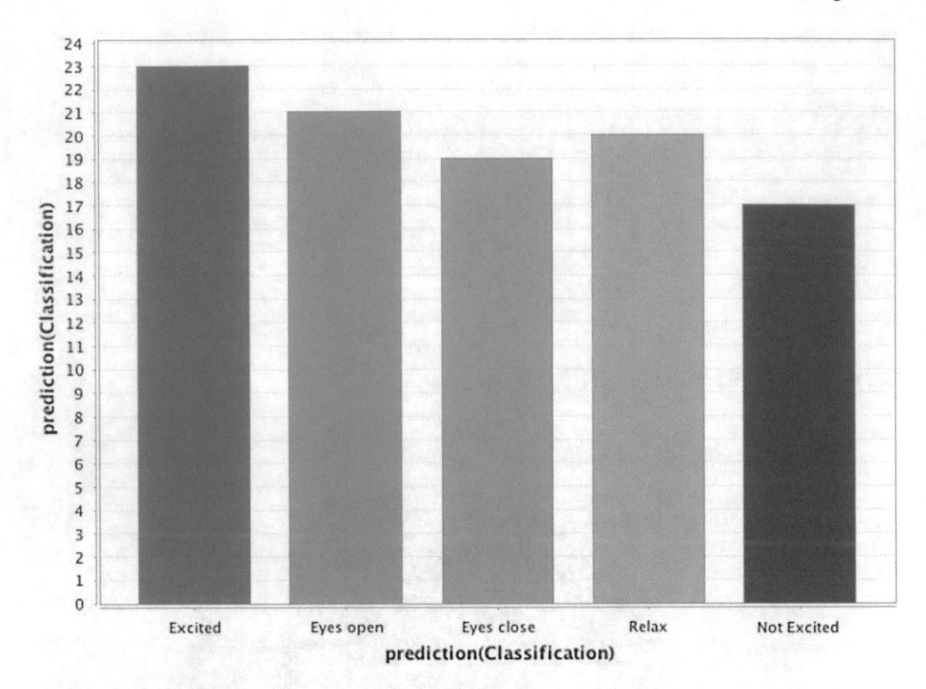

Fig. 10 Bar graph

management. This chapter only proposes wearable and bed smart health care but can be used in cars, ambulances for patient's health test while en route hospital, or can be used as a point of treatment in small hospitals in absence of doctors. Applying technologies like artificial intelligence and machine learning alongside the proposed model can help people on masses (Fig. 10).

References

1. Bhandari T (2013) Health system research: development, designs and methods. J Health Allied Sci, Pokhara University
2. Zhang H, Li J, Wen B, Xun Y, Liu J (2018) Connecting intelligent things in smart hospitals using NB-IoT. IEEE Internet Things J 5(3):1550–1560
3. Singh R, Deep V, Mehrotra D (2018) Electricity generating and monitoring system using IoT. In: IET conference proceedings, p 17 (6 pp)-17 (6 pp). https://doi.org/10.1049/cp.2018.1385
4. IET Digital Library. https://digital-library.theiet.org/content/conferences/10.1049/cp.2018.1385
5. Ramasamy P, Sivapatham S (2016) Assessment of factors associated with early and late stage diagnosis of buccal mucosa carcinoma. J App Pharm Sci 6(08):079–082
6. Sorg MH, Greenwald M, Wren JA (2016) Patterns of drug-induced mortality in Maine, 2015 update. Maine Policy Rev 25(1):34–46. https://digitalcommons.library.umaine.edu/mpr/vol25/iss1/8
7. https://www.cdc.gov/media/releases/2014/p0501-preventable-deaths.html

8. Zhang H, Liu J, Li R, Le H (2017) Fault diagnosis of body sensor networks using hidden Markov model. Peer-to-Peer Netw Appl 10(6):1285–1298
9. Andrzejak RG, Lehnertz K, Mormann F, Rieke C, David P, Elger CE (2001) Indications of non-linear deterministic and finite-dimensional structures in time series of brain electrical activity: dependence on recording region and brain state. Physical Review E, 64(6):061907
10. Dharmawan Z (2007) Analysis of computer games player stress level using EEG data. Man-Machine Interaction Group, Delft University of Technology, Delft, Netherlands
11. Kharb L (2018) A perspective view on commercialization of cognitive computing. In: 2018 8th international conference on cloud computing, data science & engineering, IEEE
12. www.gacovinolake.com/practice-areas/medical-malpractice/injury-related-to-delayed-diagnosis/
13. Salem O, Guerassimov A, Mehaoua A, Marcus A, Furht B (2013) Sensor fault and patient anomaly detection and classification in medical wireless sensor networks. IEEE ICC 2013:4373–4378

Rashbir Singh is a young innovator, developer, and technology enthusiast who loves to research and learn continuously. He did his B. Tech (IT) from Amity University, Greater Noida, India. He wishes to pursue MS Program from Australia. He has strong interest in the field of Data Science and Machine Learning and has written and presented two papers in International Conferences sponsored by Springer. He has a special interest in working with live data through biomedical sensors (EEG, ECG, EMG) and natural language data. He found a start-up named LAZADO in 2017. He did internship as Research and Development Intern at DRDO in 2018, and is working as Data Analyst at CRMNEXT, Delhi.

Prateek Singh is a final year student of Masters in Computer Science Program at Jagan Institute of Management Studies (JIMS), Delhi, India. He is currently working as an Intern with IT Department of Religare Health Insurance Company Ltd. He has strong interest in the field of Data Science and Machine Learning and has written and presented two papers in International Conferences sponsored by Springer. He has written book chapters for Emerald, Springer, AAP, and IGI Global (in press).

Latika Kharb is currently a Professor at Jagan Institute of Management Studies (JIMS), Delhi, India. Her research for the past 13 years has been directed in the areas of Software Engineering, Artificial Intelligence, and Data Analytics. She served as a reviewer and advisory board member of IEEE, Springer, Elsevier, and IGI Global journals and conferences. She has been Editor of two books with title "Communications in Computer and Information Science with Springer. Five conferences have been organized by Dr. Kharb with Springer sponsorship. She has published over 137 technical papers in various national/international journals and conferences. She is also a member of Editorial Board/Review Board by the Board of Governors of International Association of Scientific Innovation and Research (IASIR-United States), CSTA-ACM Computer Society, International Association of Computer Science and Information Technology (IACSIT-Singapore), SCIence and Engineering Institute (SCIEI-USA), The Society of Digital Information and Wireless Communications (SDIWC), International Journal of Computer Applications (IJCA-USA), International Association of Computer Science and Information Technology (IACSIT), Global member of Internet Society (USA/Switzerland), and International Association of Engineering (IAENG).

A Fog-Based Approach for Real-Time Analytics of IoT-Enabled Healthcare

G. Jeya shree and S. Padmavathi

Abstract In recent years, the number of Internet of Things (IoT) devices/sensors has been increased to a great extent. IoT makes use of connected intelligent devices to gather the data using embedded sensors and actuator. The IoT devices generate huge amount of data which are currently being processed using cloud computing. Considering real-time patient monitoring in the healthcare industry, there is a delay caused by sending data to the cloud and receiving back to the application which causes high latency. To address this issue, fog computing plays a major role in computation, analytics, and storing sensitive data of the patient with the advantages of reduced latency, quick decision-making, improved energy efficiency, and reduced network congestion. With real-time monitoring of the critical health condition in-place by means of a smart medical device connected to a smartphone application can save a life on time. In this chapter, a fog-based scenario is considered where health data from patients are collected and transferred to the fog nodes. These data are filtered, preprocessed, and analyzed, and dynamic decisions are made using intelligent methodologies that are incorporated in the fog. The decisions are made based on the current patient state and stored continuously for long-term analysis, while abnormality alone is notified to people via mobile apps and other linked devices. Thus, we have compiled this chapter with the introduction of sensors in healthcare, key advantage of processing them in fog instead of cloud, their evolution, and future directions.

Keywords Fog computing · Cloud computing · Internet of Things · Healthcare · Sensors/actuators

G. Jeya shree (✉) · S. Padmavathi
Department of Information Technology, Thiagarajar College of Engineering, Madurai 625015, India

S. Padmavathi
e-mail: spmcse@tce.edu

R. Raj et al. (eds.), *Internet of Things Use Cases for the Healthcare Industry*,
https://doi.org/10.1007/978-3-030-37526-3_3

1 Introduction

The sophisticated lifestyle of the current generation has led to a different perspective and a lot of advancements in today's technology. Automation is present almost in every day to day activities of human life. This has led to rapid growth in the number of Internet of Things (IoT) and it thereby enormously increased the amount of data being generated (big data). IoT is a network of connected devices (sensors/actuators) that captures data from the users and is connected to the cloud. This technology has been greatly adopted in various sectors and it ensures betterment in the lifestyle and well-being of mankind [1, 2]. The adoption of IoT technologies in various sectors like large-scale industries, healthcare, agriculture, smart home, and smart cities improved the quality of service by automating the tasks and reduced human interventions. For hosting IoT applications, cloud infrastructure is often used [3]. Cloud offers various scalable and elastic services (PaaS, IaaS, and SaaS) in a pay-as-you-go model and has its own advantage in terms of large data centers suitable for hosting complex and computation-intensive applications.

Healthcare is conventionally an important sector as it deals with the overall well-being of the people in terms of physical as well as mental health. An efficient healthcare system can contribute to a significant part of a country's economy, development, and industrialization [4]. The various types of healthcare such as medical, psychology, physiotherapy, public health, and allied health are differentiated depending upon the disciplinary perspectives of the people. Healthcare at any level is a process which is important and it can be either public (in groups, societal health) or private (individual, personal health). Healthcare services [4] are generally subdivided into three categories such as primary care, secondary care, and tertiary care.

a. **Primary care**

Primary healthcare deals with services such as elderly patient monitoring, chronic disease monitoring, and so on. Chronic diseases like asthma, depression, hypertension, COPD, diabetes, back pain or anxiety may be usually treated in primary care. Primary care also includes many basic maternal and child healthcare services, such as family planning services and vaccinations. Continuity is a key characteristic of primary care, as patients usually prefer to consult the same practitioner for routine checkups and preventive care, health education, and every time they require an initial consultation about a new health problem. This recommends the healthcare system to maintain their health histories for providing better services to the patients.

This chapter focuses mainly on primary care as it deals with the real-time yet vital factors to monitor. Monitoring an elderly or a chronic illness patient may arise situations where they witness an unexpected, critical condition that has to be taken utmost care and to be responded immediately. The effectiveness of the proposed approach is discussed based on a case study, considering primary care services.

b. **Secondary care**

Secondary care covers the required treatment for a brief limited period of time where acute care is necessary but does not cover the serious illness, injury, etc. The healthcare services usually provided by the emergency department in the hospital fall under this secondary care type. The secondary care also encompasses skilled turnout during labor and delivery, conscientious care, and medical visual diagnosis. Medical analyst, pulmonologist, occupational therapists, speech pathologist, and nutritionist are some healthcare professionals who work under secondary care.

c. **Tertiary care**

The tertiary care involves its services in complex care in the field of radiation therapy for cancer, surgical treatment for the nervous system, cardiovascular surgery, plastic surgery, and treatment of deeper skin tissues damage, advanced pediatrics services during childbirth, and other complex remedy and medical intercession. It is expert advisory healthcare, generally for inpatients and to those who look up for guide after a primary or secondary health professional's referral. In such a case, tertiary care is able to provide facilities that have both personnel and intense medical care for the patients to manage conflict disease or any serious disorder, such as a tertiary mentioned clinic.

Healthcare industry has acquired a lot of advancements due to the evolution of IoT into it. IoT has helped healthcare sector with several services like monitoring elderly or chronic patients, remote monitoring, detecting and predicting fall, telemedicine, mobile or m-health, activity tracking, physiological attribute monitors, smart pills, smart beds, and so on. The connected devices continuously monitor and considers even a small detail in the patient's health that enables the possibility to make the right decisions at the right time thus improves patients' overall health. This is more helpful for people with chronic diseases or elderly people who have problems in their Activities of Daily Living (ADL). The IoT in healthcare can be detailed as a combination of technology (wearables), analytics and connectivity. It has the benefits for both patients to stay safe and healthy as well as physicians to deliver good care. The concept of IoT in Healthcare entails the use of sensors (wearables) or any other electronic devices to capture and monitor data from the patient. These devices are connected to the cloud (public/private) and analyzed to trigger actions on certain abnormal conditions. The abnormal condition is subjected to individual patients who are being monitored based upon their own health condition.

Not just healthcare, nowadays, the Internet of Things (IoT) has been adopted by a large number of organizations and enterprises, where a large amount of data is generated. So, the demand for quick access to such enormous amounts of data is kept on increasing. The characterization of big data is along three dimensions such as volume, velocity, and variety [5]. But IoT use cases like smart transportation, smart cities, and smart grid are generally distributed in nature. Hence, this needs a fourth dimension to the characterization of big data, i.e., geo-distribution.

2 IoT Analytics

IoT Analytics is the next important topic to be studied. The analytics of data plays a major role in healthcare as it all deals with the life of people. IoT analytics is an art and science of finding out hidden patterns, identifying abnormalities, and bringing out insights from the massive quantity of data generated by connected IoT devices. Enterprises highly rely on their IoT platforms for various services. First, they need to deploy various platform analytics services and then test the analytics configuration processes and also it is important to evaluate the following three types of analytics capabilities [6] such as:

- **Descriptive Analytics**—It will be used to describe and aggregate incoming IoT data.
- **Predictive Analytics**—By analyzing historical data, it will be used to model its future data and behaviors.
- **Prescriptive analytics**—With the uses of advance techniques, it helps to optimize a solution that has to be taken in the future.

To better understand the analytics on the IoT health data, let us detail the overall architecture of the IoT. Figure 1 shows the comprehend architecture of IoT across any application sectors.

The bottom-most layer is the **edge** where the devices collect data from smart and non-smart devices. The second layer is the **gateway** layer where the devices represent cloud near the edge devices. The third layer is the **cloud**, a repository that bears storage and computes for the underlying devices. The fourth layer is the **consumption** layer where mining of required data out from the repository. The fifth layer is the **insight** layer where the knowledge is derived from the data consumed and the final layer is the **application** layer that contains software performing user services with the support of edge devices using the processes data from the previous layer.

The sequence of processes generally carried out in IoT analytics across the various industry (Google, Microsoft, Amazon, IBM, etc.) platforms is [7]:

- Data generation,
- Data gathering,
- Data consumption,
- Real-Time data stream processing,
- Data storing, and
- Data visualizing.

Figure 2 describes the abovementioned steps that are being followed across various industry platforms

a. **Data gathering and Consumptions**

This is the first step in this IoT analytics. By using different option, the data is collected from the IoT sensors such as Apache NiFi, Direct ingestion from MQTT

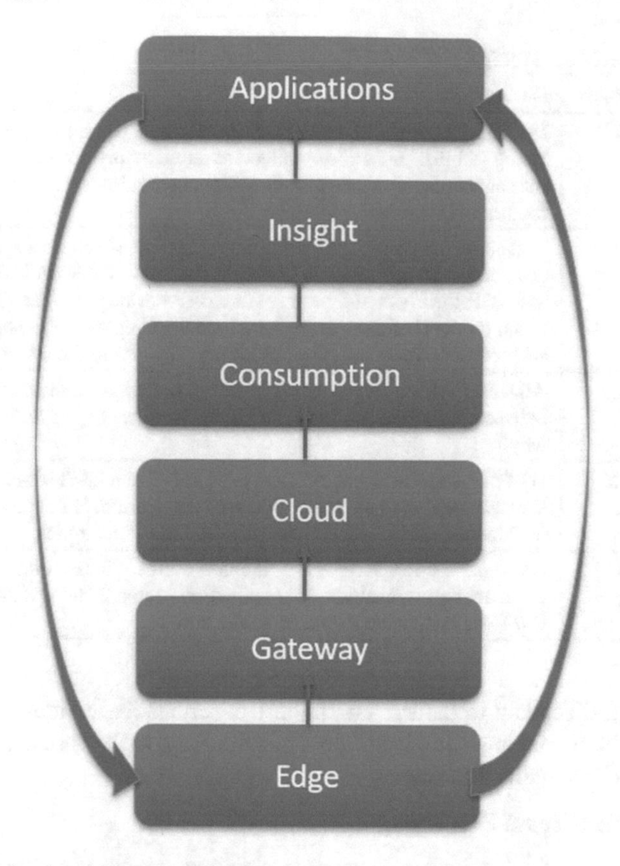

Fig. 1 Comprehend architecture of IoT

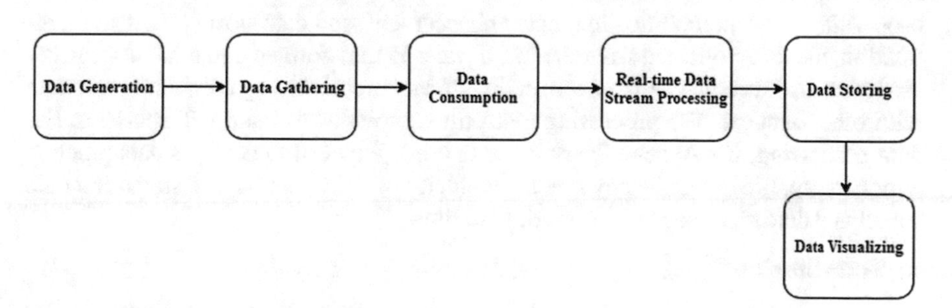

Fig. 2 Stages in IoT analytics

Broker, Stream sets. Using Apache MiNiFi on raspberry is a low consuming agent, and hence, data can be easily collected and route it to the Apache NiFi and also to multiple destinations. Direct ingestion from MQTT broker is one way to ingest data directly from MQTT broker where we need to build a data flow pipeline using a different processor. Stream Set data collector edge is an ultralight agent, used to

Table 1 Protocols used for IoT platform

S. no.	Protocols	Description
1	MQTT	Message Queuing Telemetry Transport is a machine-to-machine protocol. It uses publish/subscribe architecture based on broker model and useful for connecting with a remote location where minimum bandwidth/code footprint is required
2	CoAP	Constrained Application Protocol is a web-based protocol specially designed to connect with lightweight devices IoT device. Unlike HTTP and TCP, the flows of the packet in CoAP are very smaller. CoAP works based on the client/server model where the client makes a request to the server and server send a corresponding response to the client
3	AMQP	Advanced Messaging Queuing Protocol is an open standard for messaging between organizations and applications in an encrypted and interoperable way
4	HTTP	HTTP is a standard web services protocol. The RESTFul architecture style is extensively used in mobile and web application. HTTP is a document-centric protocol and still used in IoT analytics
5	DDS	Data Distribution Service is a standard protocol for real-time analytics. It is a machine-to-machine communication protocol and this can be used in low footprint device as well as in the cloud

collect data and sends it to the stream. Table 1 describes the various protocols that are used in direct data ingestion from sensor devices and to forward them for further processing and visualization stages.

b. **Real-Time Stream Processing**

The real-time stream processing means carrying out processing while the data is still being produced from the IoT device. The steps involved in the real-time stream processing are data modification, data enhancement, and data storing. In data modification, the data collected from the IoT devices is transformed and ready for further analytics. In data enhancement, the quality of data is enriched by combining raw data with other data set. The processing platform is provided to build IoT analytics. For data processing, the Apache Spark is being used. We need to design a data pipeline which is capable to handle any size and velocity of data because IoT streaming data speed and data size may vary from time to time.

c. **Data Storing**

The various industries provide platforms such as HBase, HDFS, ElasticSearch for storing of data. The data storage is another important step as all the intelligent systems might need historic data for training the system to commit efficient decision-making.

d. **Data Visualizing**

It is the most important part where the data presentation lies. The industry solutions offer a custom dashboard for the visualization of the data. Visualizing helps to learn the performance of the whole system at the end.

Table 2 Various IoT analytics platforms

Steps	Google IoT architecture	AWS IoT architecture	Microsoft Azure IoT architecture
Consumption	• Cloud Pub/Sub is used to collect data from AQTT broker • The advantage of using Cloud Pub/Sub is to natively connect to other cloud platform service and also handle real-time stream data	• In AWS IoT architecture Kinesis stream is used for data consumption	• The Event Hub is connected to MQTT • The data consumption is published by Raspberry pi on the MQTT broker
Processing	• Once the data is digested from Cloud Pub/Sub then it further sends to cloud dataflow for processing	• Data is collected from MQTT and sent to Kinesis Analytics for future processing	• The data is processed using Stream Analytics
Storing and processing	• After processing the cloud dataflow pipeline sends the processed data to the BigQuery. And further DataLab is used for data visualizing	• Once processed, the data is sent to Amazon Redshift and Amazon s3 • In AWS the data is represented using Amazon QuickSight that can build visualization dashboards	• The data after processing is sent to Azure CosmoDB and visualized on power BI

Table 2 shows how IoT analytics is followed across various industries. In all the IoT analytics platform, the same steps are followed as mentioned above.

3 Fog Computing

Fog computing is an emerging paradigm that extends cloud computing and services to the network edge. Fog computing has been discussed as a platform to provide support for Internet of Things (IoT) [8]. In contrast to the cloud, fog computing is aimed at deploying services in a widely distributed manner whereas it is centralized in the cloud [8]. Fog provides storage and computation resources as well as application services to the users, like cloud [9]. The low-latency and geo-distributed applications that do not fit well in the cloud can be addressed through fog computing [5]. Generally, the IoT data in latency-sensitive applications have a very less life span. By the time the data reaches the cloud for its analysis, the actual need for that data might be lost

[8] hence it must be processed fast. A MIST-Fog-based analytics scheme for cost-efficient resource provisioning for IoT application is presented in [10] in which the data consumer association, task distribution, and virtual machine placement problem are also considered in minimizing the overall cost while the QoS requirement is still satisfied [10]. The processing of data is generally carried out in the nodes present in the fog layer called fog nodes. A fog node can be any device with storage, computing, and network connectivity. Fog layer acts on IoT data in a fraction of seconds and analyzes the most time-sensitive data at the edge close to the end users where it is generated. This reduces the cost, time, and effort in outsourcing them to the cloud. The fog has been emerged as a powerful platform to deploy various applications like energy, healthcare, traffic, and so on [5]. Thus, fog computing outperforms cloud by creating a distributed framework for IoT to cope up with the needs of sensors and embedded systems such as data processing and storage.

Figure 3 shows the basic architecture of fog computing layer. Fog computing layer is generally capable to carry out tasks such as gathering, filtration, and aggregation of data. Fog cannot perform independent of cloud and hence cannot be its replacement. One key aspect of this new era is that both computation and production are heavily distributed and are at the network's edge or closer to where data generated. Fog computing applications that have low-latency requirements cannot rely on the cloud for its data and processing support. Also, the centralized data centers in the cloud

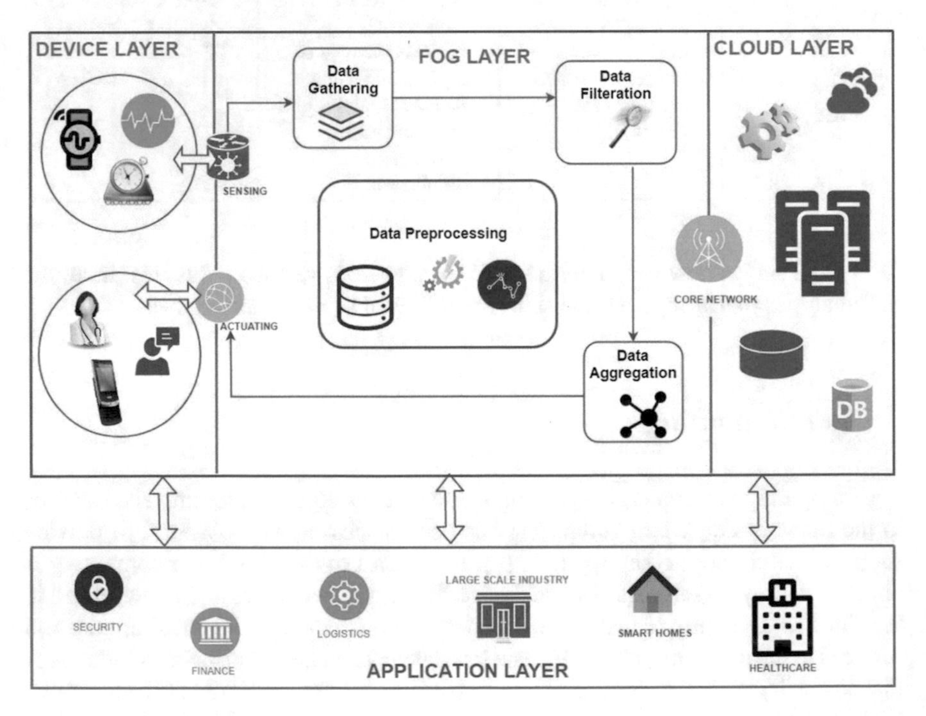

Fig. 3 Fog computing architecture

do not support mobility, and hence, the heavily distributed IoT applications need distributed support for data and processing at the edge [11]. The IoT layer can be connected to the fog layer through low-level connectivity like Zig-Bee, Bluetooth, Wi-Fi, etc., and fog layer is connected to the cloud through a gateway with high-level connectivity. The gateway performs operations such as protocol translation between sensor and cloud layer. Exploiting such gateways at the edge provide a better overall enhancement in the system such as energy efficiency, mobility, performance, reliability, and security [12].

a. **Characteristics of fog computing**

The open fog consortium is a group of high-tech industries and academic institutions worldwide who provide the standard architecture for fog computing. The general characteristics of fog computing imposed by open fog consortium are described in [13]. Further, many literatures have presented various characteristics of fog computing such as real-time application support, large-scale application support, mobility support, virtualization support, and heterogeneity support. In this section, we describe the specific characteristics and benefits of fog computing which should be considered predominantly with respect to the healthcare industry.

i. **Low latency**

Most of the healthcare applications like monitoring patients in Intensive Care Units (ICU), remote monitoring of isolated patients in home or hospital, elderly or chronic patient's monitoring involves critical analysis of patient's condition and notify via automatic alarms once criticality is detected. So, the criticality must be informed within seconds or less. Hence, this implies the real-time properties such as response time [14]. Latency cannot be tolerated in such emergency conditions. This shows the importance of "low-latency requirement". Since fog is available at a one-hop distance, low-latency requirement will be satisfied.

ii. **Mobility**

Healthcare applications like remote monitoring of patients in hospitals or home may involve a change of environment. The processing and decision-making in fog is subjected to user geo-location. The location is based on the behavior of the system or human interventions [10]. Thus, user behavior decides the time and place of the computing device, and it is distributed. Hence, centralized cloud will not be suitable for this kind of applications and hence we need fog like distributed architecture.

iii. **Energy efficiency**

The fog nodes are generally constrained devices, while it encounters some of the tasks like surveillance systems, where data comes in a continuous stream and makes it intensive. In such cases, the tasks can be offloaded to nearby fog nodes, and thus, the computational complexity can be reduced [15].

iv. **Network Bandwidth**

The IoT layer keeps sending the raw sensed data to the fog nodes. The bit rates of data differ based on physiological attributes. For example, the transmission of body temperature requires only low sampling frequency whereas attributes like Electroencephalogram (EEG) or Electrocardiograms (ECG) may require a high sampling frequency [14]. The amount of data that is being generated is ever-increasing ever since the IoT is popularized and it cannot always make up to send data to the cloud for analysis and retrieve back from them. Hence having the fog at a nearby distance, part of processing and analysis can be done there and a significant amount of network traffic can be reduced [15].

v. **Security**

Since the patient data are highly sensitive and any potential attack or tampering of data can happen to the personal data of patients, the security requirement in healthcare is really high [14]. Several mechanisms are invoked in the fog layer to enhance the security as the association between sensor nodes and fog computing nodes are highly dynamic.

b. **Comparison of fog, cloud, and edge**

Table 3 shows the comparison of fog with other infrastructures such as the cloud and edge to demonstrate the significance of fog computing in various sectors. The different computing paradigms have different features and the following table differentiates fog based on the attributes that are important to consider in healthcare.

Table 3 Difference between cloud, fog, and edge

Attributes	Cloud	Edge	Fog
Architecture	Hierarchical, large centralized data centers located in a remote place	Distributed and localized devices at the edge	Small devices such as routers, access points, gateways, setup boxes, or even the end device itself
Connectivity	Always needs to be connected to the network core, e.g., WAN	Can work with intermittent internet connectivity, e.g., WAN, LAN, Wi-Fi	Can work with low or no Internet connectivity, e.g., Zig-Bee, Wi-Fi Bluetooth
Services access	Global (through core)	Local (at the edge of the network)	Less global (through connected devices from edge to the core)
Availability of computing resource	High	Moderate	Moderate
Latency	High	Low	Low
Virtualization support	Available	Not available	Available
Mobility support	Not available	Not available	Highly available

4 Role of Fog Computing in Healthcare

The involvement of fog computing in the healthcare sector is to make it easier for patients to stay connected to their medical experts, and for the medical personnel to provide quality, value-based care to their patients. Fog computing has come up as an effective infrastructure for transforming the healthcare IoT from novelty to reality. In order to completely realize the true potential of fog computing in the healthcare industry, the three major challenges need to be addressed: the difficulty in converting big data into smart data, the mobility nature of the patients/providers and their lack of interoperability, and the security issues in maintaining the sensitive health data. This section describes various healthcare applications and the involvement of fog computing in such applications.

Luiz et al. [10] described two classes of applications as latency-sensitive and latency-tolerant. Latency-sensitive applications generally involve critical analysis and require a quicker response like healthcare where it deals with the life of a patient (e.g., emergency situation of a patient who needs immediate hospitalization), and latency-tolerant applications involve one's conveniences and sophistication (e.g., smart environment to ease patient's daily activities such as smart pillbox, online appointment for doctors through mobile app, and so on). Though both latency-sensitive and latency-tolerant applications can be handled through the fog. However, in this chapter, we mainly focused the latency-sensitive applications.

Even critical healthcare applications can be categorized as emergency and nonemergency applications. To analyze the adversity of emergency events, techniques like temporal mining are used [16]. Kraemer et al. [14] categorized the applications in healthcare into five major classes such as data collection, data analysis, critical analysis, critical control, and context management. The data collection deals only with the collection of data, and it is later examined by medical professionals when needed. Data analysis also deals with the collection of data followed by some automatic analysis and help patients. Even when the system fails, the patients are safe in both data collection and data analysis classes, the criticality is very low. Whereas, in critical analysis classes, data is analyzed to find the criticality and it has real-time properties such as maximum response time limits. Cardiac patient monitoring, COPD patient monitoring, Diabetic patient monitoring [17] are examples of critical analysis classes. COPD means Chronic Obstructive Pulmonary Disease, which refers to a group of diseases that causes blockage in airflow and causes problems related to breathing [18]. The critical control classes involve alerting the personnel on finding some criticality and context management is simply to improve the healthcare system by efficient planning and by taking the right decisions.

Since the Fog computing works on data at the network's edge, i.e., close to where the data being generated, this significantly improves the response time otherwise reduced latency and also reduced network traffic. Several literatures have used fog computing in healthcare for predicting and preventing specific diseases like chikungunya [19], Zika virus attack [20] and monitoring patients' health in smart homes [16], providing Emergency system for smart enhanced living environments [21], and also for incorporating intelligence in the fog layer for data analytics [22]. Vijayakumar et al. [23] designed an intelligent healthcare system for detecting and preventing mosquito-borne diseases, where similarity coefficient is used to differentiate various mosquito-borne diseases based on symptoms of the patient, then it is classified into infected or uninfected using fuzzy K-nearest neighbor. Considering the patient monitoring applications, a lot of work has come up with assisting the patients through smart pills [24], early sign detection of an attack and so on. Monitoring diabetes patients is described in [17] where a decision tree is employed to predict the risk level and it shows greater accuracy. By monitoring healthy/less-critical patients continuously, they can be kept away from the hospital as much as possible, and it is described as shifting from reactive to proactive otherwise preventive in [25]. Several literatures also employed Body Area Networks (BANs) to collect traces of patient's action and made to pass through gateways. Fall detection [26] is one of the major competent research problems, as 80% of the elderly adults who live alone fall unexpectedly due to various factors like giddiness, a sudden drop in blood pressure or deviations in their ECGs. Castillo et al. [27] propose many techniques to detect fall and notify immediately through alarms. To enforce fault-tolerant healthcare systems, pattern-matching algorithms were employed in [28] to avoid false alarms.

5 Deployment of Healthcare Applications

a. Cloud-IoT Environment

There are many IoT-related healthcare applications that exist uses cloud computing for its deployment. A Cloud-Based Intelligent Health Care Service (CBIHCS) is proposed in [29] to perform real-time monitoring of a user's health data for diagnosis of the diabetic patient. Similarly, a cloud-based mobile system is presented in [30] to support people suffering from respiratory diseases and to improve homecare for them. These applications rely on the cloud infrastructures for their processing, computing, and storage requirements. WSNs based sensor-cloud architecture [31] is proposed which uses cloud servers to remotely monitor patients. The implementation of cloud-based healthcare system often uses cloud servers and data centers for processing the IoT data.

IoT data are generally unstructured which makes them difficult in analyzing with traditional analytics platforms/tools that are designed to process structured data. Due to the distributed nature of the IoT technologies, the current computing paradigm which uses the cloud as its centralized data center becomes unsuitable to support many of the IoT applications like finance, large-scale industry, and healthcare, which are highly latency-sensitive. These kinds of applications cannot tolerate delay caused during the transmission of data to the cloud for analysis since it requires a faster response to make timely decisions. Network traffic is another drawback that can happen in the cloud as a huge amount of data is being transmitted to and from the cloud simultaneously.

These challenges in cloud raised the need for new computing and hence is the fog computing, a distributed platform for managing the distributed computing, networking, and storage resources at the edge. Bonomi et al. [5] defined Fog computing as a computing paradigm that extends the cloud to the network edge. Fog act as an intermediate layer between the cloud and devices and it reduces the amount of data to be stored locally. By performing the data analysis locally before sending to cloud, latency can be reduced. Also having the fog at a single hop distance, bandwidth can be reduced.

b. **Edge/Fog Deployments**

Fog computing is closely related to IoT as it is generating an enormous amount of data day by day. The emerging trends in the Smart application are to use Fog computing over the cloud for its processing of IoT data. Fog computing empowers the edge node devices to carry out the Local data processing, Cache data management, Dense geographical distribution, Local resource pooling, Load balancing, local device management, latency reduction for better QoS and edge node analytics. The critical aspect considered in fog computing is Time. The most time-critical tasks in the applications are locally analyzed and it results in the lowest latency and prevents major damage before it may even occur (e.g., alarm status, device status, fault warnings). On the other hand, the less time-critical tasks are sent to the central mainframe and it results in persistent, periodical storage and can be retrieved as and when required (e.g., files, reports for historical analysis, device logs). Table 4 describes some of the healthcare applications that have used fog or edge for its computations. These implementations utilize constrained devices like gateway devices, routers, base stations, etc., for the computation purpose.

6 Case Study: A Real-Time Fog Healthcare Scenario

In this section, the environmental setup is done for implementing a heart patient monitoring system using sensors, fog nodes, and cloud platform. The fog computing layer consists of a number of fog nodes and each fog node takes responsibility for the processing of data. The fog nodes here are Raspberry pi and Arduino. One of the main advantages of fog computing is its support for mobility which is not supported in cloud computing. These features of fog computing make it efficient for real-time applications as the users tend to move from one place to another. The novel aspect of this architectural framework is the ability of the decision-making system to adapt to the dynamically changing requirements of the applications

Figure 4 shows the architecture with the three layers such as application, fog, and cloud layer. The bottom-most layer is the application layer that captures data from sensors and transmits them through low-level networks such as Bluetooth, Wi-Fi,

Table 4 Fog involved application scenarios

S. no.	Application	Computation	Deployment	Implementation
1	COPD patient monitoring system [11]	Analysis of patient's vital signs and detection of dramatic changes using BAN- and GPS-based location prediction	Mobile devices with network interface	Edge/fog computing
2	ECG monitoring [33]	Analysis and processing of EEG and ECG data based on the transformation of the wave and notifying the classification based on ML	Intelligent Power over Ethernet (PoE) gateway	
3	Fall detection [26]	Local analysis of fall using accelerometer data with filtering based on trained data	Mobile devices with backend web services	
4	Vital signs monitoring [34]	Prediction of location and activity along with physiological parameters (ECG, body temperature, heart rate) by preprocessing and merging data from the smart shirt	Hospital with WSN systems	
5	Activity monitoring [35]	Analysis of movement data in the context of the location and analysis of heart rate, acceleration, and activity like sitting, driving, and walking	Mobile and ProWare middleware	

LAN. This is one main advantage of fog computing. The middle layer is the fog layer, where the data is processed on fog nodes. A cloudlet is a group of fog nodes intended to collaboratively divide the tasks and process them in parallel. The IoT data is gathered and distributed across the fog nodes. The AI methodologies and decision-making system are deployed on those fog nodes based on its capability.

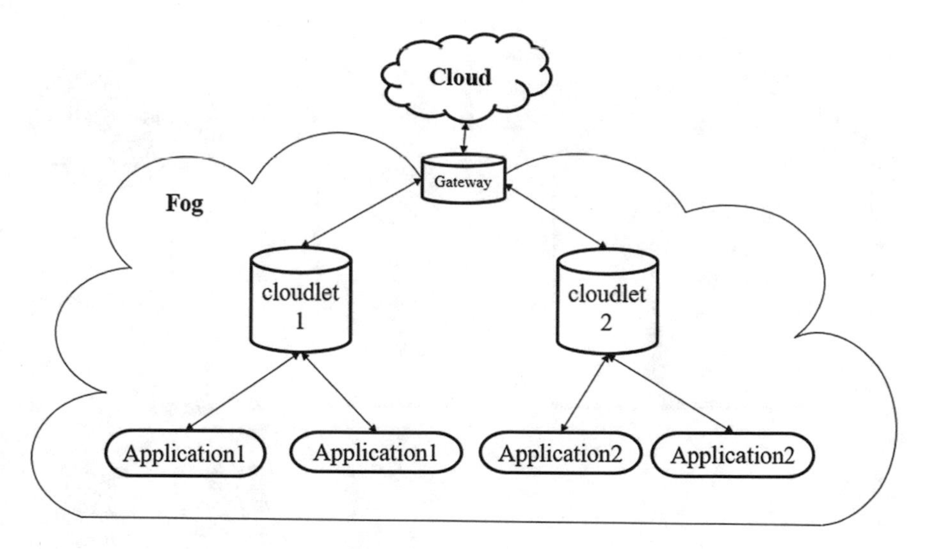

Fig. 4 Fog computing application deployments

Based on the results of processing, the alert or notification kind of output is delivered through actuators and data for the long term and periodical analysis is sent to the cloud layer which is at the topmost layer. As familiar through various studies, the cloud computing layer comprises the centralized data centre.

In this work, an environment for heart patient monitoring in addition to pills monitoring has been designed. The results are evaluated using the Raspberry Pi and Arduino and data are gathered using sensors like DHT 11, Pulse rate, Load cell, HX711. The DHT 11 is used to collect Temperature and Humidity data. The collected data are analyzed in the fog node itself and alert notification are sent through the Android application to both physician and caretaker. The data are visualized using an open-source cloud platform.

Figure 5 explains the environment that is proposed in this chapter for the patient monitoring system. The load cell and HX711 are used to monitor whether the patient has taken their pills or not based on the weight of the capsules in the pillbox. Let X1 be the weight of the pillbox with pills and X2 be the weight of pillbox without pills. If weight = X1, it considered that the patient has not taken the pills yet else they have taken it. This is the way of monitoring whether the patient has taken their pills or not.

The DHT 11 and Load cell are connected to the Raspberry pi which is one of the fog nodes, the pulse rate is connected to Arduino which is another fog node. Both fog nodes are connected to the cloud through the open-source cloud platform. Once the environment is set, the sensor starts to read the values from the patient and

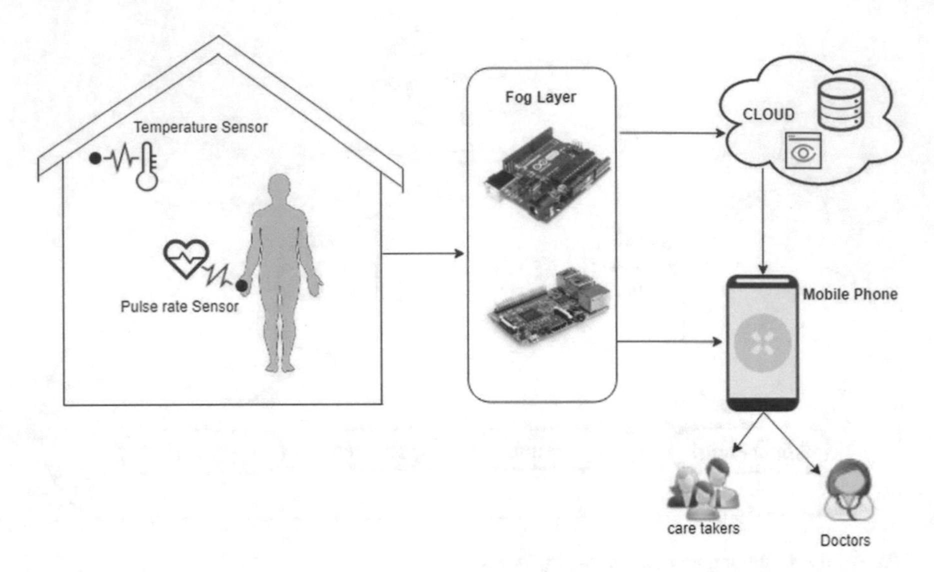

Fig. 5 Patient monitoring system

processed in fog node itself rather sending them to cloud to reduce the latency, energy consumption, and bandwidth. For the processing of data in fog node, we used the generalized algorithm given below. The threshold value is set on each sensor based on the medical standards of each sensor. For example, the average medical standard of heart rate is 60–100. If there are any abnormalities found in the values then the alert notification is sent to the Physician and Caretaker through in-app notification to Android application, created for the physician and caretakers. And the real-time data have also been visualized through the open-source cloud platform.

Algorithm 1: Emergency Notify
This algorithm is generalized and it is applied to the abovementioned sensors. The threshold defined in the algorithm is different for different sensors. Each sensor plays a vital role in monitoring the heart patient. For any heart patient, the following three parameters are very important, namely**, environment, physiological, and activity** based on the three sensors used for each parameter.

The temperature and humidity sensor monitors the environmental parameter, pulse rate sensor monitors the physiological parameter, and load cell sensor monitors the activity parameter.

INPUT: Real values from sensors

1. Temperature and Humidity
2. Pulse rate
3. Load cell

OUTPUT: Notification during critical situations

STEPS:

1. Create an environment with the sensors, fog nodes, and cloud connectivity
2. Initialize the threshold values for temperature sensor as **T_Threshold** and Pulse rate as **P_ Threshold.**
3. Assume weight X1 be the weight of the pillbox with pills and X2 be the weight of the pillbox without pills.
4. Read the real input values from the sensors and process them in fog node.
5. If (Temperature <T_ threshold || Temperature >T_ threshold) || (weight==X1(the weight of the pillbox with pills)) then,
   a. Notification is sent to **caretaker** via in-app notification to the Android application that we created

   Else if (Pulse rate <P_ threshold || Pulse rate> threshold)

   b. Notification is sent to the **physician as well as caretaker** via the in-app notification to the Android application

   Else

   c. Data are stored in the cloud for future analysis.
6. Data visualization is done in an open-source cloud platform.

The Raspberry Pi and Arduino are used to gathering the real-time data of temperature, pulse rate, pills monitoring with respect to a sensor like DHT11, Pulse rate, Load cell, HX711. The data gathered are visualized using thing speak platform and they are sent to the firebase for real-time data storage.

Figure 6 is the output for pills monitoring which is calculated based on the weight of the pillbox. This is done with the help of Load cell and HX711. As the Raspberry does not support direct analog signals, they are converted to digital signals using HX711 which is given as input to the raspberry pi. Let X1 be the weight of the pillbox with pills and X2 be the weight of pillbox without pills. If weight = X1, it considered that the patient has not taken the pills yet else they have taken it. This way whether the patient has taken their pills or not can be monitored.

Figure 7 is the output of the pulse rate of a patient. The BPM is the expansion of Beats Per Minute. If the beat is sensed then it results as "**A Heartbeat Happened**" else "**No HeartBeat Happened**".

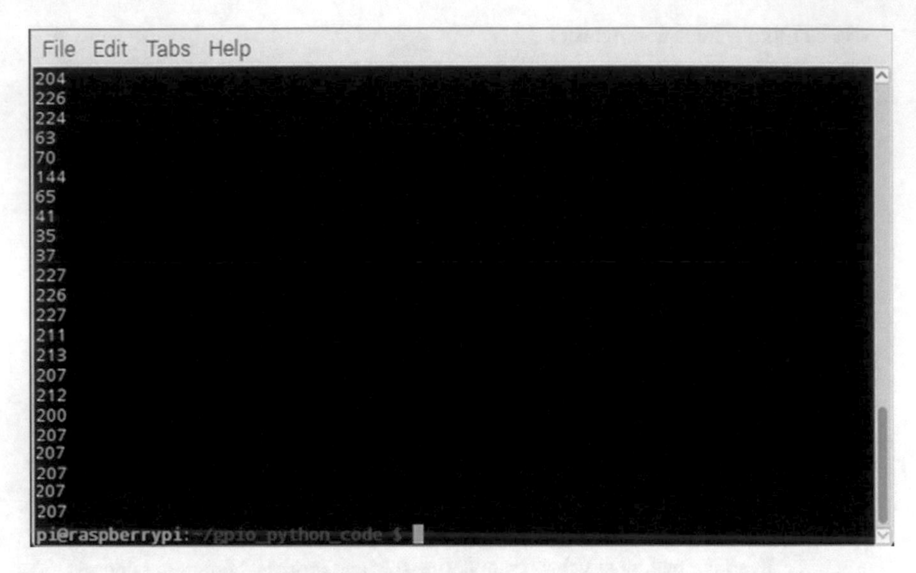

Fig. 6 Pill monitoring based on weight calculation

Figure 8 infers the pulse rate of a patient at a certain time. Patient heart rate is normal over some period and has a sudden deviation at some point and back to normal in a few seconds. Hence, the visualization of values helps us in monitoring the abnormalities in pulse rate of the patient.

Figures 9 and 10 are the visualization of the environment parameter, which shows a gradual increase and decrease in the temperature and humidity and provides us in a better way to keep tracking the environment.

Figure 11 is the results for temperature and humidity which is taken using DHT 11 sensor with the help of Raspberry pi. The environmental condition of heart patients such as a temperature and humidity is important. If it is normal, then the patient will be more comfortable in their activities. In turn, the fall in temperature also causes the heart patient to have some breathing troubles which may lead to abnormalities. Hence, temperature and humidity are considered to be one of the important factors.

7 Notification Through Android Application

An Android app is developed in case of any emergency, the alert notification is sent to the caretaker and the physician. The caretaker can monitor Heart patients by monitoring the pulse rate. They can also monitor whether the patient has taken the pills. Any critical situation like less heartbeat or no beat, the notification is sent to the caretaker and Physician. Both caretaker and physician have their own login with their username and password as the credentials. They can view the current status of

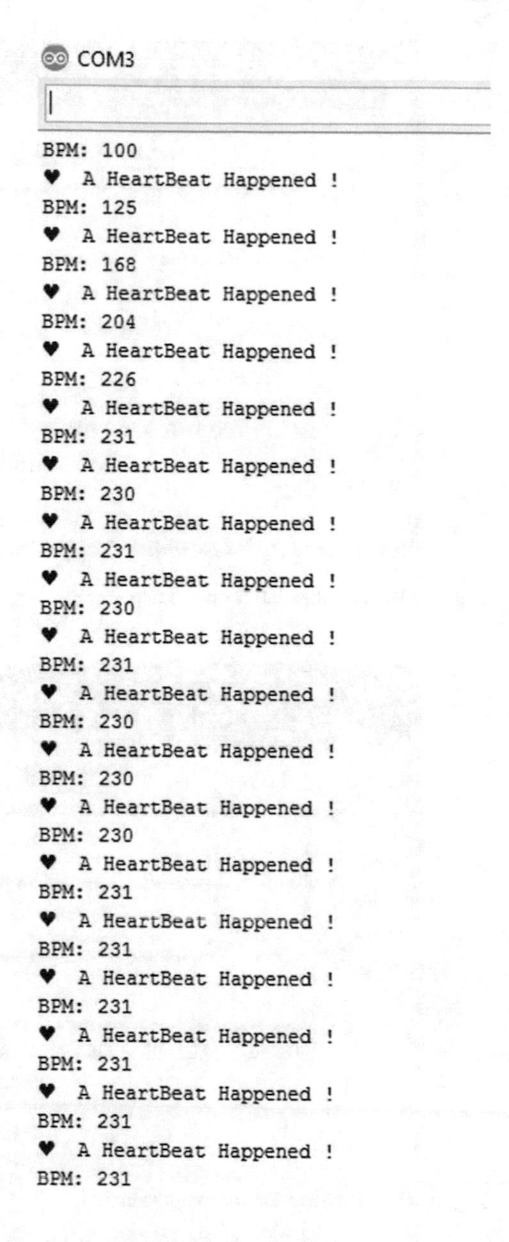

Fig. 7 Pulse rate monitoring using the sensor

the heart patient. The physician can also suggest the caretaker about the medications or change in medications.

Figure 12 shows the application that has been created for the heart patient monitoring system and it has a login for authenticated Physician and Caretaker. The user interface is created to monitor temperature and humidity, pulse rate, and pills monitoring and through which we can use in-app notification to send alert notification to the Physician and Caretaker.

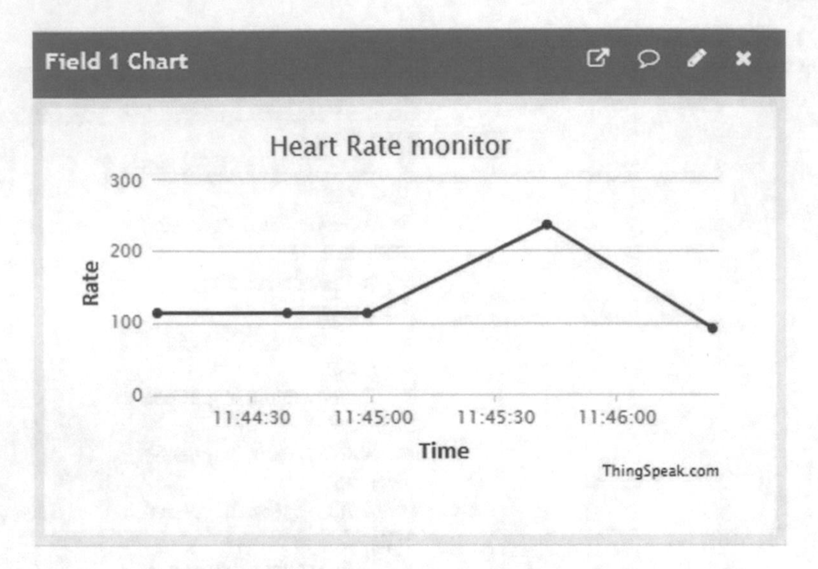

Fig. 8 Data visualization for pulse rate

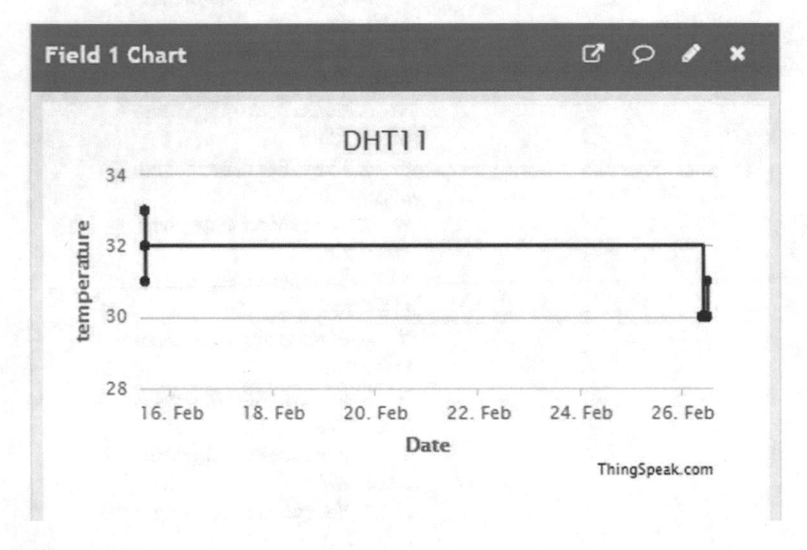

Fig. 9 Data visualization for temperature

8 Conclusion

Providing healthcare services means "the timely use of personal health services to achieve the best possible health outcomes" [32]. In this chapter, the patient monitoring framework is proposed and the environment with the use of Wireless sensors and Fog nodes (Raspberry Pi and Arduino). The main motive is to overcome the drawback

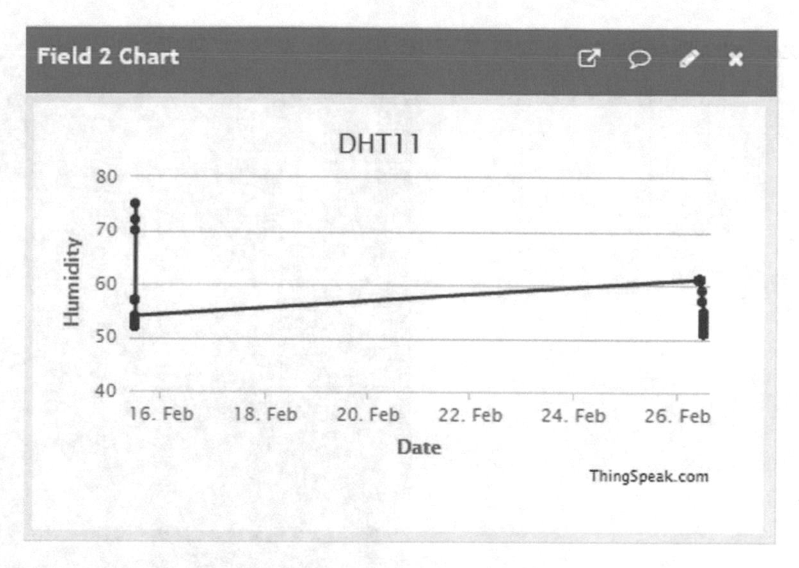

Fig. 10 Data visualization for humidity

```
pi@raspberrypi: ~/py_project
pi@raspberrypi ~/py_project $ sudo python sen_dht11.py
ERR_RANGE
pi@raspberrypi ~/py_project $ sudo python sen_dht11.py
Humidity:36%
Temperature:23C
pi@raspberrypi ~/py_project $ sudo python sen_dht11.py
ERR_RANGE
pi@raspberrypi ~/py_project $
pi@raspberrypi ~/py_project $ sudo python sen_dht11.py
ERR_RANGE
pi@raspberrypi ~/py_project $ sudo python sen_dht11.py
Humidity:36%
Temperature:23C
pi@raspberrypi ~/py_project $ sudo python sen_dht11.py
Humidity:36%
Temperature:23C
pi@raspberrypi ~/py_project $ sudo python sen_dht11.py
ERR_RANGE
pi@raspberrypi ~/py_project $ sudo python sen_dht11.py
ERR_RANGE
pi@raspberrypi ~/py_project $ sudo python sen_dht11.py
Humidity:36%
Temperature:23C
pi@raspberrypi ~/py_project $ sudo python sen_dht11.py
```

Fig. 11 Temperature and humidity sensor readings

of cloud which takes more response time. The patient monitoring is the critical application when compared to other application, so the fog layer is added as an intermediate layer for quick processing. The real-time data are stored and further, the alert notification is sent to the Android application during an emergency to the Physician and Caretaker. The proposed approach can be extended by monitoring

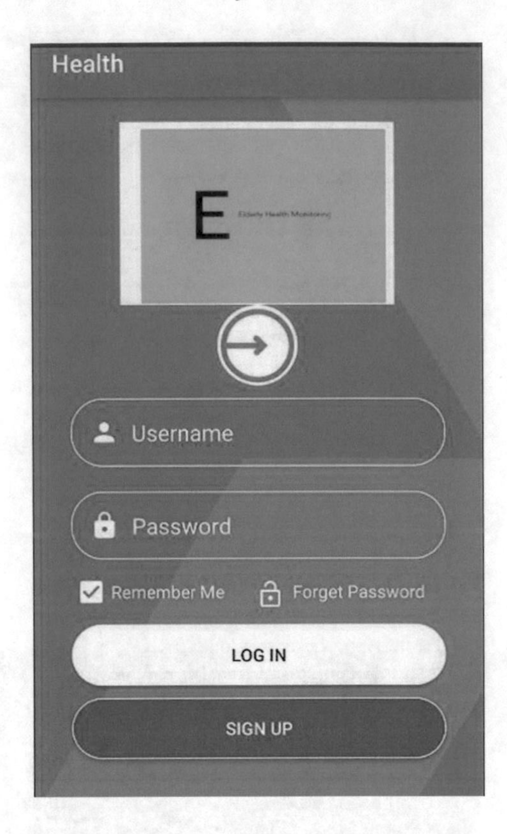

Fig. 12 Android application home page

the additional physiological status of the patient and monitor the patient 24 × 7 by placing the camera which can be pushed to the fog layer for analytics and decision-making. Thus, fog computing is a major role player in real-time healthcare and further research is essential for a healthy future.

References

1. European Commission Information Society (2009) Internet of things strategic research roadmap. http://www.internet-of-things-research.eu/. Accessed 14 Jul 2015
2. European Commission Information Society (2008) Internet of things in 2020: a roadmap for the future. http://www.iot-visitthefuture.eu. Accessed 14 Jul 2015
3. Botta A, De Donato W, Persico V, Pescapé A (2016) Integration of cloud computing and internet of things: a survey. Futur Gener Comput Syst 56:684–700
4. https://en.wikipedia.org/wiki/Health_care
5. Arkian HR, Diyanat A, Pourkhalili A (2017) MIST: fog-based data analytics scheme with cost-efficient resource provisioning for IoT crowdsensing applications. J Netw and Comput Appl 82:152–165
6. https://www.networkworld.com/article/3324238/3-types-of-iot-platform-analytics.html
7. https://www.xenonstack.com/blog/iot-analytics-platform/

8. Kang QK, Cong W, Tao L (2016) Fog computing for vehicular ad-hoc networks: paradigms, scenarios, and issues. J China Univ Posts Telecommun 23(2):56–96
9. Stojmenovic I, Wen S (2014) The fog computing paradigm: scenarios and security issues. In: 2014 IEEE federated conference on computer science and information systems, pp 1–8
10. Bittencourt LF, Diaz-Montes J, Buyya R, Rana OF, Parashar M (2017) Mobility-aware application scheduling in fog computing. IEEE Cloud Comput 4(2):26–35
11. Wac K, Bargh MS, Bert-jan F, Bults RGA, Pawar P, Peddemors A (2009) Power-and delay-awareness of health telemonitoring services: the mobihealth system case study. IEEE J Sel Areas Commun 27(4):525–536
12. Rahmani AM, Gia TN, Negash B, Anzanpour A, Azimi I, Jiang M, Liljeberg P (2018) Exploiting smart e-Health gateways at the edge of healthcare Internet-of-Things: a fog computing approach. Futur Gener Comput Syst 78:641–658
13. http://denver.chapters.comsoc.org/files/2017/06/OpenFog-Consortium-Reference-Architecture-Summary-presentation-for-Denver-Summit.pdf
14. Kraemer FA, Braten AE, Tamkittikhun N, Palma D (2017) Fog computing in healthcare–a review and discussion. IEEE Access 5:9206–9222
15. La QD, Ngo MV, Dinh TQ, Quek TQS, Shin H (2018) Enabling intelligence in fog computing to achieve energy and latency reduction. Digit Commun Netw
16. Verma P, Sood SK (2018) Fog assisted-IoT enabled patient health monitoring in smart homes. IEEE Internet Things J 5(3):1789–1796
17. Devarajan M, Subramaniyaswamy V, Vijayakumar V, Ravi L (2019) Fog-assisted personalized healthcare-support system for remote patients with diabetes. J Ambient Intell HumIzed Comput 1–14
18. Centers for Disease Control and Prevention, CDC 24/7: Saving lives, Protecting people, National Center for Chronic Disease Prevention and Health Promotion, Division of Population Health
19. Sood SK, Mahajan I (2017) A fog-based healthcare framework for chikungunya. IEEE Internet Things J 5(2):794–801
20. Sareen S, Gupta SK, Sood SK (2017) An intelligent and secure system for predicting and preventing Zika virus outbreak using Fog computing. Enterp Inf Syst 11(9):1436–1456
21. Nikoloudakis Y, Panagiotakis S, Markakis E, Pallis E, Mastorakis G, Mavromoustakis CX, Dobre C (2016) A fog-based emergency system for smart enhanced living environments. IEEE Cloud Comput 6:54–62
22. Tang B, Chen Z, Hefferman G, Pei S, Wei T, He H, Yang Q (2017) Incorporating intelligence in fog computing for big data analysis in smart cities. IEEE Trans Industr Inf 13(5):2140–2150
23. Vijayakumar V, Malathi D, Subramaniyaswamy V, Saravanan P, Logesh R (2018) Fog computing-based intelligent healthcare system for the detection and prevention of mosquito-borne diseases. Comput Hum Behav
24. Minaam DSA, Abd-ELfattah M (2018) Smart drugs: improving healthcare using smart pill box for medicine reminder and monitoring system. Futur Comput Inform J 3(2):443–456
25. MacIntosh E, Rajakulendran N, Khayat Z, Wise A (2016) Transforming health: shifting from reactive to proactive and predictive care. https://www.marsdd.com/newsand-insights/transforming-health-shifting-from-reactive-to-proactive-andpredictive-care/
26. Cao Yu, Chen S, Hou P, Brown D (2015) FAST: a fog computing assisted distributed analytics system to monitor fall for stroke mitigation. In: 2015 IEEE international conference on networking, architecture and storage (NAS), pp 2–11, IEEE
27. Castillo JC, Carneiro D, Serrano-Cuerda J, Novais P, Fernández-Caballero A, Neves J (2014) A multi-modal approach for activity classification and fall detection. Int J Syst Sci 45(4):810–824
28. Mirchevska V, Luštrek M, Gams M (2014) Combining domain knowledge and machine learning for robust fall detection. Expert Syst 31(2):163–175
29. Kaur PD, Chana I (2014) Cloud based intelligent system for delivering health care as a service. Comput Methods Programs Biomed 113(1):346–359
30. Risso NA, Neyem A, Benedetto JI, Carrillo MJ, Farías A, Gajardo MJ, Loyola O (2016) A cloud-based mobile system to improve respiratory therapy services at home. J Biomed Inf 63:45–53

31. Mohapatra S, Rekha KS (2012) Sensor-cloud: a hybrid framework for remote patient monitoring. Int J Comput Appl 55(2)
32. Access to Health Care in America (1993) The National Academies Press. US National Academies of Science, Engineering and Medicine
33. Granados J, Rahmani A-M, Nikander P, Liljeberg P, Tenhunen H (2014) Towards energy-efficient healthcare: an Internet-of-Things architecture using intelligent gateways. In: 2014 4th international conference on wireless mobile communication and healthcare-transforming healthcare through innovations in mobile and wireless technologies (MOBIHEALTH), pp 279–282, IEEE
34. López G, Custodio V, Moreno JI (2010) LOBIN: E-textile and wireless-sensor-network-based platform for healthcare monitoring in future hospital environments. IEEE Trans Inf Technol Biomed 14(6):1446–1458
35. Preden JS, Tammemäe K, Jantsch A, Leier M, Riid A, Calis E (2015) The benefits of self-awareness and attention in fog and mist computing. Computer 48(7):37–45

Ms. G. Jeya shree received her B.E. (Computer Science and Engineering) and M.E. (Computer Science and Engineering) from Anna University, Chennai, Tamil Nadu, India. She is currently pursuing her Ph.D. (Information and Communication Engineering) at Anna University, Chennai, Tamil Nadu, India. Her research interest centers around fog computing, cloud computing, and the Internet of things.

Dr. S. Padmavathi received her B.E. (Electrical and Electronics Engineering) from Madurai Kamarajar University, Madurai, Tamil Nadu, India; and M.E. (Computer Science and Engineering) and Ph.D. (Information and Communication Engineering) from Anna University, Chennai, India. Currently, she is working as a Professor in the Department of Information Technology, Thiagarajar College of Engineering, Madurai, Tamil Nadu, India. Her current research interests cover free-space and adaptive optics, scheduling algorithms, cloud computing, and parallel computing.

Applications of IoT in Indoor Air Quality Monitoring Systems

Jagriti Saini and Maitreyee Dutta

Abstract This book chapter explores the applications of the Internet of Things (IoT) in the Indoor Air Quality (IAQ) monitoring systems. Indoor air pollution is an important area of concern for most developing countries as it is directly related to mortality and morbidity. Around 3 billion people throughout the world use coal and biomass (crop residues, wood, dung, and charcoal) as the primary source of domestic energy. Moreover, humans spend 80–90% of their routine time indoors, so indoor air quality leaves a direct impact on overall health and work efficiency. This book chapter provides insights into the implementation of high-performance IAQ monitoring systems using IoT. Being the most emerging technology in the world, IoT has huge potential to mitigate the challenges associated with designing efficient and reliable real-time monitoring systems. The ultimate goal of this extensive analysis is to provide a detailed study on factors associated with indoor air pollution, public health, the current status of research, associated challenges, and possible research recommendations from the IoT world. After going through this chapter, readers will gain a deep understanding of the development of feature-rich and cost-effective IAQ monitoring systems using IoT.

Keywords Indoor air pollution · Internet of things · Work efficiency · Developing countries · Public health

J. Saini (✉)
Electronics and Communication Engineering Department, NITTTR-Chandigarh, Panjab University, Chandigarh 160019, India
e-mail: jagritis1327@gmail.com

M. Dutta
Computer Science and Engineering Department, NITTTR-Chandigarh, Panjab University, Chandigarh 160019, India
e-mail: d_maitreyee@yahoo.co.in

P. Raj et al. (eds.), *Internet of Things Use Cases for the Healthcare Industry*,
https://doi.org/10.1007/978-3-030-37526-3_4

1 Introduction

The Internet of things, or in short IoT, is all about extending the potential of the Internet beyond smartphones and computers to cover the entire range of processes, things, and environments. Those wirelessly connected things can share information both ways by working as a transmitter and receiver as well. In general, IoT provides a network to people and businesses to stay connected with the world around them while producing more meaningful results.

Getting connected through the Internet is probably the most wonderful thing for the current generation. It gives us plenty of benefits that were beyond imagination before. Although IoT appears a pretty simple concept: "connecting the world to the Internet", it has the potential to make the world act smartly and being smart is always good. There are unlimited applications of IoT, the most amazing ones are in the field of disaster management, health care management, smart farming, smart energy management, smart transport facilities, and smart homes as well.

In this chapter, we are mainly focusing on using IoT for Indoor Air Quality (IAQ) Monitoring, one of the essential applications for occupational health and pollution control. Human beings spend 80–90% of their routine time indoors, so IAQ leaves a direct impact on overall health and work efficiency as well. Moreover, 90% of the rural households in the most developing countries and around 50% of the world's population makes use of unprocessed biomass for open fires and poorly functioning cooking stoves indoors. Indoor Air Pollution (IAP) is an important area of concern for most developing countries as it is directly related to mortality and morbidity. This chapter presents an in-depth study on the development of Indoor Air Pollution Monitoring (IAPM) system using IoT technology.

The first section of this chapter covers the basics of IoT. It will provide readers with some valuable insights about the history of IoT along with its potential to serve almost every sector with advanced applications in the coming years. The second section introduces factors affecting IAP and associated medical health issues. It will also describe the motivation behind the development of IAPM systems. The third section provides an in-depth survey on existing IAQM systems along with the gap in the literature. This section will help readers to understand new opportunities and challenges in the field of IAPM system development.

This chapter is focused on developing a clear understanding among new age researchers about the development of IAPM systems using IoT technology.

2 Basic Concepts of IoT

Well, defining Internet of things is the real challenge; probably due to the newness of this domain and the wide range of possibilities associated with it. IoT is not just about any one type of hardware; rather it represents a unique combination of a variety of hardware units that are otherwise existing as unconnected units in the world. Some experts define it as a system of some interrelated computing devices, objects, people, animals, and digital and mechanical machines that communicate through Unique Identifiers (UIDs). The things connected through this network have the potential to communicate data without requiring any human to a computer or human-to-human interaction. Note that a "thing" in teams of IoT can be a person carrying heart monitor implant in his body, a farm animal with some biochip transponder, some vehicle with built-in sensors that send alert signals to the driver on road or any other man-made as well as natural object. However, in order to transfer data over a dedicated network, the object or thing is desired to have an IP address [1].

In most cases, communication through IoT networks is completed through RFID tags, although the goal can be also accomplished through QR codes and other wireless technologies. IoT has more significance in our life because it gives a different ability to the nonliving objects as well by assigning them a digital identity. When many such objects in the IoT world act in unison, they are supposed to have ambient intelligence.

2.1 History of IoT

The term IoT was coined in the year 1999 by the executive director and co-founder of Massachusetts Institute of Technology's Auto-ID Center, Kevin Ashton. The organization was later replaced by research-oriented Auto-ID Labs in the year 2003. The term Internet of things was seen for the first time as the title of a presentation that Ashton made for Procter and Gamble when he was working as a brand manager in that company. Before presenting his work to the senior executives of the Procter and Gamble, Ashton came to know that certain shade of lipstick from the list of cosmetics that he was supposed to launch got sold out at a fast rate from local stores. With that incident, Ashton started thinking hard about how the products in the line can be made trackable so that one can get an instant update about their availability at a specific time. At the same time, the market was getting influenced by the efficiency of RFID tags that could transfer data wirelessly to the dedicated systems. Ultimately, the project that Ashton presented to Procter and Gamble proposed the idea of using RFID tags to manage the supply chain of the corporation so that stock, as well as store location of all items, can be monitored with higher accuracy [2].

With a simple analysis of the product line, Ashton gave the world an idea about developing a technology that can build direct connections between almost anything around. After getting inspired through this idea, LG Electronics in the year 2000 designed a refrigerator with a connection to the Internet. This product was named as Internet Digital DIOS Refrigerator, and it was capable enough to keep perfect track of all the food items stored inside. By scanning the respective RFID tags of each item inside the refrigerator, the system was even able to provide direct insights about the quantity as well. Sadly, the company was not able to make considerable profits for this product as people found it much expensive to buy at that time. But this advanced and feature-rich refrigerator provided a way to connect various household objects and gadgets together to the Internet [3]. Since then, IoT technology experienced huge growth in the market starting from the connections between few hosts to a network of billions of interconnected devices. As per the current scenario, the number of closely connected things to the Internet is quite high as compared to the numbers of people connected on this planet. By the year 2020, this connectivity is believed to experience the estimated growth of 24 billion devices.

2.2 IoT: Everywhere Around Us

There is no doubt to say that IoT has revolutionized our lifestyles—it is working actively almost everywhere in this world. In simple terms, IoT is a new wearable, portable, implantable, and connected universe that transforms various physical objects into a potential ecosystem of valuable information. IoT technology has changed the way we used to perform our routine work a few years ago; today, it is showing its impact on almost every industry [4] (Fig. 1).

Below is the list of impressive applications of IoT from the world around us:

- IoT technology is the most efficient solution to design smart parking with the ability to monitor all parking spaces in the city.

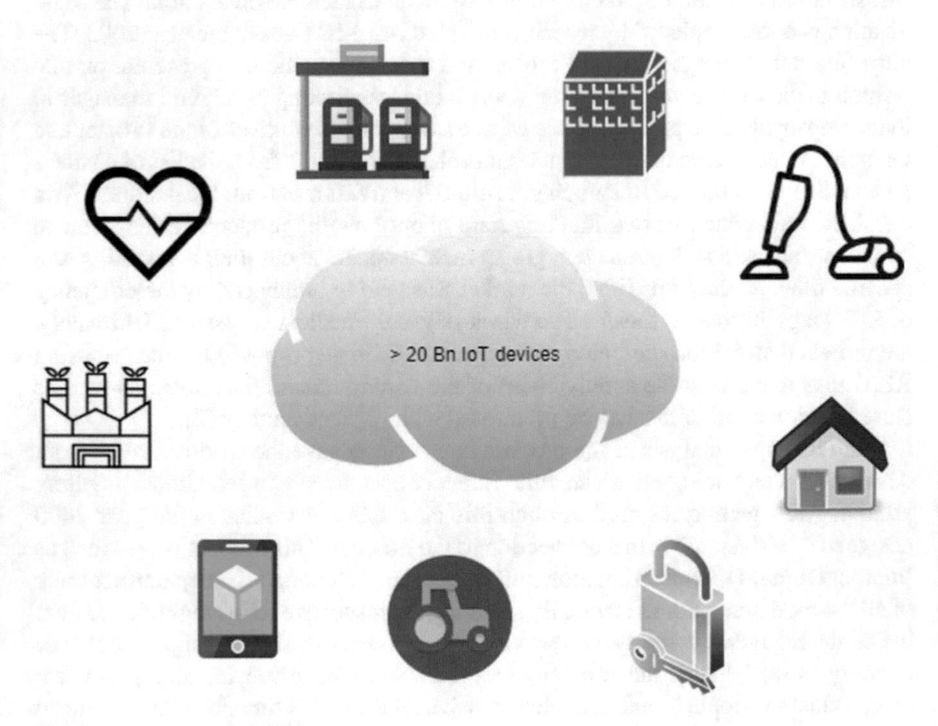

Fig. 1 Applications of IoT [5]

- It works for structural health improvement by monitoring material conditions and vibration levels in buildings, historical monuments, and bridges as well.
- Real-time sound monitoring applications at centric zones and bar areas.
- Detect any Android device, iPhone, or any other gadget that works with Bluetooth and Wi-Fi interfaces.
- Easy measurement of radiations from Wi-Fi routers and cell stations.
- Efficient monitoring of pedestrian levels and vehicles on the road to optimize walking routes and driving tracks.
- Smart lighting solutions for streets with weather adaptive and intelligent features.
- Automated waste management systems with highly optimized trash collection routes.
- Intelligent highways with quick alert systems for adverse climate conditions, diversions, and traffic jams to improve transportation experience.
- Monitoring of preemptive fire conditions and combustion gases to define alert zones in forests.
- Air pollution management by controlling CO_2 emissions, farm generated toxic gases, and vehicle pollution as well.
- IoT systems can monitor avalanche conditions and quality of ski tracks to ensure higher safety.
- Monitoring land conditions to detect dangerous patterns related to vibrations, soil moisture, and earth density as well.
- Early detection of the earthquake so that losses can be minimized or avoided at target locations.
- Ability to monitor the quality of tap water in overcrowded cities.
- A detection system for factory generated wastes and leakages into rivers and sea areas.
- Controlling swimming pool conditions from remote locations to ensure a safe experience to the community.
- Monitoring and detection of liquid outside tanks to avoid water leakage while controlling the pressure variations within the pipes.
- Active monitoring of variations in water level at reservoirs, dams, and rivers as well.
- Smart grid designs to lead efficient monitoring and management of energy consumption.
- Radiation measurement at nuclear power stations to generate leakage alert from time to time.
- Detection of hazardous and explosive gases around chemical factories and mines as well.
- Ability to track products in the supply chains to ensure proper inventory in the big industries.
- IoT leads to awesome shopping experience as per unique customer habits, preferences, likes, and dislikes.
- Temperature controlling in an industrial environment, health centers, and sensitive merchandise.

- IAQ monitoring to ensure safe work conditions without deteriorating health of occupants.
- Greenhouse development with efficient control of micro-climate conditions to maximize the production of vegetables and fruits.
- Product quality testing systems to ensure quality designs.
- Animal tracking, offspring care, and monitoring of toxic gas levels with smart farming solutions.
- Smart home design with remote controlled appliances, intrusion detection systems, energy, and water consumption monitoring.
- Advanced patient surveillance systems, fall detection, sportsmen care, and measurement of ultraviolet radiations to create healthy living conditions.

In short, IoT is everywhere around us, and it has the potential to automate our life with the highly efficient interconnection of objects to the Internet.

2.3 Extensively Growing IoT Market: The Stats

The wide range of applications draws attention to the market share of IoT that has an extensive growth rate in coming years. In the year 2011, the market value of IoT technology was observed somewhere around $44.0 billion. However, the comprehensive market research performed by RnRMarketSearch reveals that IoT and M2M market share will grow beyond $498.92 billion by the end of 2019 and this market is expected to hit $1423.09 billion in the year 2020. Moreover, the Internet of Nano Things (IoNT) is also playing an impressive role in the market and is expected to hold the value of around $9.69 billion by the end of the year 2020. Furthermore, the information-sharing practices and cooperation among leading companies in the IoT sector such as Ecobee Inc., Fujitsu, ARM, Intel, Cisco, Samsung, Google, IBM, and Microsoft along with the small business communities are expected to boost the market growth and IoT adoption rate by a great extent. Reports reveal that the numbers of connected devices in the year 2014 were only 6033.63 million; in the year 2017, this count reached 13,142.30 million and the growth is expected to cross the range of 27,858.35 million connected devices by the year 2020 [4].

3 Indoor Air Quality

3.1 Background

Several decades ago, when human beings first moved to the temperate climates, the problem of IAP started affecting the lifestyle. In the prehistoric times, during the growth stage of humanity, people started feeling the importance of comfortable shelters. They also started using fire for cooking, warmth, and light; however, it was later observed that soot found in various prehistoric caves is the primary cause of environmental pollution [6]. Today as well, more than 90% of people in the rural areas of developing countries or even approximately 50% of the world's population use unprocessed biomass for open fires and poorly functioning cooking stoves. These inadequate methods of cooking lead to IAP while affecting the overall health of women and young children who spend much of their routine time in the polluted environment [7]. Biomass and coal smoke carry various harmful pollutants such as Particulate Matter (PM), Sulfur Oxides (SO_x), Nitrogen Dioxide (NO_2), polycyclic organic matter, Carbon Monoxide (CO), and formaldehyde [8, 9]. Routine combustion of solid fuels causes repeated exposure to IAP, and it is considered as the common cause behind harmful diseases in developing countries. Some of the most common diseases spread by IAP are Acute Respiratory Infections (ARI), Chronic Obstructive Pulmonary Disease (COPD), asthma, otitis media, tuberculosis, low birth rate, lung cancer, cancer of larynx and nasopharynx, perinatal conditions, and severe eye diseases that can further lead to permanent blindness [6, 10].

The impact of modernization leads to a significant shift in cooking and heating practices. Instead of using biomass fuels such as petroleum products and wood, people are now buying electricity-based appliances. In the early 1900s, biomass fuels used to drive approximately 50% of global energy proportion. However, in the year 2000, it was significantly reduced to only 13%. It is believed that the types of fuels typically used for household needs can become more efficient and cleaner only if people start moving upward on the energy ladder. Note that animal dung is the lowest level of this ladder and the successive steps are built with crop residues, wood, charcoal, kerosene, gas, and electricity [9]. The energy ladder diagram is shown in Fig. 2. People try to move upward on this energy ladder with the changing socioeconomic conditions and lifestyle habits, but it is observed that poverty is the principal hurdle in shifting toward cleaner fuels. Sadly, the slower development cycles in many corners of the world show that the consumption of biomass fuels will continue in poor households even for the decades ahead.

One of the essential factors associated with the measurement of IAQ is ventilation; in general, it can be defined as the circulation of air into the closed structures from the outside world. In the case of poor ventilation arrangements within buildings, the IAQ levels fall below the threshold, and the indoor premises become unhealthy to live. Studies reveal IAP associated with poor ventilation arrangements is observed as the primary cause of increasing health issues. Approximately 66 percent of households in the rural and 44 percent of households in the urban areas are suffering from poor ventilation arrangements. Some stats about IAP are shown in Fig. 3. One of the prime reasons for the improved housing conditions in the urban areas as compared to the rural ones is the better educational and occupational status. These conditions have a direct relationship with the fuel selection for cooking and consequently leave a considerable impact on IAQ.

Stats reveal that poor IAQ is the second major cause behind the higher mortality rate in India. It leads to more than 1.3 million deaths per year in the country. Note that almost 70% of the population in India belongs to rural areas, out of which almost 80% are dependent on biomass fuel to fulfill their routine household requirements. Clearly,

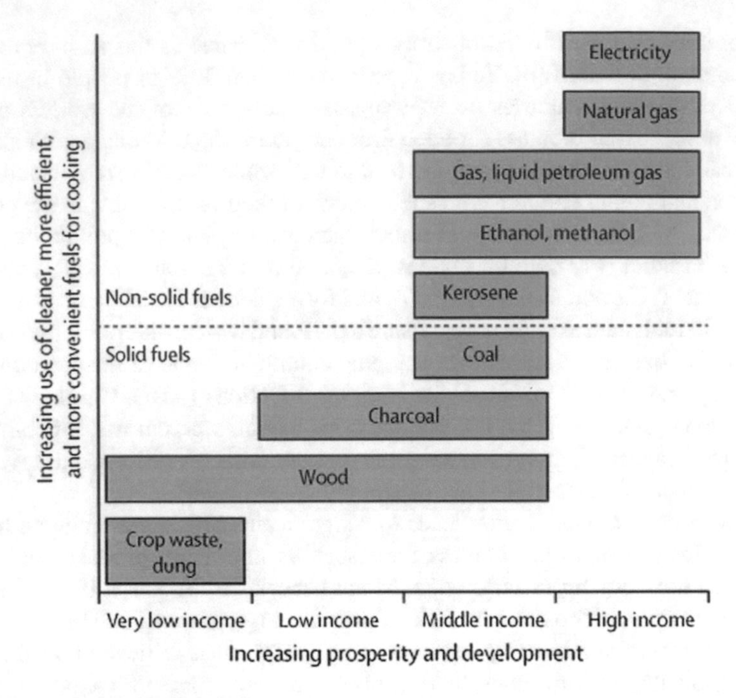

Fig. 2 Energy ladder diagram [11]

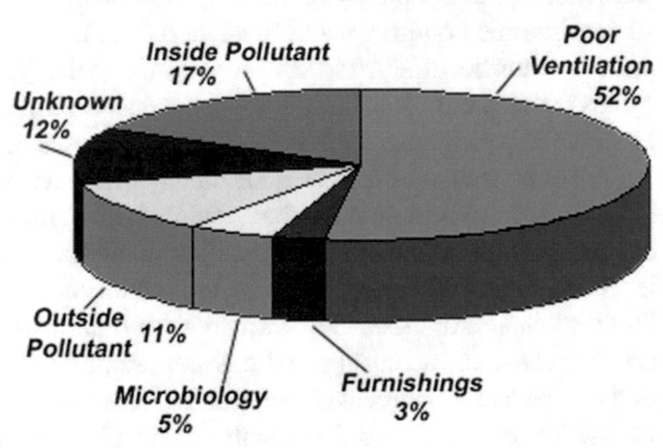

Fig. 3 Stats about indoor air quality [12]

the largest population in the nation lacks access to efficient sources of fuel to meet their cooking needs. In developing countries, excessive use of kerosene and biomass fuels is the prime reason behind stillbirth. In India itself, it is possible to reduce cases of stillbirths by 12% by just switching to cleaner fuel consumption in the household. Similar studies conducted in other developing countries such as Bangladesh, Kenya, Nepal, and Peru reveal that IAP is leading to serious health hazards. Hence, it is important to address the challenges, especially for indoor cooking practices in rural areas. As a lack of awareness about the benefits of cleaner cooking solutions is the main cause of adverse health conditions, it is important to train the affected sectors to improve their lifestyle. At the same time, experts need to work for the development of some efficient and affordable household cooking solutions so that traditional stoves can be avoided. Note that it can be done only if we study the behavioral patterns of the low-income population in the affected parts of the world.

The upliftment in economic conditions contributes to a reduction in IAP caused by harmful biomass fuels. However, there are few adverse effects of the modern lifestyle as well. It is observed that with the improvement in the living standards, instead of using natural ventilation systems, modern homes are furnished with indoor heating and cooling systems [9]. This scenario is further contributing to Sick Building Syndrome (SBS), and terribly, the cases of SBS have increased from 30% to 200% in just a few years [13]. Some of the most common factors affecting the indoor environment in the buildings include the rate of air exchange, temperature, humidity, ventilation, particle pollutants, biological pollutants, and gaseous pollutants. The modern homes are more airtight and packed with advanced insulation materials. Although they help to reduce the energy losses and may save on electricity bills, sadly, it leads to a reduction in the fresh air circulation in the premises. At the same time, the increasing consumption of synthetic materials and chemical products in residential and commercial buildings give rise to Volatile Organic Compounds (VOC). It is also considered as the principal causes of compound hypersensitiveness [14]. Hence, it is fair to say that even with the improved lifestyle and economic conditions, we are still unsafe from hazards associated with IAP.

Numerous researchers around the world these days are working for the development of efficient IAQM systems to deal with the increased cases of mortality and morbidity due to IAP. As the maximum population in the world spend 80% to 90% of their time indoors while working at home or in offices; it is necessary to take immediate steps to improve the IAQ. The idea is to identify some healthy solutions that can contribute to enhancement of living environment while reducing the chances of medical health consequences.

3.2 *Medical Health Consequences*

When we talk about health hazards associated with indoor air environment, it relates to every unusual suspended material that may interfere with the normal functionality of organs; all such elements are termed as air toxicants. Also, the estimation for IAP and health hazards cannot be determined by just calculating pollution levels; rather it is greatly affected by the average time that a person spends indoors while breathing in the polluted air. Medical health professionals and researchers have reported the occurrence of several harmful diseases due to IAP. Hence, in order to improve building environment and health conditions for occupations, it is important to work on the ultrafine indoor particles, their impact on the environment as well as on the living beings. The sections below describe some of the most common health hazards associated with IAP.

- *Respiratory illness*

It is well understood that most of the air pollutants find their way to the human body through airways; the respiratory system is on high risk due to poor IAQ. Depending upon the level of exposure to the pollutants and their deposition on the target cells, they may cause severe damage to the respiratory system. Acute lower respiratory infections are the main cause of mortality in kids; stats reveal that almost 2 million children below 5 years age group die per year just because of poor IAQ. Also, the repeated exposure to IAP in households in developing countries leads to several cases of acute law respiratory infections per year [15–17]. Biomass fuel smoke is another common cause of acute respiratory illness in kids; it leaves a major impact on the upper respiratory tract. It further leads to some disturbances in voice. Studies reveal that middle ear infection is an uncommon fatal symptom of this disease; however, it can also lead to morbidity, and deafness, etc. If this health issue is not treated on time; it may even cause mastoiditis [18], lung cancer and asthma [19]. The potential air pollutants such as PMs and many other respirable chemicals as like O_3, dust, benzene, etc., can cause serious trouble to the respiratory tract.

- *Cardiovascular dysfunctions*

Numbers of epidemiologic and experimental studies have proven a direct connection between IAP and cardiac-related illness [20, 21]. These harmful air pollutants also cause some unwanted alterations in the count of white blood cells that ultimately affect the normal functionality of the cardiovascular system. On the other hand, the studies conducted on animal models describe a close relationship between IAP and hypertension [22]. The higher concentration of NO_2 in the building environment hampers left and right ventricular hypertrophy. Various findings report the high risk of potential diseases due to repeated exposure to combustion of kerosene/diesel; however, such issues can be easily eliminated by using a clean cooking solution in the households. As per the experiments conducted in the rural households, the estimated increase of 10% was observed for cardiovascular mortality in 10 years; however, it was reduced to 6% in the areas where primary sources of cooking are gas or cleaner fuel [23].

- *Neuropsychiatric complications*

There is a strong relationship between air suspended toxic materials and nervous system performance; these harmful substances cause long-term damage to the nerves. People who spend more time in the toxic indoor air are likely to suffer psychiatric disorders and neurological complications. Some of the most common psychiatric disorders include aggression, antisocial behaviors, and stress, whereas neurological impairment includes some devastating consequences that are more common among infants. Terribly, IAP also leads to age-inappropriate behaviors, neurological hyperactivity, the risk of neuroinflammation [24], Parkinson's disease, and Alzheimer's disease [25].

- *Chronic pulmonary disease*

As per a study conducted on indoor biomass smoke pollution in New Guinea, communities were observed to report higher cases of chronic pulmonary disease [26]. Chronic Obstructive Pulmonary Disease (COPD) can be defined as a progressive inflammatory condition of pulmonary vessels, lung parenchyma, and airways; it is reported as a third common cause of death and fifth most reported the cause of disability worldwide. People who breath more often in the areas with higher combustion of solid fuels are likely to suffer severe damage to the lungs. That is why woman and kids that spend more time indoors are found to be at higher risk of COPD [18].

- *Cancer*

One of the main causes behind increasing cases of lung cancer worldwide is the repeated exposure to tobacco smoke. But as per studies carried by health professionals, even nonsmokers, especially woman, in the developing countries are also affected by lung cancer. Around two-thirds of female lung cancer patients in India [27], Mexico [28], and China [29] were nonsmokers. The Chinese population is highly affected by lung cancer. As per a study conducted in the year 2008, the estimated number of deaths in China due to lung cancer were 452,813, whereas the newly reported cases were somewhere around 522,050 [30]. The major cause behind woman suffering from lung cancer in China was observed to be the repeated and excessive exposure to coal smoke while cooking. Low-income population in China make use of smoky coal, and it is found to be highly carcinogenic as compared to wood smoke and cleaner coal. One study shows that cooking for three hours in biomass smoke exposes a woman to an equal amount of benzo[a]pyrene that is otherwise caused by smoking of two packets of cigarettes per day [18].

- *Pulmonary tuberculosis*

A recent study carried on approximately 200,000 Indian adults; researchers found a close association between wood smoke exposure and self-reported tuberculosis [31]. Generally, people who use biomass for burning needs are at higher risk of tuberculosis as compared to those who make use of cleaner fuels; the ratio of odds for this study is 2:58 (1.98–3.37) with appropriate adjustment of socioeconomic factors. These findings are quite similar to the studies carried on North India that describe a direct connection between biomass fuel and tuberculosis.

- *Low birth rate and infant mortality*

As per a recent study carried on rural areas of Guatemala with adequate adjustment of various maternal and socioeconomic factors, women that spend more time in wood fuel conditions were observed to deliver babies with 63 grams lesser weight as that of the women that use electricity and gas for cooking needs. Although there are limited evidence in support of this fact, some researchers observed that tobacco smoke and increased exposure to carbon monoxide are the prime reasons behind this condition. It is well proven that the concentration of carbon monoxide usually goes higher in households where biomass fuels are commonly used. Some evidence also links ambient air pollution to lesser birth weight [32, 33]; however, only one study shows a direct relationship with carbon monoxide [34]. The worldwide burden of mortality attributes to the IAP; stats collected in the year 2012 reveal almost 4.3 million deaths along with 7.7% of global mortality.

- *Cataract*

Biomass fuel combustion is the primary cause of eye irritation, and the excessive exposure may even lead to cataracts [35]; cases of cataracts are quite high in developing countries where most of the population is dependent on solid fuels for their routine cooking and heating needs [36]. Various epidemiological studies from India and Nepal also demonstrate poor indoor cooking standards as the main cause of blindness and cataracts. A recent study carried out in the hospital at Delhi evidenced a direct relationship of liquid petroleum gas with the development of nuclear, cortical, and mixed cataract; however, most cases of posterior subcapsular cataracts are reported due to repeated exposure to wood and cow dung [37]. In developing countries, the main cause of increasing cases of cataracts is the lack of awareness and knowledge about factors that have a direct impact on vision. During a study on 89,000 households in India, the estimated odds ratio of 1:3 was observed for blindness in females who use biomass fuel in the home [18].

- *Sick building syndrome*

As people spend most of their time indoors, IAQ has a direct connection with Sick Building Syndrome (SBS); commonly, it happens due to insufficient ventilation arrangement in the living spaces. Chemical contaminants that lead to considerable emission of VOCs in the building environment include upholstered furniture, cleaning agents, carpeting, adhesives, and paint. VOCs are considered as a primary cause of SBS with symptoms like mental fatigue, dizziness, headache, skin irritation, nausea, eye irritation, and difficulty in concentrating as well. Other than this, factors that contribute to SBS are dust, mold, harmful organisms, toxic gases, bacteria, chemical vapors, harmful compounds, etc. [38].

It is observed that rural women suffer more due to IAP than urban women due to the improved quality of living standards. The lack of knowledge and the unavailability of essential resources make it difficult for the rural woman to improve health conditions.

3.3 Motivation for the Design

As described in Sect. 3.3, poor IAQ is the major cause behind increasing cases of serious medical health consequences. As human beings spend most of their routine time indoors, it is important to ensure a healthy building environment to avoid risks associated with occupational and building health. The IAQM systems are the best solution to deal with such issues, and the IoT technology has huge efficiency in providing the most reliable and feature-rich solution to the world. The high-performance IAQM systems can generate alerts for bad indoor air levels so that appropriate ventilation arrangements can be made on time. It is a thought for the development of healthy work conditions for the coming generations as well.

4 IoT for Indoor Air Quality Monitoring

By considering the huge potential of IoT technology, researchers these days are working on the development of IAQM systems to improve the indoor work environment. This section highlights the contribution of early researchers in this field while describing the gaps and challenges for the future.

4.1 Survey on IoT-Based IAQ Monitoring Systems

Idrees et al. [39] investigated the computational complexity, infrastructure, issues, and procedures for designing real-time IAQ monitoring systems. The prototype for this study was designed using the IBM Watson IoT platform and Arduino board. The sensing module used eight different sensors: humidity, temperature, O_3, SO_2, NO_2, CO, $PM_{2.5}$, and PM_{10}. The major advantage of this system was its ability to reduce the computational burden of the sensing nodes by almost 70% leading to longer battery life. Authors used automatic calibration setup to ensure higher accuracy of sensors and a data transmission strategy was used to minimize the power consumption along with redundant network traffic. This model reported a reduction of 23% in the overall power consumption and the performance was validated by setting the system in different environments.

Kang and Hwang [40] introduced an air quality monitoring system to test the relevance of the Comprehensive Air Quality Index (CAQI) for accurate IAQ indication. Authors also proposed a real-time Comprehensive Indoor Air Quality Indicator (CIAQI) system that can work effectively against all dynamic changes and is quite efficient in processing ability along with memory overhead. In order to develop the experimental setup for realistic indoor air environment monitoring, the authors used VOC, PM_{10}, CO, temperature, and humidity sensors. Authors also compared the proposed system performance with section average (AVG) used for ambient AQI as well as with Simple Moving Average (SMA) scheme and observed that proposed CIAQI system is more adaptive to real-time changes in the IAQ. Also, this system utilized small memory, and hence, it was proven to be the best solution for the Internet of Things (IoT) based and budget-friendly air quality monitoring.

Firdhous et al. [41] proposed an IoT-based IAQM system for tracking concentrations of ozone near the photocopy machine. Researchers designed an experimental system using semiconductor sensors that were capable enough to monitor ozone concentrations in the area surrounding a high-volume Xerox machine. The interconnected IoT devices were programed for efficient collection and transmission of data for the estimated duration of 5 min over the Bluetooth network. Sensors transmitted data to a gateway node that further makes use of Wi-Fi LAN to communicate with the processing nodes. Note that all the sensors for this system were calibrated using proven calibration techniques. The proposed IAQM system was also able to generate warnings for the exceeding range of pollution levels in the indoor environment.

Benammar et al. [42] presented an end-to-end IAQM system for measuring relative humidity, ambient temperature, Cl_2, O_3, NO_2, SO_2, CO, and CO_2. The prime role of the gateway in this study is to process the IAQ data and perform reliable dissemination via a web server. This system was adapted to open source IoT web server platform, named as Emoncms to ensure long-term storage as well as live monitoring of IAQM data. Seamless integration of smart mobile standards, WSN, and many other sensing technologies is performed to design the ultimate scalable smart system to monitor IAP.

Srivatsa and Pandhare [43] proposed a system containing a sensor network that was connected through IoT to provide efficient IAQM services. The system had three prime sections that work together to provide complete analysis; the first one is a wireless sensor network that collected PPM reading for CO_2 from the dedicated room; at the second level, this information was passed to the wireless access point, and details were stored on the server machine. Finally, the server side containing user interface and notification system functionalities processes this data to provide alerts for IAP.

Panghurian et al. [44] developed an IAQM system based on the measurement of PM2.5, CO_2, CO, humidity, and temperature. The communication was performed over IEEE 802.11 b/g wireless network. The prime focus for development of this system was to reduce power consumption of the sensor network so that the network can also function better in emergency situations like fire, etc. The monitoring for this system was done remotely through a web application.

Marques and Pitarma [45] proposed iAQ as an advanced system based on IoT technology for monitoring air quality in the indoor environment. The system incorporates Xbee technologies, ESP8266 and Arduino for data processing and transmission whereas microsensors were utilized for data acquisition. In this system, it was possible to collect data through mobile application and web system as well; even doctors can access this data instantly to lead effective medical diagnostic procedures. Researchers in this study focused on five natural parameters: glow, carbon dioxide, carbon monoxide, moistures, and air temperatures as well.

Cynthia et al. [46] proposed an IAQM system for monitoring live air quality in the area using IoT technology. This system makes use of air sensors to collect information about harmful compounds and gases, and the data was further processed through PIC16F877A microcontroller. The microcontroller transmits this data over the Internet, and the gas level variations can be monitored over a web page from any corner of the world.

4.2 Challenges

Although it is possible to use conventional analytical instruments for measurement of pollutants affecting IAQ, they are not considered a practical solution due to a few potential reasons:

- They are too bulky and hence are not a feasible solution for practical measurement.
- These sensors are noisy so are an inadequate solution for indoor use.
- These sensors are expensive to install.
- The operation often goes quite complicated; they demand experienced professionals to handle the process.
- They consume more power.

At present, researchers need to find some low-power, battery-operated devices that can be readily deployed at various locations. The great news is that recent advances in the technologies have presented a wide range of measuring units for the indoor air pollutants such as PM, SO_2, NO_2, O_3, CO_2, CO, and VOCs. In ideal conditions, these sensors are expected to have a fast response time, ensure high performance in the practical environment and are robust solutions for the real-time measurements. With time, these devices are also becoming lightweight, compact, and inexpensive while ensuring great performance for selectivity, sensitivity, and measurement efficiency. A wide range of sensors in the market are wearable and mobile, and they allow data transfers over Wi-Fi and Bluetooth networks as well.

The real-time data collection systems are managed by ATmega microcontroller; however, Raspberry Pi is another common choice for setting up a sensor network in the target environment. WSN is an ad hoc network, where sensor networks consume huge energy while transmitting data in multiple hops. At the same time, the time taken by sensors to send a signal to the monitoring unit was observed to be considerably high. In such situations, researchers needed to work on battery power management to improve overall system performance. The prime limitation of gas sensors is that they suffer from short life span. Considering the battery life expectancy and reliable single-hop communication abilities, IoT monitoring systems are known as the most reliable solutions for IAQ measurement. With lower latencies and lesser power consumption, these systems also demand lesser efforts on maintenance procedures. IoT-based real-time monitoring systems are known as smart systems; hence, most of the researchers and industrial manufacturers are more attracted to this technology. Experts reveal that IoT systems have the ability to monitor a large number of parameters even without compromising system performance.

One of the prime concerns in the development of IAQ systems is the higher cost and huge power consumption of sensor nodes. If we consider the real-time applications of IAQ systems, the sensor units are usually installed in an industrial environment, inside homes, offices, and outdoor areas as well. But in all these cases, the design of the sensor unit demands more focus on size, design cost, power consumption, communication protocol, and performance dependence on changes in temperature and humidity. Sensor calibration is currently the biggest challenge in front of future researchers to ensure accurate real-time monitoring. Although Metal Oxide Semiconductor (MOS) sensors are cheaper when compared to the optical and electromechanical sensors (some examples are TGS 2442 and TGS416), they work on the resistive heating; hence, consume loads of energy from limited battery unit of wireless motes. As a result, it reduces the overall lifetime of the network. A considerable solution to solve this problem is placing motes in sleep mode when they are not working actively in the system. Some studies also reveal that high-quality micro-gas sensors are able to perform better in variable humidity and temperature conditions. One advanced solution to air quality monitoring is MAQS—personalized mobile sensing system that is gaining huge popularity due to its portable, energy-efficient, and inexpensive design. Most of the researchers have used ZigBee to establish a communication network between sensor nodes and controller unit, but its prime disadvantages of ZigBee modules are short communicating range and low network stability with high maintenance cost. The highly efficient IoT systems bring a new scope to this field; the best idea is to combine them with a Raspberry Pi controller that comes with the in-built Wi-Fi communication module ensuring fast data transfer. Note that Arduino boards do not offer direct network connectivity; users need to add one extra chip for Ethernet port that also demands extensive coding for connection development. One preferably used Wi-Fi module for Arduino boards is ESP8266 chip, but it needs an external converter for 5-3 logic shifting and cannot even handle complex data inputs. Moreover, it leads to additional cost and energy consumption. Also, the clock speed of Arduino is approximately 40 times lesser than Raspberry Pi, and the RAM for the later unit is 12,800 times larger than the Arduino.

Beyond these technical challenges, another major point of concern for IAQ management is social issues. Although several systems are already designed by early researchers to address this problem, not all of them are accessible to the sufferers, especially those who live in rural areas and have limited financial sources. Moreover, the lack of awareness about IAP and associated hazards brings millions of people under risk of serious medical health consequences. In order to improve the quality of building environment and living conditions of occupations, government agencies, health care experts, and researchers need to work together. New policies must be designed to focus on all socioeconomic sectors, especially the rural population in the developing countries. The efforts should not be limited to planning rather ground level implementations for all aspects must be ensured. Then only the latest technologies like IoT can be actually useful to address problems associated with IAP.

4.3 Requirements of Future IAQM Systems

The above sections of this chapter must have cleared most of your doubts regarding the development of IAQM systems, but before you move ahead to the designing world, it is first important to understand the requirements of future IAQM systems. In order to design the best equipment to serve the community, first of all, one must consider the common preferences and needs of the buyers. This analysis can help in making more appropriate decisions at each level during the entire design process, and the ultimate product will ensure more efficient outcomes in the real-time environment.

Below are a few essential points that must be considered for designing a new age IAQM system:

- *Accuracy of the system*:

Indeed, this is the prime concern for the development of a future system to measure IAQ. People will buy equipment only when it can ensure reliable results and can keep them safe from hazardous variations in the IAQ levels. The accuracy of an IAQM system relies on three factors:

i. Precision: The ability to deliver consistent output.
ii. Calibration: The device must be adjusted to achieve maximum accuracy in all variable environments.
iii. Resolution: The sensitivity of the sensor system to minute changes in the measured parameters.

Other than this, researchers need to set an appropriate range for their monitoring systems by indicating clear thresholds for the performance.

- *Convenient to use*:

The standard IAQM systems are required to be easy to use, and they must be accessible to all. IAQ affects 90% of the world's population; hence, it is important to design a system that can fit the universal needs. It must be simple to use, efficient in producing results and convenient to access as well. The thoughtfully designed system can ensure an intuitive experience to the end users.

- *Portable and power-efficient design*:

In this fast pacing world, immobile systems are of no use. People need IAQM systems for home, office, and probably for their cars as well but it does not mean that they must buy separate equipment to address issues all these places. Rather, future researchers need to design mobile, lightweight, and portable solutions to meet the requirements of coming generations. While making a portable system, it is also important to work on the battery life of the equipment. It must be capable enough to serve people for long hours without risking their lives in emergency situations.

- *Essential features and qualities*:

Well, there is no specific list of features that an IAQM system must have because it varies from user to user as per their individual needs. However, in general, one needs to consider response time, connectivity, and noise as prime concerns for designing process. *Response* time indicates that the sensor can display readings faster without compromising for accuracy. *Connectivity* is a measure of making your device suitable for modern smart homes. The new-age equipment must provide easy access to output on web portals, mobile apps while the alerts can be sent through e-mails as well. Also, the system must be less noisy so that it can be used by sensitive sleepers as well.

5 Conclusion

This chapter presents an in-depth study of IoT-based IAQM systems by focusing on several design aspects. A smart approach in designing high-performance systems can provide reliable results to address the serious medical health consequences associated with IAP. Although there are several open research challenges to work in this direction, a systematic approach can provide a considerable solution. As IoT has huge potential to serve design requirements of highly efficient monitoring and control systems in every field, it is possible to address the issues in the IAQ management as well.

References

1. Internet of Things. In: Wikipedia [Internet]. 2019 [cited 2019 Apr 11]. https://en.wikipedia.org/w/index.php?title=Internet_of_things&oldid=891691444
2. Ashton K, That "Internet of Things" Thing 1
3. Smart refrigerator. In: Wikipedia [Internet]. 2019 [cited 2019 Apr 11]. https://en.wikipedia.org/w/index.php?title=Smart_refrigerator&oldid=882811110
4. Dastjerdi AV, Cloud Computing and Distributed Systems (CLOUDS) Laboratory Department of Computing and Information Systems The University of Melbourne, Australia Manjrasoft Pty Ltd., Australia. Internet of Things, p 53
5. IoT, a solution of Astellia [Internet]. Astellia [cited 2019 Apr 11]. https://www.astellia.com/solutions/technologies/harness-the-business-potential-of-iot/
6. Bruce N, Perez-Padilla R, Albalak R (2000) Indoor air pollution in developing countries: a major environmental and public health challenge. Bull World Health Organ 15
7. Arungu-Olende S (1984) Rural energy. Nat Resour Forum 8(2):117–126
8. Koning HWD, Smith KR, Last JM, Biomass fuel combustion and health, p 16
9. Smith KR (2000) Indoor air pollution in developing countries and acute lower respiratory infections in children. Thorax 55(6):518–532
10. Ezzati M, Kammen DM (2001) Quantifying the effects of exposure to indoor air pollution from biomass combustion on acute respiratory infections in developing countries. Environ Health Perspect 109(5):8
11. Roser M, Ritchie H (2013) Indoor air pollution. Our World in Data [Internet] [cited 2019 Apr 7]; https://ourworldindata.org/indoor-air-pollution
12. Invest in a healthy future with certified air quality testing in Northern Virginia—Envirotex [Internet]. [cited 2019 Apr 11]. https://www.environmentalinspectionsite.com/learning-center/certified-air-quality-testing-northern-va.html
13. Fisk WJ, Faulkner D, Palonen J, Seppanen O (2002) Performance and costs of particle air filtration technologies. Indoor Air 12(4):223–234
14. Wang Z, Bai Z, Yu H, Zhang J, Zhu T (2004) Regulatory standards related to building energy conservation and indoor-air-quality during rapid urbanization in China. Energy Build 36(12):1299–1308
15. Collings DA, Sithole SD, Martin KS (1990) Indoor woodsmoke pollution causing lower respiratory disease in children. Trop Doct 20(4):151–155
16. Armstrong JR, Campbell H (1991) Indoor air pollution exposure and lower respiratory infections in young Gambian children. Int J Epidemiol 20(2):424–429
17. Robin LF, Less PS, Winget M, Steinhoff M, Moulton LH, Santosham M et al (1996) Wood-burning stoves and lower respiratory illnesses in Navajo children. Pediatr Infect Dis J 15(10):859–865

18. Fullerton DG, Bruce N, Gordon SB (2008) Indoor air pollution from biomass fuel smoke is a major health concern in the developing world. Trans R Soc Trop Med Hyg 102(9):843–851
19. Weisel CP (2002) Assessing exposure to air toxics relative to asthma. Environ Health Perspect 110(Suppl 4):527–537
20. Nogueira JB (2009) Air pollution and cardiovascular disease. Rev Port Cardiol 28(6):715–733
21. Andersen ZJ, Kristiansen LC, Andersen KK, Olsen TS, Hvidberg M, Jensen SS et al (2012) Stroke and long-term exposure to outdoor air pollution from nitrogen dioxide: a cohort study. Stroke 43(2):320–325
22. Sun Q, Yue P, Ying Z, Cardounel AJ, Brook RD, Devlin R et al (2008) Air pollution exposure potentiates hypertension through reactive oxygen species-mediated activation of Rho/ROCK. Arterioscler Thromb Vasc Biol 28(10):1760–1766
23. Samet JM, Bahrami H, Berhane K (2016) Indoor air pollution and cardiovascular disease: new evidence from Iran. Circulation 133(24):2342–2344
24. Calderón-Garcidueñas L, Solt AC, Henríquez-Roldán C, Torres-Jardón R, Nuse B, Herritt L et al (2008) Long-term air pollution exposure is associated with neuroinflammation, an altered innate immune response, disruption of the blood-brain barrier, ultrafine particulate deposition, and accumulation of amyloid beta-42 and alpha-synuclein in children and young adults. Toxicol Pathol 36(2):289–310
25. Calderón-Garcidueñas L, Mora-Tiscareño A, Ontiveros E, Gómez-Garza G, Barragán-Mejía G, Broadway J et al (2008) Air pollution, cognitive deficits and brain abnormalities: a pilot study with children and dogs. Brain Cogn 68(2):117–127
26. Master KM (1974) Air pollution in New Guinea: cause of chronic pulmonary disease among stone-age natives in the highlands. JAMA 228(13):1653–1655
27. Gupta RC, Purohit SD, Sharma MP, Bhardwaj S (1998) Primary bronchogenic carcinoma: clinical profile of 279 cases from mid-west Rajasthan. Indian J Chest Dis Allied Sci 40(2):109–116
28. Medina FM, Barrera RR, Morales JF, Echegoyen RC, Chavarría JG, Rebora FT (1996) Primary lung cancer in Mexico city: a report of 1019 cases. Lung Cancer 14(2–3):185–193
29. Gao Y (1996) Risk factors for lung cancer among nonsmokers with emphasis on lifestyle factors. Lung Cancer 1(14):S39–S45
30. Mu L, Liu L, Niu R, Zhao B, Shi J, Li Y et al (2013) Indoor air pollution and risk of lung cancer among Chinese female non-smokers. Cancer Causes Control 24(3):439–450
31. Mishra VK, Retherford RD, Smith KR (1999) Biomass cooking fuels and prevalence of tuberculosis in India. Int J Infect Dis 3(3):119–129
32. Wang X, Ding H, Ryan L, Xu X (1997) Association between air pollution and low birth weight: a community-based study. Environ Health Perspect 105(5):514–520
33. Bobak M, Leon DA (1999) Pregnancy outcomes and outdoor air pollution: an ecological study in districts of the Czech Republic 1986–8. Occup Environ Med 56(8):539–543
34. Ritz B, Yu F (1999) The effect of ambient carbon monoxide on low birth weight among children born in southern California between 1989 and 1993. Environ Health Perspect 107(1):17–25
35. Ellegård A (1997) Tears while cooking: an indicator of indoor air pollution and related health effects in developing countries. Environ Res 75(1):12–22
36. Lewallen S, Courtright P (2002) Gender and use of cataract surgical services in developing countries. Bull World Health Organ 80(4):300–303
37. Mohan M, Sperduto RD, Angra SK, Milton RC, Mathur RL, Underwood BA et al (1989) India-US case-control study of age-related cataracts. India-US Case-Control Study Group. Arch Ophthalmol 107(5):670–676
38. Norhidayah A, Lee CK, Azhar MK, Nurulwahida S (2013) Indoor air quality and sick building syndrome in three selected buildings [cited 2019 Apr 8]. https://researchspace.auckland.ac.nz/handle/2292/30807
39. Idrees Z, Zou Z, Zheng L (2018) Edge computing based IoT architecture for low cost air pollution monitoring systems: a comprehensive system analysis, design considerations & development. Sensors 18(9):3021

40. Kang J, Hwang K-I (2016) A comprehensive real-time indoor air-quality level indicator. Sustainability 8(9):881
41. Firdhous M, Sudantha B, Karunaratne P (2017) IoT enabled proactive indoor air quality monitoring system for sustainable health management, pp 216–221
42. Benammar M, Abdaoui A, Ahmad S, Touati F, Kadri A (2018) A modular IoT platform for real-time indoor air quality monitoring. Sensors 18(2):581
43. Srivatsa P, Pandhare A (2016) IoT solution, Indoor Air Quality, p 3
44. Panghurian FP, Surantha N, Zahra A (2018) A low-power scenario for IOT-based indoor air quality monitoring system at workplace. IOP Conf Ser Earth Environ Sci 14(195):012048
45. Marques G, Pitarma R (2016) An indoor monitoring system for ambient assisted living based on internet of things architecture. Int J Environ Res Public Health 13(11):1152
46. Cynthia BB, Priya BD, Nandhini R, Sindhuja P, Senthilkumar MA, Raja S, Proactive indoor air quality monitoring system. Int J Recent Innovat Trends Comput Commun 6(3):6

Jagriti Saini received her bachelor's degree from Himachal Pradesh University, India in 2013 and master's degree (Electronics and Communication Engineering) from NITTTR, Panjab University, India in 2017. She was also a recipient of Gold Medal for her master's degree from Panjab University, India. At present, she is a Ph.D. candidate in the Electronics and Communication Engineering Department at NITTTR, Chandigarh. Her research interests include neural networks, image processing, environment health, artificial intelligence, and IoT. She has published many papers in reputed SCI and Scopus indexed journal.

Maitreyee Dutta is working as a Professor and Head in the ETV Department at NITTTR, Chandigarh, India. She has a Ph.D. (Engineering and Technology) with specialization in Image Processing and M.E. in Electronics Communication and Engineering from Panjab University, Chandigarh and a B.E. in Electronics Communication and Engineering from Guwahati University, India. She has over 17 years of teaching experience. Her research interests include digital signal processing, advanced computer architecture, data warehousing and mining, and image processing. She has more than 90 research publications in reputed ISI journals and conferences.

CloudIoT for Smart Healthcare: Architecture, Issues, and Challenges

Junaid Latief Shah and Heena Farooq Bhat

Abstract The integration of cloud and IoT known as CloudIoT offers a novel approach for designing coherent and structured healthcare monitoring systems. With CloudIoT, diverse IoT-based healthcare applications interconnect and exchange information for dispensing efficient clinical healthcare solutions. As sensor-based communication has seen an exponential growth in recent years, humongous amounts of data gets generated, which becomes difficult to handle with limited processing and storage available in sensor nodes. To overcome this, cloud and IoT amalgamation known as CloudIoT provides an efficient solution for bridging communication between heterogeneous devices and handling increasing data demands in healthcare applications including seamless application deployment and service rendering. In this chapter, we review the available CloudIoT literature and present a holistic vision on CloudIoT-based healthcare integration components. The chapter presents seamless applications dispensed by CloudIoT platform and contemplates discussion on factors driving CloudIoT health integration. The chapter also presents a conceptual architectural framework for healthcare monitoring system that considers a range of aspects including data collection, transmission, and processing including cloud storage. The chapter also discusses a use case scenario including a brief discussion on design considerations for healthcare architecture. The chapter highlights security issues affecting IoT layered architecture including vulnerabilities inherent in the cloud which could render healthcare services nonfunctional and critical patient information can be abused by malevolent users. Also, a brief discussion on some potential mitigation measures will be provided. The chapter also elaborates discussion on various CloudIoT platforms available. Finally, the chapter concludes by identifying some open research issues and challenges hampering CloudIoT-based healthcare adoption.

Keywords CloudIoT · Cloud · IoT · Sensor · Healthcare

J. L. Shah (✉)
Department of Information Technology, Sri Pratap College, Cluster University Srinagar, Srinagar, India

H. F. Bhat
Department of Computer Science, University of Kashmir, Srinagar, India

P. Raj et al. (eds.), *Internet of Things Use Cases for the Healthcare Industry*,
https://doi.org/10.1007/978-3-030-37526-3_5

1 Introduction

In recent years, the increase in old age population around the world has resulted in severe chronic health issues leading to rise in clinical and hospital expenditures for common people [27, 58, 82]. Monitoring health periodically plays a significant role for aged people with acute diseases in order to lower hospitalization costs and elevate the ambient quality of life [11, 19]. Conventional models for healthcare diagnosis are pretty tedious and inconvenient. These models do not suffice to the medical requirements of our aging population. This, in turn, entails for designing systematic and effective healthcare facilities which aid in reducing load on hospital organizations and healthcare systems, lower health monitoring costs and ameliorate ambient quality of life for common people.

The "Internet of Things (IoT)" refers to a novel technological innovation that permits pervasive communication of things with "physical or virtual world" via Internet [3]. As sensor devices and "radio frequency identification (RFID)" communication have seen an exponential surge in recent years, humongous amounts of data gets generated, which becomes difficult to handle with limited processing and storage available in these sensor nodes [2]. To overcome this, cloud and IoT amalgamation also known as CloudIoT provides an efficient solution for bridging communication between heterogeneous devices and handling ever-increasing data demands [24, 82]. CloudIoT framework permits seamless application deployment and service rendering using cloud service-based models [3, 22]. The integration of cloud and IoT known as "CloudIoT" provides a novel approach for designing coherent and structured healthcare surveillance systems [3]. With CloudIoT, diverse IoT applications interconnect and exchange information with each other for dispensing efficient healthcare solutions [60, 81]. A number of challenges exist in healthcare monitoring that motivates our research in this area. These include ever-increasing aging population around the world, increase in immedicable diseases and high cost of clinical healthcare [60, 61, 85]. The operation of CloudIoT model in healthcare area can generate numerous opportunities for medical infrastructure and researchers claim that it can notably ameliorate clinical healthcare system and add to its persistent and sustained innovation [24]. The application of CloudIoT in healthcare offers a novel way for patients to improvise on their quality of life by permitting them to carry on with their usual business, while the medical experts are tracking them in the back end and offering them with consultation and health advice [60]. Given the fact that new chronic diseases have been discovered in recent times, the use of enabling platforms such as cloud and IoT enact a pivotal role in their prior detection and prevention which significantly impacts healthcare expenditure and budgets of common people [40, 66]. Bridging the integration between cloud and IoT in healthcare perspective can substantially contribute in developing efficient healthcare applications for overseeing and monitoring hospitals and patients [35].

CloudIoT can streamline healthcare processes and upgrade the standard of medical infrastructure by establishing collaboration among the diverse units involved

[23]. To ease everyday work life of patients having ailments and severe medical conditions, the concept of ambient assisted living (AAL) has evolved over a period of time [7, 8]. With implementation of CloudIoT in healthcare, it has become feasible to dispense many novel applications such as employing sensor network for aggregation of sensitive patient data, transferring the data to cloud for archival storage and finally processing and analyzing the data for extracting meaningful information with data analytics by back end users [78]. One of the significant features of CloudIoT application in healthcare is its offering of quality ubiquitous medical services with minimal operational cost [24, 52]. Given the pervasive nature of healthcare systems, humongous amount of data gets generated by sensor networks that demand efficient management and handling for further data analysis [87]. The cloud presents an excellent platform for processing healthcare data and facilitates abstraction of technical details from the user [14]. Moreover, it guides to automated task of aggregating and transferring data at low cost, thereby making mobile devices self-sufficient for health information accessibility, analysis, and data processing [55]. The CloudIoT model is being implemented globally in order to connect medical infrastructures and dispense pervasive, robust, and intelligent healthcare facilities to patients with severe ailments [67, 69]. A significant progress in healthcare monitoring has indicated the productive as well as propitious future of CloudIoT in healthcare applications [24]. Use of CloudIoT in healthcare involves amalgamation of ICT technology, interconnected apps, sensor devices, and back end people that coordinate and work together as one intelligent system to monitor, track, and store including analyze the patient data [8]. Most CloudIoT-based healthcare monitoring models have primarily three major components: smart wearable and implantable sensors for data collection, data transmission which is responsible for real-time and secure transmission of captured data to the healthcare data center and cloud data storage for processing, analytics, and visualization [24, 65]. In addition, the model can also have clinical stations (e.g., doctors) who remotely extract information from cloud storage. The on-demand service model of cloud provides flawless access to medical and health experts to diverse pool of data from heterogeneous sources which include electronic medical records (EMRs), medical prescriptions and lab report data [83]. The treatment of chronic diseases like asthma or following drug regimens automatically alert medical experts in case of contrasting or missed prescriptions. Additionally, CloudIoT offers state-of-the-art data analytics that will equip doctors or healthcare community to monitor and track patients at any given point in time [23, 59, 78].

Despite visible success on ground, technical and implementation challenges question the roadmap of rapid development and systematic establishment of intelligent CloudIoT-based healthcare systems [83]. CloudIoT faces certain bottlenecks with respect to security, privacy, and reliability of patient data [3]. CloudIoT systems transact sensitive personal information over critical infrastructures which could be abused by users with malicious intent [23]. What is needed is a robust and secure system that will protect user data and privacy [57]. Also, robust CloudIoT-based services, particularly, for delay-sensitive applications such as healthcare demand low power consuming intelligent architectures. Although a reasonable number of energy-efficient architectures have evolved over time, however, most of them deal with IoT and cloud independently. Energy efficiency of CloudIoT models can improve sensor network lifetime which can increase the overall operational quality of the available services. To overcome delay-sensitiveness and energy consumption, concept of fog computing can be employed that lowers the traffic on cloud and also acts as local storage for IoT devices [2, 58]. As healthcare data is sensitive, country regulations do not permit them to be used outside the system of healthcare service providers. Therefore, fog computing forms an ideal solution to bridge this gap by steering computational processing closer to the healthcare service providers [1]. This, in turn, results in reduced latency, reduced energy consumption, data privacy, as well optimal bandwidth utilization.

In this chapter, we review the available CloudIoT literature and present a holistic vision on the CloudIoT-based healthcare integration components. The chapter also presents seamless applications dispensed by CloudIoT platform and contemplates discussion on factors driving CloudIoT health integration. The chapter presents a conceptual architectural framework for healthcare monitoring system that considers a range of aspects including data collection, transmission, and processing including cloud storage. The chapter also discusses a use case framework that identifies actors and data flows responsible for transforming sensor data into real-time transmission to cloud. Also, a brief discussion on design considerations for healthcare architecture will be provided. The work in this chapter also highlights security issues affecting IoT layered architecture including vulnerabilities inherent in the cloud. These vulnerabilities could render healthcare services nonfunctional and critical patient information can be abused by malevolent users. The chapter also presents a brief discussion on some potential mitigation measures. The chapter elaborates discussion on various CloudIoT platforms that aim at solving heterogeneity issue between the cloud and things. Finally, the chapter concludes by identifying some open research issues and challenges hampering CloudIoT-based healthcare adoption.

The entire chapter is segregated into 12 sections. Section 2 presents background work and related application areas of healthcare implementation. Section 3 presents a little background of "Internet of Things" and cloud computing-based healthcare. Section 4 introduces CloudIoT and presents a holistic vision on the CloudIoT integration components including its diverse healthcare applications. Section 5 presents CloudIoT complementary aspects and drivers for integration. Section 6 presents a conceptual architectural framework for healthcare monitoring system that considers a range of aspects including data collection, transmission, and processing including cloud storage. Section 7 discusses a use case scenario that identifies actors and data flows responsible for transforming sensor data into real-time transmission to cloud. Section 8 lays a brief discussion on design considerations for healthcare architecture. Section 9 highlights security issues affecting IoT layered architecture including vulnerabilities inherent in the cloud. Section 10 elaborates discussion on various CloudIoT platforms that aim at solving heterogeneity issue between the cloud and things. Section 11 presents some open research issues and challenges hampering CloudIoT-based healthcare adoption. Finally, Sect. 12 concludes the chapter.

2 Application Areas and Related Work

The CloudIoT technology often finds application in remote healthcare monitoring and dispenses feasible solutions to patients with severe health conditions and disabilities. Employing remote monitoring through cloud and IoT aids in proactive and prior detection of diseases and as such, suitable healthcare solutions could be provided to ensure patient convenience and comfort. The CloudIoT-based healthcare applications have seen an increasing popularity in recent times due to low cost and ubiquitous availability of sensors. A number of implantable as well as wearable medical sensors are available in the market today that performs precise and accurate sensing.

In [87], authors present a survey on IoT-based healthcare and study the application of IoT devices in various areas such as monitoring toddlers, kids as well as managing chronic diseases, motion sensors, and guidance in surgery. The work also presents a comparison of IoT healthcare devices contrasting their battery life, cloud connectivity, and other parameters. The work in [82] presents K-Healthcare model that operates with four layers which include sensing layer, networking layer, Internet layer, and application service layer. The layers work in coordination, dispensing a platform for smart and remote health surveillance using smartphones. The paper also presents comparative overview of diverse architectures and cloud-based IoT applications employed for smart health. In recent years, a lot of research has focused on developing remote monitoring systems for patients with severe health issues. Most of these systems measure essential patient signs that help in early anomaly detection and allow timely care [42]. Some of these systems are designed to measure electrocardiography (ECG) of patients, which is later on transmitted to the cloud database via Internet or other wireless mode of data communication. The recorded data is analyzed and monitored and appropriate actions are undertaken [30, 34, 47].

The researchers in [35] worked toward the integration of "body sensor networks (BSN)" hinged on cloud platform and designed a system called as "ECGaaS". The system allows monitoring and analysis of ECG data obtained from individual users or group of people living in remote areas. The other related research monitors and records key body parameters such as blood pressure, pulse rate, respiration rate which aids in triggering alarms in case any abnormal activity gets detected. This further helps in prior detection and diagnosis of diseases such as hypertension. Some systems employ a questionnaire method for measuring vital body signs and collection of patient data [78, 79]. The users found the system effective, helpful, and easy to operate. In [40], the authors present a system that monitors weight and blood pressure for heart disease patients. The system checks for patient's vital symptoms using a questionnaire and triggers an alert to the medical healthcare center in case an anomaly gets detected in recorded data values. In [79], authors present a novel critical heart failure (CHF) monitoring system which employs the use of body sensors, web-based servers, and medical databases. The application is highly effective in tracking weight changes and blood pressure reading of patients. The underlying algorithms powering these healthcare monitoring systems result in developing prediction models that result in high accuracy. The researchers in [13] developed a telemonitoring system that uses a smartphone for tracking health status of critical heart patients. The smartphone acts as a hub as well as a sensing and communication device.

Aged care monitoring using telecommunications has enabled old age patients to live an independent and ambience life [42]. The CloudIoT-powered smart homes and smart medicine has enhanced the quality of life of aged people [79]. The authors in [21] designed a "Silver Link" system that utilizes objects and human-based sensors for tracking health status and patient activities. The sensors collect the data which is analyzed and monitored for any abnormal behavior. If any such anomaly is observed, the system sends message notifications to the medical emergency team. The prototype examination has been carried and the results show a high success rate. In [12], authors propose "Help to you" (H2U) healthcare monitoring framework for dispensing advanced healthcare services to the aged people. The framework operates with varied technologies which include wearable biomedical sensors and sensor networks for tracking real-time health status. The system also has a provision for emergency medical reminders and critical symptom checks.

An IoT-powered healthcare monitoring system has been proposed by researchers in [44]. The system sends real-time alert notifications to the doctors and medical team in case any exigency arises. The notification alert rules are dynamic and can be configured at runtime. The system is agile and addition or removal of sensors from the system does not disrupt its normal operation.

Dispensing quality medical care is one of the challenging tasks among the aged people. Reminding patients of periodic checkups and scheduled medication has been the pivotal role of CloudIoT-driven healthcare. In [63], the authors designed a drug management system hinged on RFID technology to monitor medicine usage of patients. A similar research [43] proposes "Intelligent Pill box" that reminds patients of scheduled medications.

The CloudIoT integration framework also dispenses emergency applications that detect anomalies so that proactive action and emergency steps could be taken [44]. Such systems involve personal health devices that monitor collected data to detect critical situations and communicate data to the medical and clinical care systems. When an exigency occurs, the response team can quickly dispense its service and reach out to the patient. In [59], the author's present telemedicine and emergency telecare based healthcare monitoring system. Using telemedicine, the patients are provided with the disease information and its respective treatment. The emergency telecare dispenses information with respect to user location, critical information, and medical instructions for user assistance. In [41], authors propose design and working of a healthcare monitoring system used in critical emergency services. The designers have used Intel GALILEO 2nd Generation development board connected to a server to display data collection and integration as well as interoperability of IoT data. The board processes and uploads the data aggregated by the biosensors to the server. For analysis, the system converts and processes the data into statistical charts and graphs. The authors claim that the proposed design considerably reduces health risks and its associated costs as the model collects, stores, analyzes, and shares data in real time and in a regulated method.

The IoT enables support for diverse collection of medical services such as remote healthcare, AAL, and old age care. In [18], authors proposed a framework for smart hospital system for examining and tracking patients for real-time status updates. In case of exigency situations, the alerts are directly sent to the medical professionals. In [10], authors present a hierarchical based framework for monitoring old age patients. The framework model is segregated into four layers which include perception or sensing layer, gateway or networking layer, cloud layer, and device interfacing layer. Their work takes into consideration monitoring of health and nutrition, safety monitoring, monitoring localization and navigation, and encouraging social life for elderly people who may feel lonely. Some healthcare systems employ restful APIs to connect and provide seamless access to HTTP services. Authors in [25] present a monitoring system that tracks continuously and transacts medical information. The system hinges on Restful API services to drive the basic working of the system.

Given the fact that medical data gets communicated over a sensitive wireless network, enforcing security and privacy is of utmost importance. Authors in [57] suggest an end-to-end security authentication mechanism based on DTLS handshake, session control, and management. The scheme operates on hierarchical architecture reducing transmission costs and energy consumption. Their work identifies considerable security features with their implementation.

3 Background Terms

3.1 Internet of Things in Healthcare

The "Internet of Things (IoT)" provides a computing platform where every small object is deployed with sensors, microcontroller chips, and communication interface along with standard protocol stacks for interacting and communicating with the sensor network as well as with other physical objects [67, 77]. In IoT-powered healthcare systems, varied sensor nodes collect, monitor, and transfer real-time medical data to the cloud server over Internet [25]. This, in turn, enables storage, analysis, and processing of humongous volume of data and generates event-based alarms and notifications. The IoT healthcare offers a novel information generation platform that permits ubiquitous and pervasive medical information retrieval over the Internet from any connected device in the world [10]. Thus, IoT-based healthcare has enhanced quality medical care with active monitoring and reduced cost.

The title "Internet of Things" or "Internet of Objects" evolved originally in "future of Internet and ubiquitous computing" and was conceived by a British scientist "Kevin Ashton" [10]. Kevin envisioned a system where the real-world environment can be mapped or connected to virtual world using Internet-enabled sensor objects. This technological evolution varies from conventional internetworks and represents the future of ubiquitous computing. The IoT operates in an environment involving heterogeneous devices that communicate using divergent protocols [3]. The "things" in IoT represents any object or device that interconnects with other objects or devices in the network. For communication with other devices, IoT employs short-range data transmission and lower power dissipation devices which include RFIDs, "Bluetooth" and "Zigbee", etc. [84]. The IoT offers a flexible and convenient framework for humans to interact with the environment around us. Although the popularity of IoT has surged over the years, however no standard definition is yet available for the technology. In basic terms, IoT represents an internetwork of small connected devices or objects. These devices use sensors to perceive the environment around them, capture the data and transmit, or share this data over the Internet for additional tasks [41]. The IoT has allowed personalized healthcare by maintaining medical records for each patient [18]. Due to lack of ubiquitous healthcare systems, severe health issues get unexposed in traditional healthcare systems. However, due to pervasive and non-invasive systems, robust IoT systems aid in active monitoring and analysis of patient data [87]. The IoT paradigm presents a number of solutions for healthcare systems, however from the available solutions; the optimal one depends on constraints and limitations of a given application [83]. The optimal solution enables in developing cost-effective healthcare systems that augment the currently available medical services, clinical care, and remote patient monitoring [78]. For example, to measure physical data of patients in hospitals on periodic basis, the services of healthcare professionals are employed. However, using IoT banishes such requirement by dispensing pervasive monitoring systems which include sensors, gateway nodes, and cloud servers for wirelessly transmitting data to medical professionals.

3.1.1 IoT Architecture

Due to global popularity and promising future, "Intel" labeled IoT as "Embedded Internet" [3, 15]. This is due to the fact that today, embedded devices used in everyday appliances have the ability to connect and transmit information over the Internet [15]. As depicted in Fig. 1, the IoT principal architecture is segregated into four layers in a given hierarchy: "perception or physical layer", "network or transport layer", "middleware layer", and "application or service layer". Every hierarchical layer performs a defined function and services the layer above it.

This represents first layer in the hierarchy and involves the use of small physical sensors, "RFIDs", "Barcode tags", etc. The principal functionality assigned to this layer is to sense and capture information and transmit this information to the remote server node. Analogous to OSI model, the information captured by this layer is transmitted to upper layers for further operation.

"*Network Layer*"

This layer is composed of networking protocols that assist in data transfer from intended source to destination or sink node. The source and sink are usually assigned distinct IP addresses.

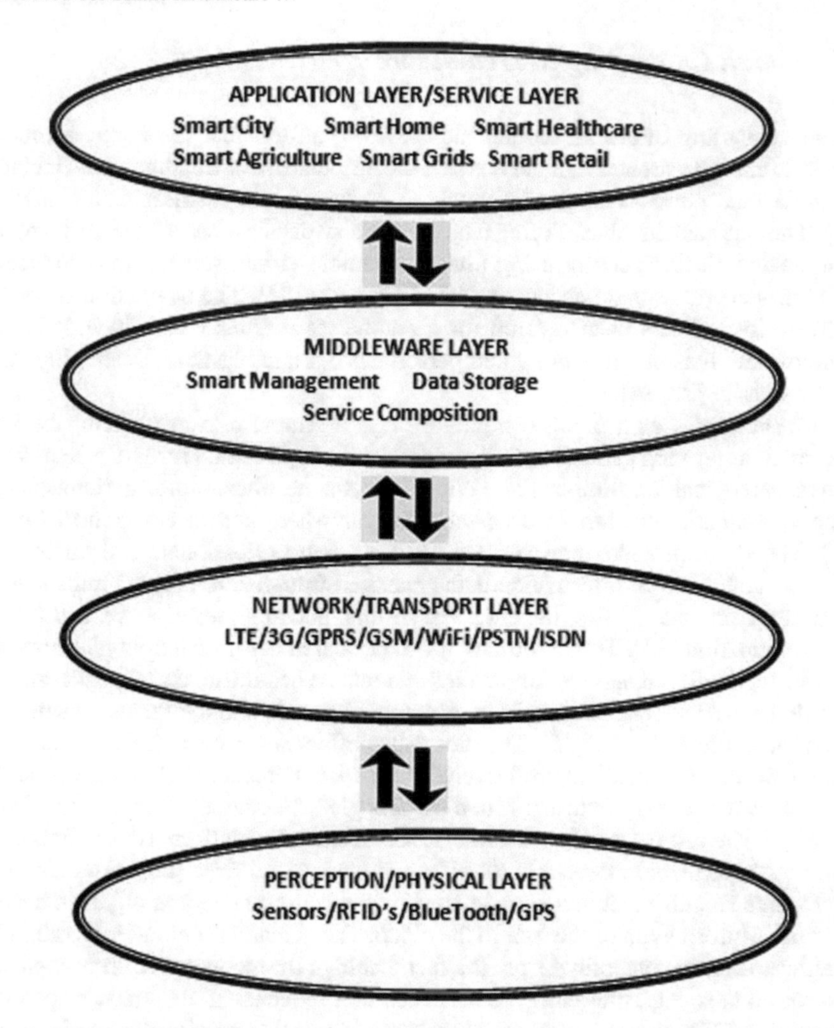

Fig. 1 IoT layered architecture "*Perception Layer*"

"*Middleware Layer*"

This is an intermediate layer between the network and application layer. This layer offers varied data management services that preprocess the data and output it to next layer.

"*Application Layer*"

This represents the uppermost layer in the hierarchy and presents application interface for user data. The layer dispenses various user application functions underpinned by below middleware layer. These services promote diverse range of application areas like industrial automation systems, automated e-healthcare, smart city, smart traffic, etc.

3.2 Cloud Computing in Healthcare

Cloud computing offers an on-demand service platform that dispenses seamless access to infinite warehouse of pervasive and distributed infrastructure which include computational power, humongous database, software, and business data analytics [15]. The approach involves storing data on a remote database server and performing computation and processing using powerful remote virtual servers, thus reducing the management tasks on account of its client users [84]. The adaptation of cloud platform for IoT has been favored for a number of reasons which include being economically feasible, reliability and performance, rapid elasticity, scalability, and robust security [22, 84].

In healthcare sector, cloud computing plays a critical role in reducing healthcare costs, improving patient's quality of service and optimizing resources that drive new technological innovations [24]. With cloud, the healthcare information is ubiquitously available and can be accessed from anywhere and in any point of time [81]. The cloud provides flawless access to medical professionals and doctors to a diverse collection of information data generated from heterogeneous information sources that include EMRs, lab data, test results, doctor's prescriptions and insurance information [34]. This information can be shared across multiple platforms to offer better quality of service for patients and reduce healthcare costs. Furthermore, it could be used for decision-making, accurate diagnosis and treatment, scheduling doctor appointments, etc. [35]. The cloud also offers state-of-the-art analytics that will aid doctors and medical professionals to track patients remotely and accurately [15]. Many technology industries such as "Google", "Amazon", "Yahoo" and "Microsoft" are investing heavily in healthcare sector and offer platforms that collaborate with health partners to develop cost-effective medical services [69]. For example, Microsoft's Health Vault and Google Health applications store and organize health and fitness information of the user in the cloud. The demand for cloud integration in Healthcare is also perceptible from the fact that high throughput platforms engaged in research labs, e.g., microarray, next generation sequencing, magnetic resonance imaging, and X-ray scans generate large data volumes that pose challenges in terms of pervasive data storage and computation, data analytics, and mining [3].

The cloud computing model offers four distinct features that differentiate it from traditional processing systems [1]. First; it offers an "on-demand service model" which allows a client to utilize server storage and processing as per his convenience and time. Second, it provides a "broader network access" by employing varied devices like smartphones, tablet computers, and also desktop machines. Third, it "pools various resources" and combines them to build a large warehouse repository which are distributed to clients on demand. Fourth, it promotes "rapid elasticity" of resources that permits a server to adjust to client request as per load and demand.

As depicted in Fig. 2, the cloud platform offers service to the clients at three distinct levels: "infrastructure as a service (IaaS)", "software as a service (SaaS)", and "platform as a service (PaaS)".

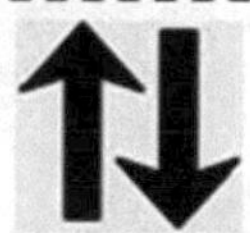

Fig. 2 Cloud service models

"*Infrastructure as a Service (IaaS)*"

The IaaS platform dispenses a virtual environment to the clients in which infrastructure resources which include virtual machines, storage, and networking are provided on subscription basis. The platform provides a billing system wherein the users pay for Infrastructure on demand. The hired infrastructure is highly scalable depending on user's processing and storage requirements.

"*Software as a Service (SaaS)*"

The SaaS model dispenses a seamless access to cloud software and database on subscription basis. The installation, up-gradation, and troubleshooting of software is managed by the SaaS platform. The user data remains secured in the cloud and failure of infrastructure hardware does not result in data loss. The applications installed on the cloud can be run remotely via Internet from anywhere in the world.

"*Platform as a Service (PaaS)*"

The "PaaS" platform offers users a coherent software design and management interface. The users can manage, develop, test, and deliver applications using this interface in addition to software and database design tools that allow direct web application

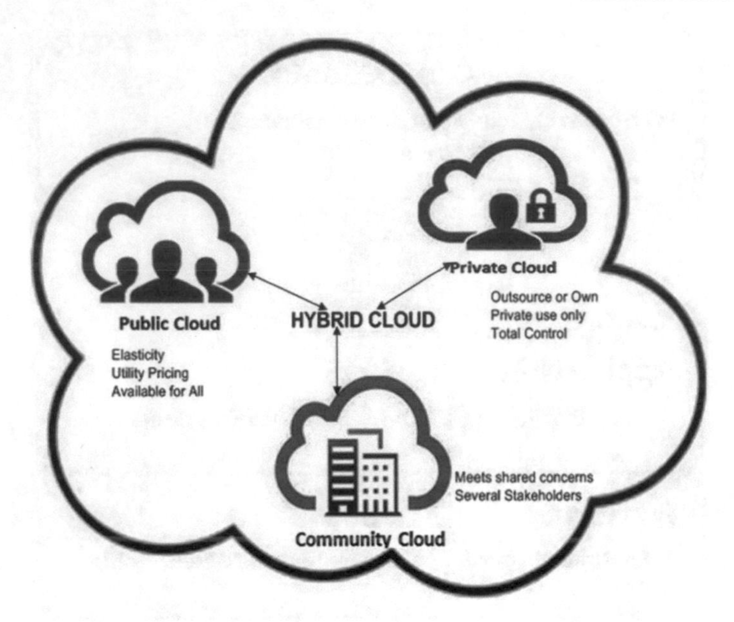

Fig. 3 Cloud deployment models

deployment. The platform also provides an efficient collaborative work environment in which different users work together remotely.

In addition to cloud service models, the technology offers four distinct deployment platforms which are discussed below and are depicted in Fig. 3.

"*Public/External Cloud*"

The "public or external cloud" offers unrestricted or public access to the cloud platform. The service provider owns the platform resources and clients pay as per service usage.

"*Private/Internal Cloud*"

The "private or internal cloud" is generally owned or hired by a company or business organization for its personalized usage. The organizations usually deploy business-critical applications on this cloud model.

"*Community Cloud*"

The "community cloud" is owned by a community of business enterprises having related interests and activities.

"*Hybrid/Virtual Private Cloud*"

This deployment platform offers a blend of private/public/community clouds.

4 Integrating CloudIoT with Healthcare

The popularity of Internet-based computation in Healthcare has increased the number of objects or things getting interconnected with each other [65]. IoT finds application in diverse areas ranging from smart healthcare, remote health monitoring, developing smart home systems, smart city, environment surveillance, and power management [15]. These application areas especially healthcare generate humongous volume of data which demand real-time processing [89]. This, however, requires flexible network architecture that would underpin high traffic volume that gets generated by heterogeneous devices [6]. As IoT devices have constrained storage space, it is not thus possible to store this data locally on interim storage devices. Also IoT suffers from constrained power and limited bandwidth which decrease its performance substantially [65]. Earlier; the sensors would transmit data to mainframe computers which were equipped with adequate computing infrastructure and resources. However, the approach had some drawbacks [75]. First, running applications and storing data on mainframes was time-consuming and not economical. Second, in case of failure, the entire system would shut down. Another approach was distributed computing wherein nodes were equipped with minimal storage and processing. However, this approach too had limitations which include cost of IoT node replacement in case of failure and cost for providing the backup power.

Thus, migrating data and computation from real-world environment to virtual platform, i.e., from "IoT to cloud" seems to be a coherent solution [15, 65]. The cloud dispenses a feasible, on-demand, pliable, and agile platform for healthcare application deployment and provides access to virtually unlimited networked computing infrastructure [22]. These computing infrastructures offer extensive processing power and substantial virtual storage that augment the constrained resources in IoT devices, hence providing robust platform for pervasive communications [31]. To define correlation and integration between heterogeneous IoT devices and cloud platform, the concept of CloudIoT or "cloud of things" (CoTs) evolved at MIT's Auto-ID Labs [3]. The IoTs are small Internet-ready devices that are distinctly pervasive and ubiquitous; however, they suffer from limited computational power and storage. These drawbacks contribute to performance bottlenecks, security flaws, and privacy affairs in IoT nodes [32].

Contrary to this, cloud offers robust, flexible, and agile platform for IoT healthcare application deployment [39]. With CloudIoT, it is envisioned that two heterogeneous technologies will integrate for dispensing efficient power and resource management, and for developing innovative healthcare solutions [16]. This technological framework can serve delay-sensitive as well as real-time applications in a reliable and secure manner. Some of the principal characteristics of CloudIoT implementation include virtually unlimited storage space and computational power for IoT nodes, pervasive and ubiquitous service model for users, cross-platform support for applications, efficient resource management, and end-to-end "quality of service (QoS)" [4].

With CloudIoT platform, the virtual resources are dispensed like a service on subscription or "pay-per-use" basis to the client users [83]. CloudIoT framework permits seamless application deployment and service rendering using cloud service-based models which are "IaaS", "PaaS" and "SaaS". Also, the framework ensures that end-to-end "QoS" is sustained in the network [68]. As an example, when service load request from client increases, the cloud must automatically augment itself to satisfy the request. Again when client request load reduces, the cloud must automatically adjust itself to accommodate the change. Thus, technological evolution of CloudIoT seems to provide a potential solution that is tangible, robust, less convoluted, and cost-effective [50, 54].

However, with numerous tangible benefits of CloudIoT platform, the integration process is somewhat arduous and not that simple [19]. The integration framework must address issues related to economic and business perspective of service providers. Other issues contemplating CloudIoT platform involves reliable as well as secure communication and data storage [22]. As CloudIoT involves private and sensitive healthcare data of patients, the platform as such is vulnerable to attacks from malevolent systems. The problem becomes more convoluted in case of hybrid clouds where the main focus should be on safeguarding confidentiality, availability, and data privacy including identity protection [57, 83]. This entails employing cryptographic techniques for data encryption and authentication. Integrating two heterogeneous technologies, i.e., cloud and IoT involves interconnection and data exchange between divergent networks. These disparate networks should be flexible, unrestricted and should underpin heterogeneous data and services [22].

5 CloudIoT Complementary Aspects and Integration Drivers

Although "cloud and IoT" are two divergent technological platforms, the current research data presents their corresponding features and attributes that underline the rationale for their amalgamation [24]. These features and characteristics as obtained from available research papers are reported in Table 1. With CloudIoT architecture, cloud layer connects underlying IoT sensor objects and end user services at the access layer. The cloud also conceals complex operations and algorithms from the client user [38].

The motivating features driving the integration and adoption of CloudIoT framework for healthcare are:

"*Storage*": The sensor nodes in IoT healthcare produce large volume of data by exploiting various information generation sources which include EMRs, lab report data, test results, doctor's prescriptions and insurance information, etc. [70]. This data is usually called as big data and is classified as either semi-structured or non-structured [1]. This big data has three well-known properties [14]: which include

Table 1 Comparison of IoT and cloud characteristics

Characteristic	IoT	Cloud
"Displacement"	Pervasive (things are everywhere)	Centralized and condensed service
Availability	Restricted	Distributed (remote access to resources)
Device nature	Things are real-world objects	Virtual infrastructure available via Internet
Computational power	Limited computational capacity	Virtually limitless processing power
Memory space	Sparse in nature	Scalable as per demand
Role of Internet	Uses Internet as convergence place	Employs Internet for delivery of service
Big data	Contributes as prime source for big data	Big data processing and management is supported

"volume" (i.e., quantity of data), "variety" (i.e., data type heterogeneity), and "velocity" (i.e., rate of production of data) [92]. To capture, store, organize, and examine such sizeable amount of data is infeasible for resource-constrained sensor nodes. Thus, cloud offers an efficient and pliable choice to manage IoT healthcare data [91]. Once the data has been preserved in cloud storage, data analytics and data mining techniques are leveraged to extract useful information. Further, it could be used for decision and policy-making, precise diagnosis and treatment, scheduling doctor appointments, etc. Also robust cryptographic procedures can be employed to secure sensitive patient data from malicious users and ensure privacy [57].

"*Computing capabilities*": Nearly all IoT nodes have limited processing capacity that restricts their ability to perform complex data processing operations online [65]. The feasible solution is to transfer the strenuous computational part to powerful and scalable server machines [67]. The on-demand cloud service platform presents virtually infinite processing power for handling data from disparate information sources such as EMRs, lab reports, and medical imaging data [6]. Additionally, the cloud also dispenses advanced data analytics service that permits doctors and physicians to remotely monitor patients from anywhere.

"*Communication*": Among the principal goals of pervasive healthcare is to permit application data sharing and provide reliable communication among sensor nodes over the Internet [10]. To supplement such communication incurs greater financial cost and as such is not feasible. Therefore, cloud offers an effective and feasible economic solution for interconnecting, managing, and personalizing applications remotely from anywhere [6]. To assist in remote healthcare administration and management of data, the cloud communications are underpinned by high-speed optical fiber Internet [67]. Although cloud considerably improves QoS in communication with sensor nodes, however in certain situations still acts as a bottleneck which limits down its computational capacity. Thus, feasible and realistic solutions need to

Table 2 Innovative services and models envisioned with CloudIoT

Acronym	Expanded form	Description of service
SaaS	"Sensing as a service"	To dispense seamless access to sensor data
SAaaS	"Sensing and actuation as a service"	To support automated control logistics with cloud implementation
SEaaS	"Sensor event as a service"	Transmitting real-time messages triggered by events perceived by a sensor
SenaaS	"Sensor as a service"	To enable remote management of distributed remote sensors
DBaaS	"Database as a service"	To enable remote database administration
DaaS	"Data as a service"	To support pervasive access to any data type
EaaS	"Ethernet as a service"	Enabling distributed layer-II access for remotely distributed devices
IPMaaS	"Identity and policy management as a service"	Dispensing ubiquitous access to management of identity and policy
VSaaS	"Video surveillance"	To enable remote video recording and performing examination and analysis on it

Source [15]

be developed to enable large volume of data transfer between sensor nodes and the cloud [15].

"*New capabilities and paradigms*": The disparity between "IoT" objects and underlying protocols make adaptability, validity, accessibility, and authenticity very arduous to attain. To address this issue, the cloud offers easy resource access, robust and strong platform for applications, and economically feasible deployment [60, 89]. The amalgamation of cloud and IoT enabled smart devices and services manage contemporary real-life situations. Table 2 (extracted from [15]) reports summary of new design models and standards evolved from this integration. Due to the lack of any standard terminology, the acronyms differ in various cases and have no coherent variance.

6 Framework for Healthcare Architecture

CloudIoT-powered health applications can be developed by collaborative integration of diverse technologies that operate on wireless communications and employ sensor networks for data collection including analysis and cloud interface for data storage

[22]. To indicate the collaborative operation, the system is usually represented by an architecture known as CloudIoT health architecture [16].

The architecture as shown in Fig. 4 normally implements three layers carrying varied functions which include data acquisition or sensing, data transmission or sending, cloud processing or storage. The data sensing or perception layer collects varied physiological parameters of patients and transmits the data to the cloud storage via transmission layer.

Data Acquisition/Sensing Layer

This layer forms the network of sensors including wearable devices that collect and record health data of patients. The sensors monitor essential signs such as body temperature, heart pulse rate, and pressure of blood, and record the data in medical

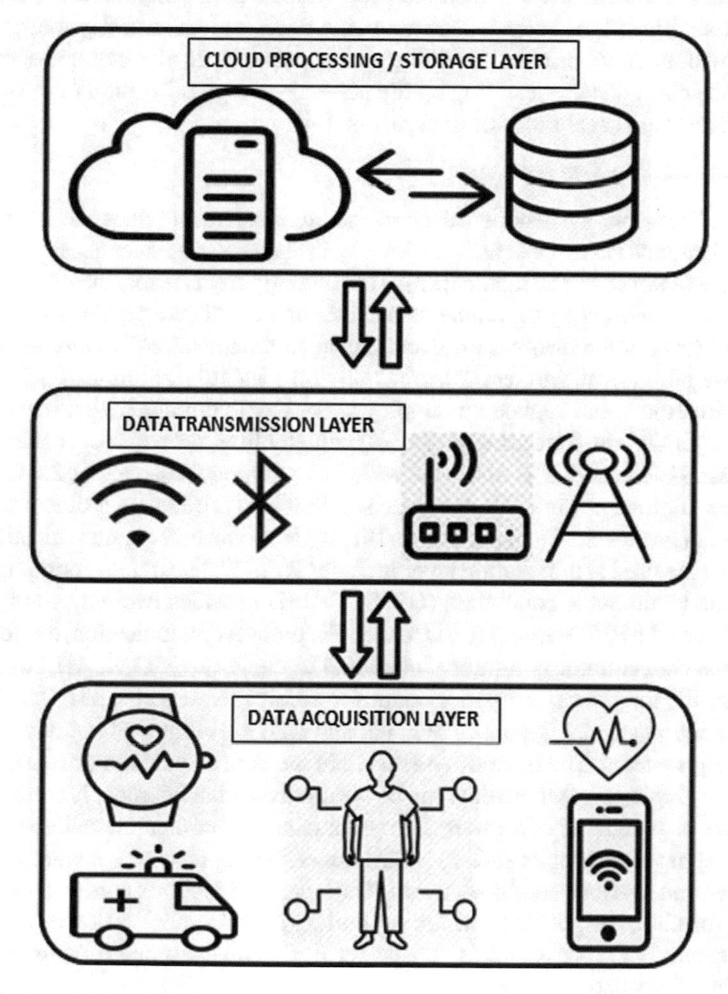

Fig. 4 Healthcare architecture framework

databases [59]. Most of these recorded parameters vary from application to application across different categories of patients. For example, in case of critical heart patients, monitoring ECG levels, oxygen saturation, and pulse rate forms a critical component in diagnosis [26]. In case of patients with diabetes, monitoring blood sugar levels are important. For the applications that underpin "AAL" for aged people, monitoring activity periodically is required [20]. Most of these applications operate with accelerometers and gyroscopic sensors for data collection and health monitoring. The sensors are segregated into invasive or noninvasive categories. Invasive sensors perform better than noninvasive counterparts; however, they are not the popular choice among the elderly people unless the issue is convoluted [37]. Some applications employ actuators for alert generation or adapting environment changes [79]. There has been lot of evolutionary development in the design of intelligent sensors which has in turn extended the capabilities of IoT infrastructure [62]. A lot of solutions hinged on body sensor networks have evolved recently that generate humongous amounts of data. To design the sensing layer, the key considerations involve the cost and size of setting up the network, energy utilization in sensing and data transmission capabilities of the sensors [64].

Data Transmission/Sending Layer

The Data Transmission/sending layer in the architecture provides the interface to communicate and share the data. Additionally, the layer also enables access to the data in existing deployed infrastructure [88]. The sending layer is responsible for transferring patient data securely to remote data center of a healthcare organization (HCO). The data transmission involves local and global communication. For monitoring and scanning environment, wireless data transmission standards are employed. Protocols such as Bluetooth and Zigbee are employed for local communication between the sensing layer and the concentrator [35, 74]. Bluetooth offers a low-cost solution for data transmission over short distances with the operating frequency of 2.4 GHz and consumes minimal power [74]. Alternate solution is to use Zigbee protocol which is however not as prevalent and popular as Bluetooth. Some other communication protocols that are used at the sending layer include "RFIDs", "near field communication (NFC)" and "ultrawide bandwidth (UWB)". RFID provides two-way communications between the RFID tag and RFID reader. For global communication, the collected data in the concentrator is further transmitted to cloud or HCO via Wifi or mobile data network for preserving patient data for archival storage [9, 53]. The mobile communication standards such as 3G, 4G, and LTE are employed in diverse health monitoring systems. The low power sensors in the data acquisition or sensing layer follow IoT architecture whose data can be acquired over the Internet via concentrator. This layer also consists of various data processing and computational applications that run on processing units such as smartphones, microprocessors including microcontrollers, and various on-chip systems. The layer also supports hardware platforms such as Arduino, Raspberry Pi which support and provide application development environment. The processed data is used for further analysis and mining including generating alerts and notifications.

Cloud Processing/Storing Layer

The CloudIoT systems interconnect diverse objects that generate large volumes of data which entail for intelligent storage mechanism [86]. The healthcare data aggregated from the sensing layer is used for further analysis and mining. The cloud processing or storing layer involves three prime elements, viz., data storage, computation on data, and data analysis [51]. The cloud presents an efficient platform for archiving patient's medical data for long-term storage as well as providing assistance to medical professionals for better diagnosis. Cloud provides data analytics that use sensor data in addition to e-health records for better diagnosis and prediction of health-related diseases [16]. Additionally, cloud also offers data visualization that presents humongous amount of data from sensors in a digestible format for physicians. A number of cloud platforms such as "Google Cloud", "OpenIoT", "Amazon", "ThingWorx" and "GENI" offer efficient storage for generated data. The complexity to manage and maintain healthcare data has been eased with the cloud technology.

To augment the storage and processing capabilities of the sensors, Cloudlet is sometimes employed which is a local processing unit such as desktop computer and can be directly accessible over Wifi whenever the local storage on sensor fails to cater the applications requirements [38]. Additionally, the cloudlet can also be used for performing time-sensitive tasks over patients collected data before transferring data to the cloud or HCO. The cloudlet also overcomes energy or connectivity limitations on the sensors.

7 A Conceptual Healthcare Scenario

The healthcare represents one of the principal challenges that world is facing today [12]. Although a lot of technological advancement occurred in recent years, yet to achieve an efficient healthcare framework is one of the challenging research problems [7]. The health organizations still rely on manual health records and paperwork for information and decision-making process [8]. The flow of digital information is isolated only between departments and healthcare applications. There is hardly any provision for sharing of patient data between departments, clinical doctors, or patients. The cloud and IoT integration provides the potential solution for driving healthcare organizations to pivot their attention on improving patient care for effective health monitoring, early diagnosis, and cost-effective treatment in a timely manner [87]. The CloudIoT augments healthcare systems by employing RFID enabled devices and sensors. This, in turn, enables real-time tracking, identification, and interaction with patients and also monitoring medical supplies including drug management. The IoT component in CloudIoT enables "machine-to-machine" (M2M) as well as "human-to-machine" (H2M) communications. The IoT efficiently connects humans, sensor nodes, and network, and ensures effective medical waste management [15]. The advancement in sensor technology has facilitated ubiquitous healthcare system [25, 41]. Wireless body area network (WBAN) is a novel field that implements the

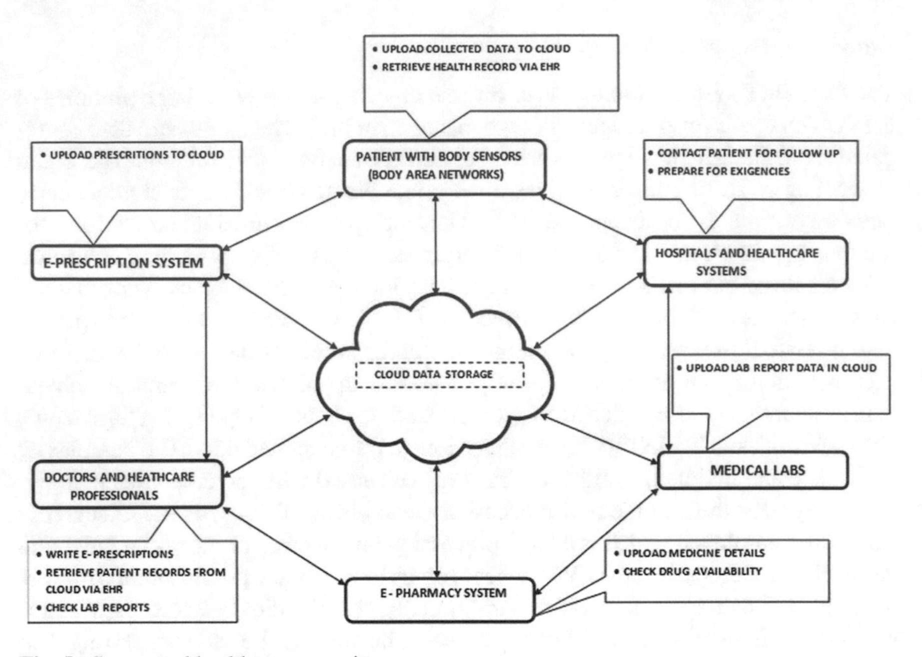

Fig. 5 Conceptual healthcare scenario

concept of e-health. A WBAN involves the use of multiple sensor nodes for health monitoring that can quantify and present the health condition of the patient. The CloudIoT health framework consists of varied applications such as e-prescription system, electronic health records (EHC), personal health records (PHC), decision systems, and drug management system. The healthcare framework offers diverse range of applications to varied stakeholders such as patients, healthcare professionals, medical labs, pharmacists, etc., across multiple platforms [69]. For example, consider a use case scenario of CloudIoT health framework as shown in Fig. 5.

The figure illustrates the various processes involved in the framework and identifies actors and the flow of data. At any given time, the patient could be wearing a monitoring device (typically a body sensor) that gathers physiological data. These biosensors are carefully placed on a human body as small implantations on skin or can be worn as jewellery or even hidden in patient's clothes or shoes. Each sensor is independently capable of sensing, monitoring, processing physical data, and transmitting it wirelessly to a remote cloud system. The sensor nodes are also capable of tracking patient location and accurately determining physical state and activity of the patient, i.e., walking, running, or sitting idle at one place. The physiological data is uploaded and stored into the cloud via an electronic health record system (EHR). For each patient, a separate medical profile is maintained in the cloud. This patient data can be shared with medical professionals and clinical healthcare systems for their analysis and opinion. Medical professionals such as physicians and doctors can dispense quick patient care by accessing the medical data on cloud and providing expert opinions. With consent of patients, the lab technicians can also upload magnetic resonance imaging (MRI) scans, X-rays, serum reports and store the information in medical profile of the patients. This profile could be shared via cloud platforms with other expert specialists around the world permitting standard diagnosis and adept recommendations in quick time frame. The medical experts can recommend life-saving drugs and medicines that need to be available in pharmacy stores. The pharmacist can check medical profile and allergic reaction of patients before issuing or recommending any medicines. Similarly, a hospital dealing with a case of an accident can check patient's blood group, whether allergic to any drugs and reactions and other preconditions before starting the treatment. This information would be available via cloud platform and accessible anywhere in the world.

By utilizing the abovementioned CloudIoT health framework, patient's e-health information such as medical history, imaging scans, blood reports, and allergic reactions could be digitized and can be ubiquitously available via a secure authentication platform. The information can flow securely through the system and can be available to every stakeholder, thus realizing the concept of pervasive healthcare.

8 Design Considerations for Healthcare

The biomedical data collected by wearable devices consist of low power sensors capable of recording patient's physiological parameters, small microcontroller or microprocessing hardware, and communication channel for data transmission [10]. Wearing these biomedical sensors leverage certain limitations on the physical design of the sensors [23, 72]. For example, the sensors should be lightweight, smaller in size, and must not restrict user's physical movement and mobility. Also, sensors need to be energy efficient because they operate on constrained battery power [15]. Although the sensor batteries can be rechargeable or replaceable, the design, however, must ensure that no data is lost during those idle periods. Therefore, it is highly recommended that sensors may be designed in such a way so that they work for extended periods of time without replacement [75]. The constrained battery power also poses limitation on the quality of data aggregated or collected from the sensor. However, the latest design of wearable devices allows sensors to be placed in close contact with the body [76, 83]. This allows measurement of patient's biomedical parameters with greater accuracy and precision [49]. A lot of research on designing low power circuits is going on with focus on improving the operational lifespan of wearable sensors [62]. Moreover, the solution could be to exploit alternate forms of energy generation and harvesting models [64].

Another efficient technique would be to program intelligent periodic sleep routines for the body sensors [16]. The sensors could go in a sleep mode if no observable perception activity occurs during a fixed time frame. Based on similar concept, an efficient energy conservation technique would be to turn on/off a sensor based on its usage importance and health status of a patient. For example, in certain situations, when energy is seriously restricted and health condition of a patient demands attention on a particular biosensor, the other sensors could go into sleep mode or be turned off to save energy and increase operational lifetime [76].

The constrained power in sensor devices demand low power communication standard and protocols, as data transmission consumes substantial amount of power in sensor nodes. Zigbee over IEEE 802.15.4 is typically employed in "low rate wide personal area networks (LR-WPANs)" to underpin data transmission between sensors that work in an estimated range of 10 meters (10 m). The Zigbee protocol offers robust mesh networking with an increased operating battery lifespan. Another significant wireless communication standard with low power short-range communication is the Bluetooth Low Energy (BLE) protocol [74]. Although the indigenous Bluetooth standard (IEEE 802.15.1) was developed to sustain short-range communication, however BLE revamps the standard by implementing prolonged sleep durations to optimize the overall power utilization. BLE obtains a reasonable accuracy and cost-effective energy utilization metrics. To further augment low power communications, "IPv6 over low power wireless personal area networks (6LoWPANs)" has evolved as a panacea for seamless connectivity of energy-constrained devices with the Internet [16]. 6LoWPAN fragments IPv6 datagram packets into a size that can perfectly fit into IEEE 802.15.4 restricted frame size for dispensing IP connectivity.

One important design consideration is to offload complex computation and decision-making process to the cloud [81]. The cloud infrastructure offers extensive processing power and substantial virtual storage that augments the constrained resources in sensors, hence providing robust platform for pervasive communications [2]. To further augment cloud capabilities, cloudlet computing can be leveraged that provides a probable solution for achieving low latency in time-critical applications such as healthcare management. Cloudlet acts as a rudimentary computing and storage platform that banishes the need to migrate complex processing tasks to the enterprise cloud.

A critical issue in designing architecture for healthcare management is maintaining privacy of the user and secure data storage in the cloud [57]. When medical records of the patients are transferred to the cloud, robust privacy protection measures need to be enforced so that data is not left vulnerable to disclosure. The data demands robust protection from unauthorized access; thus, appropriate authentication and authorization measures need to be imposed [22, 28]. The adoption of lightweight cryptographic protocols such as elliptic curve cryptography (ECC) is highly recommended that ensures low power consumption. These cryptographic protocols must be complemented with efficient key exchange mechanisms that demand minimal processing and computation [46, 48, 61].

9 CloudIoT Security Issues and Threats

The "CloudIoT" involves internetwork of connected things that drive common services ranging from smart healthcare systems, remote health monitoring, smart city and homes, intelligent traffic monitoring, environment monitoring, industrial management, as well as how these things interact with each other [39]. The cloud presents an efficient service platform for things and supports easy access to shared infrastructure which includes computational power, humongous storage space, robust applications, and seamless data analytics and mining capabilities [36]. Although CloudIoT has proven to be beneficial in ameliorating our daily health life; however, there has been no security contemplation to its practical deployment scenario [45, 73]. In case of any vulnerability abuse in CloudIoT network, the healthcare services can be rendered nonfunctional and critical patient information can be abused by malevolent users. The integration of cloud and IoT will further aggravate the scenario and as such will uncover concealed issues and vulnerabilities. The security flaws could be misused by malevolent actors to exploit CloudIoT network rendering billions of interconnected nodes vulnerable. Thus, loopholes in CloudIoT network will override its number of benefits. Also, it is not practical that deployed sensor nodes can be replaced periodically owing to its cost implications. The fundamental security architecture needs to be robust and persistent enough to work for substantial period of time without replacement and maintenance.

9.1 Security Features and Goals

CloudIoT supports data transmission between connected things and users to achieve precise goals. In order to safeguard communication in such a pervasive environment, it is essential that parameters such as authenticity, privacy, and control need to be fortified. However, given the limitations imposed by constrained infrastructure (processing capability and storage) of nodes, the framework demands fine-tuning in existing security methods in order to meet apparent security goals as shown in Fig. 6 [73].

"*Confidentiality*"

The confidentiality feature ensures authorized retrieval of the sensitive data and safeguards it from illegal access. The CloudIoT network relies on sensor nodes including RFIDs that capture and store data and this information needs to be fortified from hostile nodes as well as malevolent users. To safeguard data and preserve confidentiality, cryptographic techniques and security protocols should be designed and employed [17].

"*Integrity*"

Data integrity warrants that accuracy, consistency, and reliability of data are preserved over entire duration of data transmission. During transit between legitimate nodes, the data cannot undergo any change and steps need to be taken to prevent data fiddling or tampering. The integrity feature ensures that authentic and valid data is received by legitimate users. To enforce integrity principle, end-to-end security protocols need to be employed in data transit and reception.

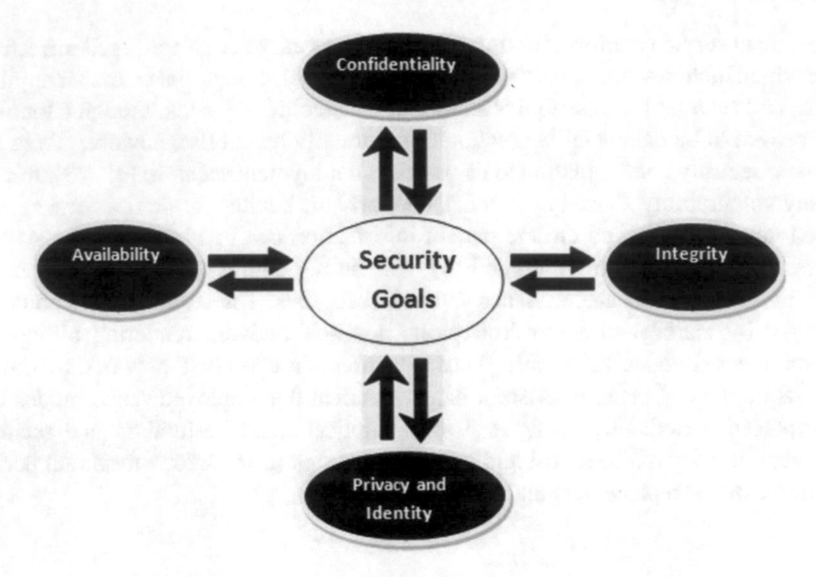

Fig. 6 CloudIoT security goals

"*Availability*"

The availability feature warrants that information and services are accessible to authorized users when required. The objects in CloudIoT network transact data in real time with minimal delays. However; failure to safeguard availability principle would result in unnecessary processing delays which would result in shutdown of network.

"*Identity and Authentication*"

The identification and authentication ratifies that valid information is transacted in CloudIoT network by authorized nodes. Though given the heterogeneity of the whole system and sensor nodes, the process becomes quite complicated [71]. The feasible and optimal solution would be enforcing strict authentication policies and protocols between the permissible entities of the internetwork.

"*Privacy*"

The privacy feature corroborates restricted information retrieval limited only to valid users. In contrast to confidentiality principle which employs encryption procedures to avert data tampering, the privacy factor permits restricted access without abstracting any other specific details.

9.2 Security Vulnerabilities

The CloudIoT security vulnerabilities include issues in both IoT network as well as those inherent in cloud data model. This section first elaborates discussion on security loopholes inherent in each layer of IoT architecture and then underlines vulnerabilities present in cloud data model.

9.2.1 IoT Issues and Limitations

The IoT's hierarchical architecture is susceptible to various attack vectors from malevolent actors. The attack vectors are primarily segregated into two categories, i.e., active and passive based on their operative signature. The active attack directly impacts normal behavior of node, thus being more hostile in nature. The passive attack works covertly in the background like a Trojan Virus [5]. The expounded security review of each IoT layer is discussed below:

Issues in Perception Layer

As the primary goal of "perception or physical layer" is to perceive and capture sensitive information from surrounding physical network, the malicious attack vectors are aimed toward node tinkering or tampering of gathered data. These sensor objects are deployed in a hostile and remote operating environment; as such remain susceptible to "node capturing attacks" in which an attacker leverages physical damage and tinkering of hardware sensors [90]. If an attacker succeeds in compromising a deployed sensor node, it therefore ensues revealing sensitive information such as cryptographic keys and authentication procedures. Also, an attacker can clone a sensor node by copying information parameters in order to authenticate itself with the IoT network. A similar attack vector known as code injection attack inserts malicious scripts into working software code of a sensor node, thereby altering its otherwise standard operating procedures. The malicious script permits attacker to control IoT network which further downgrades its normal working. Additionally, the attackers for trust exploitation can leverage Replay attack in which compromised sensor node transfers sensitive information to illegitimate destination [56]. Once trust is established, the attacker revamps authentication procedures employed in IoT system. To drain battery and deplete the operating power of sensor nodes, the attacker sometimes leverages sleep deprivation attacks. As IoT nodes are battery-powered, therefore in order to run for longer durations, they employ programmed sleep timers in order to save power utilization. The sleep deprivation attack alters sleep timers and makes nodes work continuously even when otherwise idle. This results in power loss and device shutdown [9].

Issues at Network Layer

The IoT network layer is most susceptible to abuse as most of the collected data through sensors gets transmitted at this layer. Most of the security schemes focus on accessibility of the available resources [53]. The security measures also aim at preserving node integrity as well as authentic information data that is communicated over the deployed internetwork. Some inherent vulnerabilities are highlighted below:

"Eavesdropping and interference": As underlying communication medium used by IoT devices is wireless, security threat lies in the fact that transmission medium could be intercepted by malicious actors. The quality of data exchanged between IoT nodes over wireless medium could be degraded by superimposing jamming signals [39]. Secure encryption and cryptographic procedures need to be put into place in order to uphold data accuracy.

"Denial of service (DoS) attack": This is one of the commonly executed network attack directed to render computing infrastructure in a network inaccessible to its legitimate client users. In this attack, large amount of network data traffic is redirected toward the victim node which it cannot process simultaneously, resulting in shutting down or unavailability of a server or controller node. Common attacks which gobble up resources including bandwidth, storage, node memory, and processing time include attack vectors such as "ping of death", "flooding UDP data", "ICMP flooding", etc. Common mitigation strategies implemented for thwarting the attack include implementing robust firewall rules and gateway policies.

"Spoofing attacks": These attacks are categorized into two categories: IP spoofing and RFID spoofing. Both type of attacks target and spoof control system of IoT in order to transmit malicious scripts across network [53].

"Routing attacks": In IoT architecture, routing function is performed at the network layer; therefore, these attacks fiddle with routing policy including protocols with the main aim of creating route loops that result in increased packet drop rate. This further result in increased traffic congestion and latency in network [9].

Additionally, other attacks that are directed toward network layer include "sinkhole attack", "Sybil attack", "wormhole attack", and "illegal node access attack".

Issues at Application Layer

As application layer provides interface for client requests, therefore most of the security issues in this layer are directed toward software routines. The IoT architecture is yet to be standardized; therefore, the issues related to security at application level are supreme and demand robust solutions. Diverse applications entail varied authentication and verification procedures and to homogenize these approaches is an arduous task. Application privacy and node authentication should be the primary design goal of security protocols. Some common application-level security threats include script injections such as "SQL Injections", inept coding which provide platform to XSS vulnerability, password stealing techniques such as fishing and many more [9].

9.2.2 Cloud Service Issues

The security vulnerabilities present in traditional cloud computing systems are also inherent in CloudIoT; however, the integration between two heterogeneous technologies introduces complex attack vectors that are effortless to initiate [38]. As client requests computation and data storage from cloud services, it is important that data confidentiality and data privacy is preserved. The client should be well aware about storage location of their data and its access policies offered by the service provider who manage their data. The client also demands service providers block illegitimate and unlawful access to their data. Given the on-demand cloud service model, an efficient management platform should be provided to the clients and unsanctioned and unauthorized access to this management platform needs to be blocked. The platform if left vulnerable could contribute for further attack definitions [80].The cloud also faces security threats to communication protocols at the network layer. As cloud services are distributed and pervasive in nature, most of the clients access this platform using various internetworking protocols. As majority of these interworking protocols are stateless in nature, thus security threats such "Denial of Service" attack, "man-in-the-middle" attack, eavesdropping are possible [9]. In addition to these, vulnerabilities also exist in how cloud interface is accessed. For example, mediocre authentication policies and injection attacks like "SQL injection" which directly aims at cloud system database. Also, web user interface which is accessed through a client web browser is susceptible XSS attacks. Table 3 lists some common CloudIoT vulnerabilities.

9.3 Potential Defense Strategies

It is quite obvious that amalgamation between two heterogeneous platforms, i.e., cloud and IoT will surge up security threats substantially; therefore, inviolable defense strategies need to be enforced so that vulnerabilities could be averted [9]. The defense security architecture should address both the security in IoT layers as well as in the deployed cloud model. For example, to avoid illegitimate node access in IoT perception layer, node authentication should be mandatory. Also, secure encryption techniques need to be enforced to ensure data confidentiality. To achieve this, lightweight encryption techniques and protocols like "ECC" supplemented with effective key exchange procedures should be implemented [73]. Since sensor nodes in IoT consume battery power, therefore energy-saving procedures such as sleep routines should be implemented to increase their working life span. In addition to this, providing optimal energy generation techniques, such as channelizing renewable power sources such as solar, air, and wind should be explored. To minimize physical damage to deployed sensor nodes, periodic monitoring checks and analysis should be done at the remote site. In order to avoid attacks such as "denial of service (DoS)", "distributed denial of service (DDoS)", and "man-in-the-middle" directed at IoT's network layer, the defense strategy would be to implement strong firewall policies and filtering rules. Also to avoid replay attacks, secure timestamp techniques need to be developed and employed. It is highly encouraged that cryptographic network protocols that ensure end-to-end encryption such as TLS/SSL and IPsec should be implemented. This would help in maintaining the integrity and authenticity of legitimate data [80].

To secure application layer against malicious script insertion attacks such as "cross-site scripting (XSS)" and malicious-worm attack, the defense strategy would be to practice efficient code writing and script detection techniques.

Table 3 Vulnerabilities in CloudIoT layers

	Attack/threat	Security issue	Potential solution
"Perception layer"	"Node capture attack"	Control the deployed sensor node by physical damage or change in its software routines	Effective physical site monitoring and detection of malicious script
	"Malicious code/data injection"	Inserting malevolent script into software routines of sensor node to change its working behavior	Secure code writing practices and code testing including malicious script filtering need to be developed
	"Replay attack"	Counterfeiting certification keys to gain trust of sensor device	Employing secure timestamp procedures in digital certification of keys
	"Side-channel attacks/cryptanalysis"	From plaintext/ciphertext, extract or gain illegal access to encryption keys	Secure and robust key generation and encryption procedures need to be employed
	"Signal interference"	Superimpose noise signal or data to corrupt and interfere with wireless transmissions	Robust and efficient noise removal techniques to for repairing original signal need to be designed
	"Sleep deprivation attack"	Forcibly shutdown sensor devices by altering their programmed sleep routines in order to keep them running when not required	Exploit wind, solar, and other forms of energy Secure code writing practices and code testing while designing sleep routines and procedures
"Network layer"	"Denial of service"	Directing massive traffic toward victim node to render it nonfunctional and non-serviceable	Designing robust firewall and packet examination routines in network routers and gateway
	"Spoofing attack"	Spoofs identity (IP or RFID spoofing) of legitimate user to gain illegal access to the system	Designing secure and robust authentication and authorization access procedures

(continued)

Table 3 (continued)

	Attack/threat	Security issue	Potential solution
	"Sinkhole attack"	To control data forwarding or routing, the victim node assets unusual or extraordinary power and processing capacity	Designing secure routing and data forwarding protocols and techniques
	"Man-in-the-middle"	The malevolent actor places itself between two victim nodes. Impersonates them and gains access to information without their knowledge	Designing secure and robust authentication and authorization access procedures. Also employing authentication and encryption certificates
	"Routing attacks"	This attack aims to create route loops and high congestion in the network	Designing secure routing and data forwarding protocols and techniques
"Application layer"	"Phishing attack"	To obtain authentication and authorization credentials including passwords by flooding spam mails and creating fake websites/forums	Employing robust spam filters in emails. Creating awareness among web application clients
	"Malicious-worm attack"	Infects and injects the sensor network with Worms, Viruses, and Trojans. Obtains or deletes confidential data	Designing robust firewall and packet examination routines for virus detection
	"Cross-site scripting"	To steal privileged and validation information including passwords by injecting network applications with malevolent scripts	Secure code writing practices and code testing including malicious script filtering need to be developed

This also includes rewriting the vulnerable code for sanitization. To protect cloud data, access policies and strict authentication protocols need to be designed and implemented. To prevent data leakage and theft, cloud data and files should be properly encrypted. Since cloud platform is distributed and pervasive in nature with multiple clients accessing its interface, a certain degree of concurrency control measures need to be implemented to avoid race conditions and data redundancy. Tracking cyber crimes directed at CloudIoT interface becomes arduous for forensic investigators as the data sources are heterogeneous and pervasive in nature. To detect and scan for any anomaly, the standard protocol would be that all operations on CloudIoT interface should be logged and stored in a secure file. The cyber forensic investigators can check this file at a later point in time so that appropriate corrective measures are taken. As cloud and IoT represent two disparate heterogeneous platforms, providing optimal security is a challenging task for security experts and thus requires robust security protocols.

10 Platforms and Services

10.1 Platforms

This section discusses about various available commercial as well as open-source platforms that underpin and support CloudIoT healthcare vision and its applications. The platforms discussed in this section are selected according to their suitability in distinct application domains and information about them has been obtained from the platform website as well as from surveying the available literature.

According to www.ionos.com, more than 50 CloudIoT platforms are available that cater diverse users including applications varying from healthcare, agriculture, engineering, manufacturing, and transportation. However, due to knowledge deficit about these platforms, users are unable to choose and exploit their full potential [15]. Most of these platforms focus on minimizing heterogeneity between the cloud and IoT by implementing a middleware between the two for processing and hoarding sensor data and also by dispensing an API toward applications [3]. The driving factors for the development of CloudIoT platforms include the need for facilitating machine-to-machine (M2M) communication which has seen an exponential rise in current times. Machina Research [4] forecasts that machine-to-machine (M2M) connections are anticipated to rise from one billion in 2010 to nearly 12 billion in 2020. Given such an unprecedented rise, cross-platform operation and reuse is starting to evolve [88]. Some of the existing platforms including services are discussed below:

KAA Project (https://www.kaaproject.org/) is a flexible open-source IoT middleware interface for designing robust and smart IoT solutions. It enables data exchange between connected things including data analytics and visualization services. It dispenses back end operations for IoT by employing SDKs that come prefabricated with current data processing solutions which include Hadoop, MongoDB, and others. Complete implementations already exist for platforms such as IoS, Android, and Raspberry Pi.

Sensor cloud (https://www.sensorcloud.com/) is a private IoT cloud platform dispensing platform as a service for data acquisition, visualization, monitoring, and analytics. Sensor cloud is a robust tool supporting easy data upload using open data API and csv uploader. It receives data from Lord Microstrain's wireless and wired sensors and provides efficient data encryption and security. The platform also provides efficient data visualization and mathematical tools including reminder alerts for data threshold values.

Etherios (https://www.etherios.com) is a pliable public cloud platform based on platform as a service model supporting device management, application messaging, and data storage. In addition to data visualization tools, the platform also provides APIs for time series data storage and analytics. It also provides real-time monitoring and management control of all connected devices using a single door interface.

Exosite (https://www.exosite.com/) is cloud-based software as a service platform dispensing machine-to-machine (M2M) connectivity and offering real-time data monitoring and analytics service to the users. The platform supports various development kits for designing IoT-based solutions. For example, Arduino, Microchip, Renesas boards are well supported on Exosite platform. The system also provides open API for further data processing and interoperability with enterprise based applications.

Arkessa (https://www.arkessa.com) facilitates management, monitoring, and control of remote devices using desktop computers and smartphones. The platform provides mobile Internet as well as data services for system integrators and enterprise users to command and operate remote devices and systems for users across geographical lines and applications. Arkessa follows platform as a service model to serve security, healthcare, energy, and transportation industries across Europe and America. This platform also provides Emport portal for viewing and monitoring machine-to-machine (M2M) connections with inbuilt assistance for troubleshooting and performance measurement analysis.

Axeda (http://www.axeda.com/) is a cloud-based middleware for management of connected things and machine-to-machine (M2M) applications. The platform offers Axeda machine cloud to convert machine data into precious knowledge, develop, and run machine-to-machine (M2M) including IoT applications and thus optimize varied business processes by machine data integration. APIs such as REST and SOAP further drive Axeda to initiate cloud to cloud communication using cellular as well as satellite medium. Tracking of assets, management including push notifications and alerts are some its proficient features.

Nimbits (http://www.nimbits.com/) offers "Platform as a Service" model to design software as well as hardware solutions that effortlessly integrate with the cloud and with each other. Nimbits server offers "REST Web Services" for data logging and access and also rule engine platform for ensuring machine-to-machine (M2M) connectivity. The server is driven by robust cloud platforms which include "Google App Engine" to the small Raspberry Pi device. It is capable of recording incoming data including value calculation based on which events like an alert or a push message could be triggered. The new values calculated based on the captured data can be archived to other channel triggering more cascading computations and alerts.

ThingWorx (http://www.thingworx.com/) provides an absolute end-to-end technology platform designed for enterprise IoT and offers quick and seamless development including deployment of smart objects. The platform provides integrated development tools that drive communication, connectivity, analysis, developing applications, and monitoring characteristics of IoT framework. These tools contain the "Composer", the "Mashup Builder", "Storage", and a "Search Engine". Its search engine also called as "SQUEAL (search, query, and analysis)" is employed for analyzing, searching, and filtering data. The tools also facilitate rapid business development and empowerment.

10.2 Services

In addition to above discussed platforms, number of services are available that facilitate data collection from connected things and archiving this data on the service providers cloud. These services typically present an API for data collection and sample applications to operate on such data. Xively (https://www.xively.com/) is one such platform owned by Google which offers product enterprises to connect and manage products including data and incorporate that data in other systems. Xively is based on platform as a service model and includes directory as well as data services, a trust service for security and web user interface. Its messaging system is based on MQTT which is publish-subscribe protocol. REST, MQTT, and WebSockets are supported by the API.

ThingSpeak (https://www.thingspeak.com/) is yet another platform with features very much similar to Xively and based on public cloud technology. ThingSpeak provides real-time data collection and transmits data privately to the cloud. This data could be examined and inspected using various toolkits (e.g., Matlab, Arduino) and a reaction could be triggered based on certain events. Using ThingSpeak, a user can create a sensor-logging app, track live location of objects and establish a novel social network of things. The platform API also allows mathematical processing on data such as calculating average, median, summation, and rounding.

Table 4 provides summarized view of some of the existing platforms/services including their advantages and limitations.

11 Challenges and Open Issues

It is quite evident that amalgamation of cloud and IoT in healthcare will add tangible benefits in our daily life; however, the integration also lays genesis to some perilous issues that demand robust solutions and need to be overlooked by security researchers [29].

Security and Privacy

As cloud and IoT are distributed and pervasive in nature, ameliorating underlying security and privacy infrastructure play a major role in its successful integration. To ensure authenticity, data integrity, and data availability, optimal measure needs to be designed so that critical data in cloud is preserved [22]. Failure to safeguard

Table 4 Summary of existing platforms

	Platform/service	URL	Advantages	Limitation
1	KAA Project	www.kaaproject.org	Applications using big data and NoSQL are supported Open-source middleware	Low number of hardware modules supported
2	Sensor cloud	www.sensorcloud.com	Efficient management of large number of sensor devices	Private cloud Issues with open-source devices
3	Etherios	www.etherios.com	Cloud service for devices including third-party software are enabled Trail usage period provided	Restrictions imposed on developers by some devices
4	Exosite	www.exosite.com	Easy system development Supports Arduino, Microchip, Renesas boards	Big data support lacking
5	Arkessa	www.arkessa.com	Suitable for enterprises	Does not have good visualization tools
6	Axeda	www.axeda.com	Robust M2M data management Supports REST and SOAP API	Hinges on third-party web services
7	Nimbits	www.nimbits.com	Easy platform for developers Supports REST API and Google app engine	Query processing occurs in real time
8	ThingWorx	www.thingworx.com	Supports design of data-intensive apps Offers SQUEAL for search, query, and analysis	Supports limited number of devices
9	Xively	www.xively.com	Direct support from Google Easy integration with devices using RESTful APIs	Lacks/less support for notifications
10	ThingSpeak	www.thingspeak.com	Public cloud access APIs for storing and analyzing data Mathematical operations supported	Less support for simultaneous connection for devices

these security principles could lead to data pilferage or exploitation of personal data. The issue becomes more complicated if data gets exposed to third-party vendors which could propagate it further for illegitimate activities. Thus, efficient security framework needs to be developed for heterogeneous device communication between IoT nodes as well as for protecting privacy on cloud platform.

Protocol support and Need for Standards

As no standard architecture for IoT is yet available, disparate protocols need to communicate and transact information with each other. Even if homogeneous sensor nodes are deployed in the network, the underlying communication protocols are still heterogeneous in nature which includes 6LOWPAN, CoAP, Zigbee, IEEE 802.15.4, etc. There is also possibility that data aggregation gateway would not support all of these protocols leading to incompatibility issues. The problem becomes more severe once these devices are integrated with the cloud platform. Thus, scientific community needs to develop standardized protocols and scalable platforms so that seamless integration of CloudIoT services is achieved.

Efficient Power Usage

The ubiquitous communication between cloud and IoT generates prodigious amount of data that drains battery of power-constrained sensor nodes. The problem becomes more severe if visual data (e.g., surveillance video) is involved. As sensor nodes are battery-powered, periodic and frequent replacement with silicon batteries is not feasible. The solution could be to exploit alternate forms of energy generation models such as wind and solar power [33]. Another efficient technique would be to program periodic sleep routines for the sensor nodes. The devices could go in a sleep mode if no observable perception-action occurs during a fixed time frame.

Delay and Limited Bandwidth

The distributed platform such as cloud presents limitless computing resources and varied services; however, utilizing these services with minimum latency and delay is not guaranteed. One of the prime components in achieving optimal performance is ensuring high bandwidth for data transmission. To minimize delay, a middleware layer known as "fog computing" is to be placed between cloud and IoT. The "fog computing" will achieve low latency for applications that are sensitive to delay [14, 22].

Quality of Service (QoS)

The "quality of service (QoS)" is the dominant parameter in governing aggregate performance of the internetwork. Given the prodigious data volumes that are being produced and interchanged in CloudIoT, maintaining QoS in services provided by the platform is of supreme importance. Also, considerable number of client requests demand efficient management by the cloud platform some which may be sensitive to delay. Thus, to avoid packet loss, employing QoS improvement techniques and prioritizing data packets seem to be a flawless solution. Thus utilizing next generation IP protocol (IPv6) which offers tangible features for ensuring QoS in the network is optimal choice for CloudIoT environment.

12 Discussion and Conclusion

The evolution and growing popularity of cloud and IoT has become the prime factor for enabling seamless healthcare applications influencing our everyday life. Amalgamation of cloud and IoT in healthcare systems is highly motivated by requirement for efficient computing infrastructures, limitless warehouse for data logging, optimal network performance, and availability. Also, "cloud" provides an efficient platform and solution to overcome several inherent issues (heterogeneity and resource constraints) faced by IoT systems. Majority of available research papers have surveyed cloud and IoT-based healthcare systems separately, focusing on architecture, underlying technology and affairs, however shortfall from detailed examination and in-depth exploration. To fill this research gap, this chapter carried a deep and profound review of the available research papers and presented a holistic vision on the CloudIoT-based healthcare integration components. The chapter presented seamless applications dispensed by CloudIoT platform and contemplated discussion on factors driving CloudIoT health integration. The chapter also presents a conceptual architectural framework for healthcare monitoring system that considers a range of aspects including data collection, transmission, and processing including cloud storage. The chapter presents a use case scenario that identifies actors and data flows responsible for transforming sensor data into real-time transmission to cloud. Also, a brief discussion on design considerations for healthcare architecture has been provided. The work in this chapter also highlighted security issues affecting IoT layered architecture including vulnerabilities inherent in the cloud. These vulnerabilities could render healthcare services nonfunctional and critical patient information can be abused by malevolent users. The chapter also presented a brief discussion on some potential mitigation measures. A summarized discussion on CloudIoT platforms is also presented that aim at solving heterogeneity issue between the cloud and things. Finally, the chapter concludes by identifying some open research issues and challenges hampering cloud and IoT-based healthcare adoption.

From the reviewed literature, it is quite apparent that additional research steps need to be taken to accomplish flawless and impeccable convergence of cloud and IoT-based healthcare applications. More work needs to be done on designing secure algorithms and encryption procedures so that only legitimate devices and nodes are authorized to access the patients sensitive data in IoT network and cloud. Also data privacy of patients in CloudIoT systems needs to be augmented so that integrity of the system is maintained. As sensor nodes have constrained power backup, the designed encryption protocols should be computationally light and consume minimal power. To conserve energy, the solution could be to exploit alternate forms of energy generation models. Another efficient technique would be to program periodic sleep routines for the sensor nodes. The devices could go in a sleep mode if no observable sensing activity occurs in a given time frame. For applications that are sensitive to delay, decentralizing cloud operations also called "fog computing" would ensure minimal latency and low transmission delays between cloud and IoT. Also to assure that QoS in data transmission is preserved, employing IPv6 characteristic attributes like Traffic class and Flow label are highly recommended.

References

1. Aazam M, Huh EN (2014) Fog computing and smart gateway based communication for cloud of things. In: 2014 international conference on future Internet of Things and cloud. IEEE, pp 464–470
2. Aazam M, Huh EN (2016) Fog computing: the cloud-IoT\IoE middleware paradigm. IEEE Potentials 35(3):40–44
3. Aazam M, Huh EN, St-Hilaire M, Lung CH, Lambadaris I (2016) Cloud of things: integration of IoT with cloud computing. In: Robots and sensor clouds. Springer, Cham, pp 77–94
4. Aazam M, Hung PP, Huh EN (2014) Smart gateway based communication for cloud of things. In: 2014 IEEE ninth international conference on intelligent sensors, sensor networks and information processing (ISSNIP). IEEE, pp 1–6
5. Abomhara M, Køien GM (2014) Security and privacy in the Internet of Things: current status and open issues. In: 2014 international conference on privacy and security in mobile systems (PRISMS). IEEE, pp 1–8
6. Aguzzi S, Bradshaw D, Canning M, Cansfield M, Carter P, Cattaneo G, Stevens R (2013) Definition of a research and innovation policy leveraging cloud computing and IoT combination. Final Report, European Commission, SMART 37:2013
7. Ahmed MU, Banaee H, Rafael-Palou X, Loutfi A (2014) Intelligent healthcare services to support health monitoring of elderly. In: International Internet of Things summit. Springer, Cham, pp 178–186
8. Ahmed MU, Björkman M, Čaušević A, Fotouhi H, Lindén M (2015) An overview on the Internet of Things for health monitoring systems. In: International Internet of Things summit. Springer, Cham, pp 429–436
9. Andrea I, Chrysostomou C, Hadjichristofi G (2015) Internet of Things: security vulnerabilities and challenges. In: 2015 IEEE symposium on computers and communication (ISCC). IEEE, pp 180–187
10. Azimi I, Rahmani AM, Liljeberg P, Tenhunen H (2017) Internet of Things for remote elderly monitoring: a study from user-centered perspective. J Ambient Intell Humaniz Comput 8(2):273–289
11. Baig MM, GholamHosseini H (2013) A remote monitoring system with early diagnosis of hypertension and hypotension. In: 2013 IEEE point-of-care healthcare technologies (PHT). IEEE, pp 34–37
12. Basanta H, Huang YP, Lee TT (2016) Intuitive IoT-based H2U healthcare system for elderly people. In: 2016 IEEE 13th international conference on networking, sensing, and control (ICNSC). IEEE, pp 1–6
13. Bisio I, Lavagetto F, Marchese M, Sciarrone A (2015) A smartphone-centric platform for remote health monitoring of heart failure. Int J Commun Syst 28(11):1753–1771
14. Bonomi F, Milito R, Zhu J, Addepalli S (2012) Fog computing and its role in the Internet of Things. In: Proceedings of the first edition of the MCC workshop on Mobile cloud computing. ACM, pp 13–16
15. Botta A, De Donato W, Persico V, Pescapé A (2016) Integration of cloud computing and Internet of Things: a survey. Futur Gener Comput Syst 56:684–700
16. Bui N, Zorzi M (2011) Health care applications: a solution based on the Internet of Things. In: Proceedings of the 4th international symposium on applied sciences in biomedical and communication technologies. ACM, p 131
17. Capkun S, Buttyán L, Hubaux JP (2003) Self-organized public-key management for mobile ad hoc networks. IEEE Trans Mob Comput 1:52–64

18. Catarinucci L, De Donno D, Mainetti L, Palano L, Patrono L, Stefanizzi ML, Tarricone L (2015) An IoT-aware architecture for smart healthcare systems. IEEE Internet Things J 2(6):515–526
19. Chen S, Xu H, Liu D, Hu B, Wang H (2014) A vision of IoT: applications, challenges, and opportunities with china perspective. IEEE Internet Things J 1(4):349–359
20. Cheng Y, Jiang C, Shi J (2016) A fall detection system based on SensorTag and Windows 10 IoT core. In: 2015 international conference on mechanical science and engineering. Atlantis Press
21. Chuang J, Maimoon L, Yu S, Zhu H, Nybroe C, Hsiao O, Chen H (2015) SilverLink: smart home health monitoring for senior care. In: ICSH. Springer, Cham, pp 3–14
22. Cook A, Robinson M, Ferrag MA, Maglaras LA, He Y, Jones K, Janicke H (2018) Internet of cloud: security and privacy issues. In: Cloud computing for optimization: foundations, applications, and challenges. Springer, Cham, pp 271–301
23. Darshan KR, Anandakumar KR (2015) A comprehensive review on usage of Internet of Things (IoT) in healthcare system. In: 2015 international conference on emerging research in electronics, computer science and technology (ICERECT).IEEE, pp 132–136
24. Darwish A, Hassanien AE, Elhoseny M, Sangaiah AK, Muhammad K (2017) The impact of the hybrid platform of Internet of Things and cloud computing on healthcare systems: Opportunities, challenges, and open problems. J Ambient Intell Humlzed Comput 1–16
25. Datta SK, Bonnet C, Gyrard A, Da Costa RPF, Boudaoud K (2015) Applying Internet of Things for personalized healthcare in smart homes. In: 2015 24th Wireless and optical communication conference (WOCC). IEEE, pp 164–169
26. De Capua C, Meduri A, Morello R (2010) A smart ECG measurement system based on web-service-oriented architecture for telemedicine applications. IEEE Trans Instrum Meas 59(10):2530–2538
27. Department of Economic & Social Affairs (2001) World population prospects: the sex and age distribution of world population, vol 2. United Nations Publications
28. Dhillon PK, Kalra S (2018) Multi-factor user authentication scheme for IoT-based healthcare services. J Reliab Intell Environ 4(3):141–160
29. Díaz M, Martín C, Rubio B (2016) State-of-the-art, challenges, and open issues in the integration of Internet of Things and cloud computing. J Netw Comput Appl 67:99–117
30. Dierckx R, Pellicori P, Cleland JGF, Clark AL (2015) Telemonitoring in heart failure: big brother watching over you. Heart Fail Rev 20(1):107–116
31. Distefano S, Merlino G, Puliafito A (2012) Enabling the cloud of things. In: 2012 sixth international conference on innovative mobile and internet services in ubiquitous computing. IEEE, pp 858–863
32. Dizdarević J, Carpio F, Jukan A, Masip-Bruin X (2019) A survey of communication protocols for Internet of Things and related challenges of fog and cloud computing integration. ACM Comput Surv (CSUR) 51(6):116
33. Evans D (2011) The Internet of Things: how the next evolution of the internet is changing everything. CISCO White Pap 1(2011):1–11
34. Fanucci L, Saponara S, Bacchillone T, Donati M, Barba P, Sánchez-Tato I, Carmona C (2012) Sensing devices and sensor signal processing for remote monitoring of vital signs in CHF patients. IEEE Trans Instrum Meas 62(3):553–569
35. Fortino G, Parisi D, Pirrone V, Di Fatta G (2014) BodyCloud: a SaaS approach for community body sensor networks. Futur Gener Comput Syst 35:62–79
36. Fox A, Griffith R, Joseph A, Katz R, Konwinski A, Lee G, Patterson D, Rabkin A, Stoica I (2009) Above the clouds: a berkeley view of cloud computing. Department of Electrical Engineering and Computer Sciences, University of California, Berkeley, Rep. UCB/EECS, 28(13), 2009
37. Gasparrini S, Cippitelli E, Spinsante S, Gambi E (2014) A depth-based fall detection system using a Kinect® sensor. Sensors 14(2):2756–2775
38. Grobauer B, Walloschek T, Stocker E (2010) Understanding cloud computing vulnerabilities. IEEE Secur Priv 9(2):50–57
39. Gubbi J, Buyya R, Marusic S, Palaniswami M (2013) Internet of Things (IoT): a vision, architectural elements, and future directions. Futur Gener Comput Syst 29(7):1645–1660

40. Gund A, Ekman I, Lindecrantz K, Sjoqvist BA, Staaf EL, Thorneskold N (2008) Design evaluation of a home-based telecare system for chronic heart failure patients. In: 2008 30th annual international conference of the IEEE engineering in medicine and biology society. IEEE, pp 5851–5854
41. Gupta P, Agrawal D, Chhabra J, Dhir PK (2016) IoT based smart healthcare kit. In: 2016 international conference on computational techniques in information and communication technologies (ICCTICT). IEEE, pp 237–242
42. Harper S (2006) Ageing societies: myths. Challenges and opportunities, 116
43. Huang SC, Chang HY, Jhu YC, Chen GY (2014) The intelligent pill box—design and implementation. In: 2014 IEEE international conference on consumer electronics-Taiwan. IEEE, pp 235–236
44. Jimenez F, Torres R (2015) Building an IoT-aware healthcare monitoring system. In: 2015 34th international conference of the chilean computer science society (SCCC). IEEE, pp 1–4
45. Jing Q, Vasilakos AV, Wan J, Lu J, Qiu D (2014) Security of the Internet of Things: perspectives and challenges. Wirel Netw 20(8):2481–2501
46. Jouini M, Rabai LBA (2019) A security framework for secure cloud computing environments. In: Cloud security: concepts, methodologies, tools, and applications. IGI Global, pp 249–263
47. Karthikeyan S, Devi KV, Valarmathi K (2015) Internet of Things: hospice appliances monitoring and control system. In: 2015 online international conference on green engineering and technologies (IC-GET). IEEE, pp 1–6
48. Khorshed MT, Ali AS, Wasimi SA (2012) A survey on gaps, threat remediation challenges and some thoughts for proactive attack detection in cloud computing. Futur Gener Comput Syst 28(6):833–851
49. Kim DH, Ghaffari R, Lu N, Rogers JA (2012) Flexible and stretchable electronics for biointegrated devices. Annu Rev Biomed Eng 14:113–128
50. Kovatsch M, Mayer S, Ostermaier B (2012) Moving application logic from the firmware to the cloud: Towards the thin server architecture for the Internet of Things. In: 2012 sixth international conference on innovative mobile and internet services in ubiquitous computing. IEEE, pp 751–756
51. Li N, Mahalik NP (2019) A big data and cloud computing specification, standards and architecture: agricultural and food informatics. Int J Inf Commun Technol 14(2):159–174
52. Li S, Da Xu L, Zhao S (2015) The Internet of Things: a survey. Inf Syst Front 17(2):243–259
53. Lin J, Yu W, Zhang N, Yang X, Zhang H, Zhao W (2017) A survey on Internet of Things: architecture, enabling technologies, security and privacy, and applications. IEEE Internet of Things J 4(5):1125–1142
54. Liu W, Zhao X, Xiao J, Wu Y (2005) Automatic vehicle classification instrument based on multiple sensor information fusion. In: Third international conference on information technology and applications (ICITA'05), vol 1, IEEE, pp 379–382
55. Mell P, Grance T (2011) The NIST definition of cloud computing
56. Mo Y, Sinopoli B (2009) Secure control against replay attacks. In: 2009 47th annual Allerton conference on communication, control, and computing (Allerton). IEEE, pp 911–918
57. Moosavi SR, Gia TN, Nigussie E, Rahmani AM, Virtanen S, Tenhunen H, Isoaho J (2016) End-to-end security scheme for mobility enabled healthcare Internet of Things. Futur Gener Comput Syst 64:108–124
58. Mutlag AA, Ghani MKA, Arunkumar NA, Mohamed MA, Mohd O (2019) Enabling technologies for fog computing in healthcare IoT systems. Futur Gener Comput Syst 90:62–78
59. Namahoot CS, Brückner M, Nuntawong C (2015) Mobile diagnosis system with emergency telecare in Thailand (MOD-SET). Procedia Comput Sci 69:86–95
60. Neagu G, Preda Ş, Stanciu A, Florian V (2017) A cloud-IoT based sensing service for health monitoring. In: 2017 E-health and bioengineering conference (EHB). IEEE, pp 53–56
61. Nossik M, Du L, McCulligh M (2019) US Patent 10/284,557
62. Olorode O, Nourani M (2014) Reducing leakage power in wearable medical devices using memory nap controller. In: 2014 IEEE dallas circuits and systems conference (DCAS). IEEE, pp 1–4

63. Parida M, Yang HC, Jheng SW, Kuo CJ (2012) Application of RFID technology for in-house drug management system. In: 2012 15th international conference on network-based information systems. IEEE, pp 577–581
64. Park C, Chou PH, Bai Y, Matthews R, Hibbs A (2006) An ultra-wearable, wireless, low power ECG monitoring system. In: 2006 IEEE biomedical circuits and systems conference. IEEE, pp 241–244
65. Parwekar P (2011) From Internet of Things towards cloud of things. In: 2011 2nd international conference on computer and communication technology (ICCCT-2011). IEEE, pp 329–333
66. Pollonini L, Rajan NO, Xu S, Madala S, Dacso CC (2012) A novel handheld device for use in remote patient monitoring of heart failure patients—design and preliminary validation on healthy subjects. J Med Syst 36(2):653–659
67. Rao BP, Saluia P, Sharma N, Mittal A, Sharma SV (2012) Cloud computing for Internet of Things & sensing based applications. In: 2012 sixth international conference on sensing technology (ICST). IEEE, pp 374–380
68. Rath M (2019) Resource provision and QoS support with added security for client side applications in cloud computing. Int J Inf Technol 11(2):357–364
69. Rohatgi D, Srivastava S, Choudhary S, Khatri A, Kalra V (2018) Smart healthcare based on Internet of Things. In: International conference on application of computing and communication technologies. Springer, Singapore, pp 300–309
70. Rolim CO, Koch FL, Westphall CB, Werner J, Fracalossi A, Salvador GS (2010) A cloud computing solution for patient's data collection in health care institutions. In: 2010 second international conference on ehealth, telemedicine, and social medicine. IEEE, pp 95–99
71. Roman R, Zhou J, Lopez J (2013) On the features and challenges of security and privacy in distributed Internet of Things. Comput Netw 57(10):2266–2279
72. Sharma R, Nah FFH, Sharma K, Katta TSSS, Pang N, Yong A (2016) Smart living for elderly: design and human-computer interaction considerations. In: International conference on human aspects of IT for the aged population. Springer, Cham, pp 112–122
73. Sicari S, Rizzardi A, Gricco LA, Coen-Porisini A (2015) Security, privacy and trust in Internet of Things: the road ahead. Comput Netw 76:146–164
74. Siekkinen M, Hiienkari M, Nurminen JK, Nieminen J (2012) How low energy is bluetooth low energy? comparative measurements with zigbee/802.15. 4. In: 2012 IEEE wireless communications and networking conference workshops (WCNCW). IEEE, pp 232–237
75. Soliman M, Abiodun T, Hamouda T, Zhou J, Lung CH (2013) Smart home: Integrating Internet of Things with web services and cloud computing. In: 2013 IEEE 5th international conference on cloud computing technology and science, vol 2. IEEE, pp 317–320
76. Son D, Lee J, Qiao S, Ghaffari R, Kim J, Lee JE, Yang S (2014) Multifunctional wearable devices for diagnosis and therapy of movement disorders. Nat Nanotechnol 9(5):397
77. Suciu G, Vulpe A, Halunga S, Fratu O, Todoran G, Suciu V (2013). Smart cities built on resilient cloud computing and secure Internet of Things. In: 2013 19th international conference on control systems and computer science. IEEE, pp 513–518
78. Suh MK, Chen CA, Woodbridge J, Tu MK, Kim JI, Nahapetian A, Sarrafzadeh M (2011) A remote patient monitoring system for congestive heart failure. J Med Syst 35(5):1165–1179
79. Suh MK, Evangelista LS, Chen V, Hong WS, Macbeth J, Nahapetian A, Figueras FJ, Sarrafzadeh M (2010) WANDA B.: weight and activity with blood pressure monitoring system for heart failure patients. In: 2010 IEEE international symposium on a world of wireless, mobile and multimedia networks (WoWMoM). IEEE, pp 1–6
80. Suo H, Wan J, Zou C, Liu J (2012) Security in the Internet of Things: a review. In: 2012 international conference on computer science and electronics engineering, vol 3. IEEE, pp 648–651
81. Tyagi S, Agarwal A, Maheshwari P (2016) A conceptual framework for IoT-based healthcare system using cloud computing. In: 2016 6th international conference-cloud system and big data engineering (Confluence). IEEE, pp 503–507
82. Ullah K, Shah MA, Zhang S (2016) Effective ways to use Internet of Things in the field of medical and smart health care. In: 2016 international conference on intelligent systems engineering (ICISE). IEEE, pp 372–379

83. Velte AT, Velte TJ, Elsenpeter RC, Elsenpeter RC (2010) Cloud computing: a practical approach. McGraw-Hill, New York, p 44
84. Wu M, Lu TJ, Ling FY, Sun J, Du HY (2010) Research on the architecture of Internet of Things. In: 2010 3rd international conference on advanced computer theory and engineering (ICACTE), vol 5. IEEE, pp V5–484
85. Xu S, Zhang Y, Jia L, Mathewson KE, Jang KI, Kim J, Bhole S (2014) Soft microfluidic assemblies of sensors, circuits, and radios for the skin. Science 344(6179):70–74
86. Yassine A, Singh S, Hossain MS, Muhammad G (2019) IoT big data analytics for smart homes with fog and cloud computing. Futur Gener Comput Syst 91:563–573
87. Yeole AS, Kalbande DR (2016) Use of Internet of Things (IoT) in healthcare: a survey. In: Proceedings of the ACM symposium on women in research 2016. ACM, pp 71–76
88. Yuriyama M, Kushida T (2010) Sensor-Cloud Infrastructure-Physical Sensor Management with Virtualized Sensors on Cloud Computing. NBiS 10:1–8
89. Zaslavsky A, Perera C, Georgakopoulos D (2013) Sensing as a service and big data. arXiv preprint arXiv:1301.0159
90. Zhao K, Ge L (2013) A survey on the Internet of Things security. In: 2013 ninth international conference on computational intelligence and security. IEEE, pp 663–667
91. Zhou J, Leppanen T, Harjula E, Ylianttila M, Ojala T, Yu C, Jin H, Yang LT (2013) Cloudthings: a common architecture for integrating the Internet of Things with cloud computing. In: Proceedings of the 2013 IEEE 17th international conference on computer supported cooperative work in design (CSCWD). IEEE, pp 651–657
92. Zikopoulos P, Eaton C (2011) Understanding big data: analytics for enterprise class hadoop and streaming data. McGraw-Hill Osborne Media

Junaid Latief Shah is an Assistant Professor in the Department of Information Technology, Sri Pratap College, Cluster University Srinagar, India. He completed his Bachelor's in Computer Science and Master's in Computer Science from University of Kashmir. He also obtained his Ph.D. in the field of Next Generation Networks and IPv6 from University of Kashmir. Besides this, he has qualified UGC National Eligibility Test (NET) and State Eligibility Test (SET) in Computer Science and Applications. His research areas include computer networks and security, web security, and testing.

Heena Farooq Bhat is a Research Scholar in the Department of Computer Science, University of Kashmir, India. She completed her Bachelor's in Computer Science and Master's in Computer Science from University of Kashmir. She also obtained her M.Phil. and Ph.D. in the field of Data Mining and Genome Analysis from University of Kashmir. Besides this, she has qualified UGC National Eligibility Test (NET) in Computer Science and Applications. Her research areas include artificial intelligence, genome analysis, and data mining.

Impact of IoT on the Healthcare Producers: Epitomizing Pharmaceutical Drug Discovery Process

Sudipendra Nath Roy and Tuhin Sengupta

Abstract Internet of things (IoT) emerged as a promising technology in the last decade and predicted to be ascendant in the next. Its application in the producer side of the healthcare industry is still in the nascent stage but expected to increase manifold in the near future. The purpose of this chapter is twofold; first, illuminate on the IoT applications on the pharmaceutical manufacturing and supply chain practices with real examples, and second elaborate the wide avenue of the opportunity of IoT it has in the drug discovery. Where most of the previous works argue the prospect of IoT in the conceptual or theoretical manner, we, however, intend to show the utility of automatic information processing in the context of computational drug design, which is an integral part of the drug discovery process. We integrate quantitative structure relationships with activity (QSAR), property (QSPR), and toxicity (QSTR) by utilizing an optimization technique to come up with a combined decision model. Numerical analysis has been performed with the developed optimization model considering three different cases using a simple chemical structure to test the model. Results suggest that the developed mathematical model can successfully be able to integrate QSAR, QSPR, and QSTR parameters which in terms of aid in automatic information and data capturing and lessen human efforts. This automatization can help in generating "optimal" drug candidates by considering all necessary facets. The present chapter also discusses other aspects of the healthcare producers where IoT can be proven beneficial in the near future.

Keywords IoT in pharmaceuticals · AIDC · Optimization · Computational drug design · MS-excel solver

---

S. N. Roy
Management Science, Ivey Business School, Western University, London, Canada
e-mail: sroy@ivey.ca

T. Sengupta (✉)
Department of Information Technology and Operations Management, Goa Institute of Management, Goa, India
e-mail: tuhin@gim.ac.in

Indian Institute of Management Indore, Prabandh Shikhar, Rau - Pithampur Road, Indore 453556, Madhya Pradesh, India

P. Rai et al. (eds.), *Internet of Things Use Cases for the Healthcare Industry*,
https://doi.org/10.1007/978-3-030-37526-3_6

1 IoT in the Producer Side of Health Care: Introduction

Healthcare industry functions through three main stakeholders. We can refer to them as "pillars" of the healthcare sector. These "pillars" are payers, providers, and producers [1]. Payers are the segment who are directly or indirectly responsible for the payment for the cost incurred while availing a healthcare service or affording a healthcare product. Payers can be insurance companies, public or governmental bodies, or patients in case of out of pocket expenditures. Where payers are responsible to "pay" the fee of the healthcare services or products, providers and producers are responsible for delivering them, respectively. Providers are the organizations that deliver healthcare services to the patients. Providers can vary from a small 20-bed small health clinic to an 800-bed multispecialty hospital. When producers, on the other hand, not standing on the front end of health service delivery but indispensable part of healthcare services as without required supply of products, healthcare personnel (HCP) will not be able to serve the patients in the hour of the need. Producers consist of mainly pharmaceutical, diagnostics, and medical device manufacturers.

"Internet of things" (IoT) is a much recent but popular construct in today's media and management consulting firm reports. While this book addresses IoT from multiple angles, this chapter explores the applicability of IoT concepts in the healthcare producer context, specifically in the case of the pharmaceutical industry. At the early stages of adoption of IoT in the healthcare industry, the main application was limited to the patient-centric mobility devices or wearables. Today, however, it extends to real-time patient monitoring, patient compliance or medication adherence, and HCP reporting. But practitioners still believe that the application of IoT is still in the nascent stage as a technology in the healthcare sector. Healthcare producers especially pharmaceutical companies can leverage the benefits of IoT to a great extent in the upcoming years [2].

Pharmaceutical companies retain a high-profit margin and thus has a low incentive to change. However, the situation is changing rapidly due to competition and the advent of personalized medicines. In the second case, companies need to produce a small batch of medicine which has a much low economy of scale. Currently, there is a media report suggesting that due to a $3500 broken vacuum pump, an American Pharma company lost products worth $20 million and to cater such unforeseen events in the future, the firm decided to install IoT sensors to its vacuum pumps [3]. Such an application is a classic example of how IoT can benefit pharmaceutical production environment by predicting failures way ahead. Apotex, a Canadian Pharmaceutical manufacturer, utilizes IoT-based technology to improve its solid dosage form manufacturing plant which resulted in increased productivity and improving bottom lines. Manufacturing plant floor control automation has been achieved for the Apotex due to real-time visibility of the pharmaceutical manufacturing automation and process flow tracking [4]. IoT has also benefitting pharmaceutical supply chain practices to a great extent. Drug counterfeiting is one of the main concerns for the pharmaceutical firms and to a major point for the integrity of the pharmaceutical supply chain. UK-based Eurosoft Systems Ltd. (ESL) has developed SMARTpack, an IoT-enabled product which aid to stop counterfeit of medicines by ensuring smart packaging and tracking [5].

A diverse range of IoT applications thus has the potential to alter the current healthcare system to a more accessible, quality-driven healthcare system, although proponents of the iron triangle of health care [6] can argue that this accessibility and quality probably comes with their competing issue: cost, which is the cost of the technology. We, however, need to understand that the implementation of the IoT-based mechanisms not only change the pharmaceutical manufacturing operations or supply chains but also has a much greater impact on the drug discovery process. IoT's capability to enhance R&D activities and clinical development of drug molecules is mostly unexplored and holds the potential to save financial resources to a good extent in the near future.

2 Drug Discovery Process: Current Scenario

The traditional or de novo drug discovery is a costly and time-consuming process that often contributes to the exorbitant price of a newly patented drug molecule. De novo drug discovery process contains several steps: drug target identification, screening and discovery of the molecule, optimization of the lead molecule which has the best potential to become a successful drug, testing for its in vivo properties (absorption–distribution–metabolism–excretion/ADME), preclinical and clinical trial process, and finally regulatory process. It takes 10–17 year to develop a successful drug [7], and millions of dollars were spent on the process. From the first step to final drug development, probability success is only 10% [8].

NextGen cloud-based architecture is an example that aims to reduce the cost of drug discovery by utilizing IoT concepts [2]. It intends to reduce the human effort in the process. It might seem confusing how to find a suitable drug candidate or "lead molecule" after initial screening. Here, we propose an optimization model that can reduce human effort by the help of automatic identification and data capturing (AIDC) concepts for identifying new chemical entities (NCE). Automatic identification of NCE by optimization of chemical structures for different chemical groups can aid us to automate the drug design process and opens new avenues of opportunity for finding NCE that can be prospective "lead" or drug molecules.

3 An Optimization Model for Identification of NCE

Identification of NCE or potential drug molecules can be done by various screening techniques; among them, computational drug design is a popular method of NCE screening. We try to develop an optimization model that can be integrated into the computational drug design process for automatic data serialization for identifying NCE.

3.1 Computational Drug Design for NCE Identification

Computational drug design is a three-dimensional puzzle where the drug or the "chemical molecule with the medicinal property" has been computationally designed by keeping the binding site of the biological target of the human body in mind. The drug, only with the association of the targeted biomolecule, can produce a desired therapeutic effect that alleviates a disease present in the patient body [9]. This chemical entity or drug is termed as "ligand" by the scientists. In order to come up with a successful drug, it is essential to decipher the functional groups and elements attaching to the core chemical structure of the drug [10]. The advent of computers and the use of quantitative techniques helped us to solve the enigma of finding a suitable chemical structure with all attached functional groups within a practically feasible time span [11, 12].

Quantitative structure–activity relationship (QSAR) models are quite popular and widely used techniques in the computational drug design domain. QSAR is contingent upon the assumption that the ligand molecule has several positions around its core chemical structure, and the presence of different elements/functional groups in those positions affects the activity of the ligand. With proper quantitative exercise with functional groups, researchers can suggest if a ligand can turn out to be a successful drug. However, the rationale behind a successful drug is mainly determined as the biological activity exhibited by a structure. The core structure has a certain number of elements/groups in certain positions, i.e., "most suitable" elements in "most suitable" positions of the ligand. The outcomes are represented as a numerical value, and multivariate modeling techniques are used to come up with a QSAR model for that "potential" drug molecule [13, 14]. While a desired biological or therapeutic activity is a necessary criterion to be considered as a potential drug molecule, it has to be seen that the newly designed molecule should have possessed certain necessary physicochemical properties when entering inside a human body to turn out to be a good candidate [15]. Instead of the wide popularity of QSAR models [16], consideration of physicochemical properties that affects absorption in the body, distribution throughout the body, metabolism, and excretion of the drug (ADME properties) eventually attracts the attention of the researchers. This leads to a quantitative structure–property relationship (QSPR) studies that essentially capture the relation between molecular structure and physicochemical or ADME properties of the drug molecule [17, 18]. However, even ensuring optimal biological activity and calibrated physicochemical properties does not help us to ensure the feasibility of a "good drug." As drug discovery is a costly process, initial screening has to consider one of the most important parameters of any chemical entity, i.e., toxicity produced by the chemical molecule inside the human body. Researchers conducted quantitative structure–toxicity relationship (QSTR) studies to determine how the combination of functional groups/elements in a chemical structure can determine its toxicity potential in the environment [19, 20] and inside the human body [21]. QSTR has been also adopted by other researchers to determine the toxicity profile of any new chemical molecule even if it is not a drug and just a solvent [22] of novel material [23] to bolster greener practices of the planet.

Initially, researchers tried to use QSPR as a validation of QSAR model before finalizing the multilinear regression model [24] and some researchers conducted QSTR studies in parallel with the QSAR studies. Later, many researchers advocated the need for a model that considers activity, property, and toxicity together [25]. A correct form of model that ensures optimal biological/therapeutic activity, ensures desired physicochemical or ADME properties, and confirms toxicity to be under the specified level is absent in the current literature. This motivated us to develop a model ensuring all the three main parameters of a suitable drug candidate using mathematical optimization technique. The objective of this chapter is to consider QSAR, QSPR, and QSTR parameters and come up with a combined quantitative structure relationship model for a chemical structure.

4 The Mathematical Model

We present the summarized table of notations below:

Notation	Description
n	Number of elements/groups to be tested for the structure
N	Number of positions in the structure
X_{Ni}	Choice of ith element in the Nth position (Decision Variables)
A	Therapeutic property of the drug (Parameter)
B	Toxicity property of the drug (Parameter)
M	Physicochemical/ADME property of the drug (Parameter)
α	Lower permissible bound for therapeutic property (Parameter)
β	Upper permissible bound for toxicity property (Parameter)
NU	The net utility of the drug

The mathematical problem shown below is the mathematical model to determine the optimal mix of elements in the chemical structure subject to the therapeutic and toxicity parameter of the drug. We also incorporate the physicochemical/ADME property into our mathematical model. ADME is an acronym in pharmacology for "absorption, distribution, metabolism, and excretion," thereby explaining the kinetics and pharmacological traits of the compound as a drug. The ADME property is represented by M, and the values range from 0 and 1 to capture the proportion of ADME property in the given chemical composition. We assume that there are N positions in the structure where n elements can be placed as a chemical bond to enhance the net utility of the drug. It is therefore important to incorporate a model which simultaneously decides the positions of n elements in N positions of the chemical structure. Additionally, the model incorporates that a particular element can sit in different positions of the structure to enhance the net utility. To enhance the relevance of the model, the lower and upper bounds of therapeutic and toxicity property, respectively, have been incorporated. In addition, the model ensures that no element is being considered where the utility, i.e., the difference between therapeutic and toxicity, is always positive. Non-negativity constraints have been ensured as per the practical relevance. The given model is a binary integer programming model, where the decision is to fix the choice of n elements in N positions, given that the individual properties (parameters) in each combination are known to the user.

$$\textbf{Maximize } NU_{X_{ij}} = \sum_{i=1}^{N} \sum_{j=1}^{n} X_{ij} M_{ij} (A_{ij} - B_{ij})$$

subject to

$$A_{ij} \geq \alpha,$$

$$B_{ij} \leq \beta$$

$$A_{ij} - B_{ij} \geq 0$$

$$\sum_{i=1}^{n} X_{Ni} = 1$$

$$\alpha, \beta, A_{ij}, B_{ij}, M_{ij}, n, N, X_{ij} \geq 0; X_{ij} = \textbf{Binary}$$

5 Numerical Validation of the Model

We provide empirical validation of our model by testing the same with different parametric values. To ensure the flexibility of the model, we tested the same in e different cases. **Case 1** represents a balanced problem where there are six positions in the chemical structure ($N = 6$) and there are six elements which need to be tested for each position ($n = 6$). The results, shown in Table 1, ensure that the model works N x n cases where both N is equal to n. In each of the models, we assumed $\alpha \geq 20$ and $\beta \leq 40$. However, the structural model holds for different values of α and β. Values of different parameters have been taken in such a fashion where there are elements with both high and low ADMEs, therapeutic and toxicity property in order to test the model in different scenarios. A careful examination reveals that the designated second element is favorable for position 6 and substantiated the earlier claim that

Table 1 Excel solver optimal solutions for $N = 6$ and $n = 6$

Net Utility = (A-B)*M*X					
0	0	0	0	0	11.25
M11	**M12**	**M13**	**M14**	**M15**	**M16**
0.4	0.45	0.39	0.59	0.55	0.75
A11	**A12**	**A13**	**A14**	**A15**	**A16**
24	32	20	35	29	42
B11	**B12**	**B13**	**B14**	**B15**	**B16**
31	21	12	22	20	27
X11	**X12**	**X13**	**X14**	**X15**	**X16**
0	0	0	0	0	1
POSITION 1					

Net Utility = (A-B)*M*X					
0	0	6.8	0	0	0
M21	**M22**	**M23**	**M24**	**M25**	**M26**
0.6	0.43	0.4	0.65	0.72	0.49
A21	**A22**	**A23**	**A24**	**A25**	**A26**
35	26	35	27	29	32
B21	**B22**	**B23**	**B24**	**B25**	**B26**
30	40	18	26	21	24
X21	**X22**	**X23**	**X24**	**X25**	**X26**
0	0	1	0	0	0
POSITION 2					

Net Utility = (A-B)*M*X					
6.75	0	0	0	0	0
M31	**M32**	**M33**	**M34**	**M35**	**M36**
0.75	0.56	0.52	0.68	0.32	0.41
A31	**A32**	**A33**	**A34**	**A35**	**A36**
27	34	30	28	30	21
B31	**B32**	**B33**	**B34**	**B35**	**B36**
18	31	19	25	20	30
X31	**X32**	**X33**	**X34**	**X35**	**X36**
1	0	0	0	0	0
POSITION 3					

(continued)

Table 1 (continued)

Net Utility = (A-B)*M*X					
0	8	0	0	0	0
M41	**M42**	**M43**	**M44**	**M45**	**M46**
0.52	0.5	0.47	0.65	0.34	0.7
A41	**A42**	**A43**	**A44**	**A45**	**A46**
25	28	21	32	36	28
B41	**B42**	**B43**	**B44**	**B45**	**B46**
14	12	19	26	21	20
X41	**X42**	**X43**	**X44**	**X45**	**X46**
0	1	0	0	0	0
POSITION 4					

Net Utility = (A-B)*M*X					
0	0	11.96	0	0	0
M51	**M52**	**M53**	**M54**	**M55**	**M56**
0.35	0.72	0.46	0.67	0.61	0.57
A51	**A52**	**A53**	**A54**	**A55**	**A56**
38	34	39	21	19	26
B51	**B52**	**B53**	**B54**	**B55**	**B56**
20	29	13	30	9	13
X51	**X52**	**X53**	**X54**	**X55**	**X56**
0	0	1	0	0	0
POSITION 5					

Net Utility = (A-B)*M*X					
0	7.28	0	0	0	0
M61	**M62**	**M63**	**M64**	**M65**	**M66**
0.45	0.52	0.39	0.67	0.8	0.48
A61	**A62**	**A63**	**A64**	**A65**	**A66**
35	30	26	21	38	28
B61	**B62**	**B63**	**B64**	**B65**	**B66**
26	16	20	11	35	21
X61	**X62**	**X63**	**X64**	**X65**	**X66**
0	1	0	0	0	0
POSITION 6					

the same element can be bonded at different positions to improve the net utility. The same logic is applicable for the third element which sits on both positions 2 and 5.

Case 2 represents a scenario where the number of elements is less than the vacant positions in the structure. We present the results in Table 2. Here, we purposefully eliminated element 6 from the previous case to observe the changes in the structure as element 6 was the optimal choice for position 1 in the previous case. We observe that the revised optimal solution suggests that element 4 is most suitable for position 1 given the absence of element 6. A different perspective can be brought in with regard to the elimination strategies of the elements. If we start decreasing the gap between therapeutic and toxicity parameter bounds (α and β), automatically desirable elements will be removed from the model and revised optimal solutions will start appearing.

Similar results are shown for **Case 3** in Table 3 where an additional element has been introduced from Case 1 with relatively higher ADME structure. We observe that due to high ADME parameter values, the newly inserted element is the optimal choice for positions 1, 2, 3, and 4, respectively, indicating the relevance of chemical structure with high ADME quotient.

It takes a huge amount of financial resources and scientific efforts to come up with a potential drug candidate. As an optimal therapeutic activity, the correct set of physicochemical properties or ADME properties and low toxicity profile are the characteristics of a drug molecule that cannot be compromised under any circumstances; a drug design study focused only on the QSAR, QSPR, or QSTR model, is likely to generate huge amount of drug candidates that can turn out to be erroneous, and is the synthesis and testing phase. Utilizing this mathematical model ensures "best" choice drug candidate and most preferable element/functional group choice for each position in the chemical structure. This reduces the chances of occurrences of false positive drug candidates.

This study although explained each possible scenario or cases hypothetically is consistent with the literature which suggests that we need to maintain one structure for testing. As a proper validation of a known core chemical structure, studies on QSAR, QSPR, and QSTR have to be completed under the same "testing" condition. This is to test how this optimization model helps us to come up with a suitable new chemical entity with a new incoming chemical group. We took simplistic aromatic ring, i.e., benzene where entry of the new element is restricted for six positions of the carbon and numerical analysis is done for cases where five, six, and seven new elements entered into the structure. This shows that this model is capable to handle number if new entrant groups are less, equal, and more than the available position.

For the readers of the chapter, we provide a separate tutorial section at the end of the chapter as appendices so that one can cross-verify their own optimization model with the current one in a step-by-step manner.

Table 2 Excel solver optimal solutions for $N = 6$ and $n = 5$

Net Utility = (A-B)*M*X				
0	0	0	7.67	0
M11	**M12**	**M13**	**M14**	**M15**
0.4	0.45	0.39	0.59	0.55
A11	**A12**	**A13**	**A14**	**A15**
24	32	20	35	29
B11	**B12**	**B13**	**B14**	**B15**
31	21	12	22	20
X11	**X12**	**X13**	**X14**	**X15**
0	0	0	1	0
POSITION 1				

Net Utility = (A-B)*M*X				
0	0	6.8	0	0
M21	**M22**	**M23**	**M24**	**M25**
0.6	0.43	0.4	0.65	0.72
A21	**A22**	**A23**	**A24**	**A25**
35	26	35	27	29
B21	**B22**	**B23**	**B24**	**B25**
30	40	18	26	21
X21	**X22**	**X23**	**X24**	**X25**
0	0	1	0	0
POSITION 2				

Net Utility = (A-B)*M*X				
6.75	0	0	0	0
M31	**M32**	**M33**	**M34**	**M35**
0.75	0.56	0.52	0.68	0.32
A31	**A32**	**A33**	**A34**	**A35**
27	34	30	28	30
B31	**B32**	**B33**	**B34**	**B35**
18	31	19	25	20
X31	**X32**	**X33**	**X34**	**X35**
1	0	0	0	0
POSITION 3				

(continued)

Table 2 (continued)

Net Utility = (A-B)*M*X				
0	8	0	0	0
M41	**M42**	**M43**	**M44**	**M45**
0.52	0.5	0.47	0.65	0.34
A41	**A42**	**A43**	**A44**	**A45**
25	28	21	32	36
B41	**B42**	**B43**	**B44**	**B45**
14	12	19	26	21
X41	**X42**	**X43**	**X44**	**X45**
0	1	0	0	0
POSITION 4				

Net Utility = (A-B)*M*X				
0	0	11.96	0	0
M51	**M52**	**M53**	**M54**	**M55**
0.35	0.72	0.46	0.67	0.61
A51	**A52**	**A53**	**A54**	**A55**
38	34	39	21	19
B51	**B52**	**B53**	**B54**	**B55**
20	29	13	30	9
X51	**X52**	**X53**	**X54**	**X55**
0	0	1	0	0
POSITION 5				

Net Utility = (A-B)*M*X				
0	7.28	0	0	0
M61	**M62**	**M63**	**M64**	**M65**
0.45	0.52	0.39	0.67	0.8
A61	**A62**	**A63**	**A64**	**A65**
35	30	26	21	38
B61	**B62**	**B63**	**B64**	**B65**
26	16	20	11	35
X61	**X62**	**X63**	**X64**	**X65**
0	1	0	0	0
POSITION 6				

Table 3 Excel solver optimal solutions for $N = 6$ and $n = 7$

Net Utility = (A-B)*M*X						
0	0	0	0	0	16.4	0
M11	**M12**	**M13**	**M14**	**M15**	**M1New**	**M16**
0.4	0.45	0.39	0.59	0.55	0.82	0.75
A11	**A12**	**A13**	**A14**	**A15**	**A1New**	**A16**
24	32	20	35	29	52	42
B11	**B12**	**B13**	**B14**	**B15**	**B1New**	**B16**
31	21	12	22	20	32	27
X11	**X12**	**X13**	**X14**	**X15**	**X1New**	**X16**
0	0	0	0	0	1	0
POSITION 1						
Net Utility = (A-B)*M*X						
0	0	0	0	0	12.48	0
M21	**M22**	**M23**	**M24**	**M25**	**M2New**	**M26**
0.6	0.43	0.4	0.65	0.72	0.78	0.49
A21	**A22**	**A23**	**A24**	**A25**	**A2New**	**A26**
35	26	35	27	29	42	32
B21	**B22**	**B23**	**B24**	**B25**	**B2New**	**B26**
30	40	18	26	21	26	24
X21	**X22**	**X23**	**X24**	**X25**	**X2New**	**X26**
0	0	0	0	0	1	0
POSITION 2						
Net Utility = (A-B)*M*X						
0	0	0	0	0	14.4	0
M31	**M32**	**M33**	**M34**	**M35**	**M3New**	**M36**
0.75	0.56	0.52	0.68	0.32	0.8	0.41
A31	**A32**	**A33**	**A34**	**A35**	**A3New**	**A36**
27	34	30	28	30	39	21
B31	**B32**	**B33**	**B34**	**B35**	**B3New**	**B36**
18	31	19	25	20	21	30
X31	**X32**	**X33**	**X34**	**X35**	**X3New**	**X36**
0	0	0	0	0	1	0
POSITION 3						

(continued)

Table 3 (continued)

Net Utility = (A-B)*M*X						
0	0	0	0	0	12.07	0
M41	**M42**	**M43**	**M44**	**M45**	**M4New**	**M46**
0.52	0.5	0.47	0.65	0.34	0.71	0.7
A41	**A42**	**A43**	**A44**	**A45**	**A4New**	**A46**
25	28	21	32	36	35	28
B41	**B42**	**B43**	**B44**	**B45**	**B4New**	**B46**
14	12	19	26	21	18	20
X41	**X42**	**X43**	**X44**	**X45**	**X4New**	**X46**
0	0	0	0	0	1	0
POSITION 4						

Net Utility = (A-B)*M*X						
0	0	11.96	0	0	0	0
M51	**M52**	**M53**	**M54**	**M55**	**M5New**	**M56**
0.35	0.72	0.46	0.67	0.61	0.84	0.57
A51	**A52**	**A53**	**A54**	**A55**	**A5New**	**A56**
38	34	39	21	19	40	26
B51	**B52**	**B53**	**B54**	**B55**	**B5New**	**B56**
20	29	13	30	9	27	13
X51	**X52**	**X53**	**X54**	**X55**	**X5New**	**X56**
0	0	1	0	0	0	0
POSITION 5						

Net Utility = (A-B)*M*X						
0	7.28	0	0	0	0	0
M61	**M62**	**M63**	**M64**	**M65**	**M6New**	**M66**
0.45	0.52	0.39	0.67	0.8	0.61	0.48
A61	**A62**	**A63**	**A64**	**A65**	**A6New**	**A66**
35	30	26	21	38	38	28
B61	**B62**	**B63**	**B64**	**B65**	**B6New**	**B66**
26	16	20	11	35	30	21
X61	**X62**	**X63**	**X64**	**X65**	**X6New**	**X66**
0	1	0	0	0	0	0
POSITION 6						

6 Discussion on the Scope of Optimization in Automatic NCE Identification

The previous section of the chapter contributes to the application of the mathematical optimization technique in the domain of computational chemistry. Till now, the computational design of drugs mainly utilizes statistical techniques like regression to come up with a successful model. However, in this study, we demonstrate why a regression model considering only QSAR or QSPR or QSTR parameters is not a good model to proceed with chemical experimentation. Rather, using the optimization technique, we can come with a more accurate and theoretically correct model. Numerical analysis of a simple six-carbon core structure shows the utility of the model in realistic scenarios with a different number of entrant groups in the core structure. This study contributes to the novel application of optimization in a completely new domain which has a lot of opportunities to explore further by future researchers.

Since validation with the real-life experimental data for computationally developed QSAR models is an integral part for scientific robustness [26, 27] which is absent in this chapter, a practical example for the validation is the main limitation and a potential future direction for this study. Future academicians may opt to "validate" this model with different core chemical structures and can come up with the findings that for what type of structure relationships this mathematical model holds correct and illuminate on the limitation of the model with the experimental data.

Scope of optimization in automated NCE identification is immense as it can aid to reduced human effort, effective discovery process handling, and the reduced timeline for the development of the new drug molecule.

7 IoT: The Road Ahead for Healthcare Producers

It is clear that standing in the era of Industry 4.0, the utility of IoT technologies will increase exponentially over the coming decade as IoT can both contribute to cost-cutting and increased productivity in the context of healthcare producers [5].

The following are the avenues of implementation of IoT-based technologies for a healthcare producer firm:

- Application of radio-frequency identification (RFID) technologies may aid us to real-time monitoring of the medicines that drastically reduce drug counterfeiting, managing quality inventory, and improving production planning and distribution mechanism by using itemized data obtained from the sensor.
- Item-wise automatic traceability will be the advantage for the pharmaceutical supply chain managers while making any decision. IoT helps us to develop this context-aware RFID-based drug-tracing mechanism [28, 29].
- IoT-based technologies can help us to identify if any combination of medicines has any interactions or if the patient condition (e.g., pregnancy, liver, or renal disease) is not suitable for any medicines to be prescribed and delivered accordingly. Item-wise medicine data aid the prescription for any patients [30, 31].

- Identification of medicine interaction reduces malaise in patients due to the avoidance of all medicine combination that has an interaction. This improves patient compliance with medicine [31]. Also, IoT technologies are implemented to deliver medicines in an intelligent box (iMedBox), which, like a personal pharmacist, aid a patient for the dose and medicines [32]. IoT-based wearables have immense potential for delivering patient-centric care as well [33].
- Real-time diagnostics with the help of IoT technologies have been explored by the Sysmex, a global leader in the diagnostics services [4].

Where it is clear that IoT technologies have immense prospect to emerge as a dominant adoption concept in the upcoming years, it also has limitations. First, the security of itemized data for the pharmaceutical supply chain must be protected data security practices; otherwise, it can be traced by the illegal people/organization who might be interested in some specific chemical item to produce illegal substances such as narcotic substances. Second, the advent of IoT-based manufacturing may further automate the pharmaceutical manufacturing process which might lead to unemployment of semiskilled or skilled workers. Social impact of the same must be kept in mind before implementing the IoT-based automation practices.

Despite the limitation, it is evident that IoT-based technologies will reduce cost, improve productivity, and generate new avenues of employment in the future.

8 Conclusion

This chapter is intended to emphasize the application of IoT in the healthcare producer side. First, it introduces the IoT applications in pharmaceutical manufacturing and supply chain management with real-life contexts. Next, it describes how the introduction of IoT-based technologies has the promise to revolutionize the pharmaceutical drug development procedure and reduce the involvement human efforts, and thus significantly bolster efficient discovery of designed drug candidate within a lesser time span. However, in order to achieve profuse usage of IoT, we must be able to conceptualize the aspects of the drug discovery where IoT can be utilized. Computational drug design seemed to be a relevant context where automatic identification and data capturing principles can be helpful. We deduce a simplistic linear mathematical optimization model that will integrate the principles of current computational drug design concepts such as QSAR and QSPR and can be tested through a simplistic chemical structure to verify the prowess of suggested mathematical model. Finally, the chapter discussed the utility of such models to build a cost-effective and the potential IoT for the healthcare producers. The chapter concludes with the current state of developments with relevant references and challenges such as security of data generated by RFID-based itemization in a pharmaceutical firm.

In a nutshell, the chapter elaborates the impact that IoT can bring to the producer side of the healthcare industry, point out the present state of developments, and provide a mathematical model with numerical validation to bolster the argument that use of IoT in the pharmaceutical drug discovery process is beneficial. Then, it explains the current challenges and future avenues of IoT on the producer side.

Appendix: Tutorial for Building Optimization Model in Excel Solver

We have provided a step-by-step procedure to prepare the excel solver input–output analysis for solving the linear optimization model. After each step, readers are advised to check their formulated model in the excel file with the figures provided for the proper reproducibility. However, it is a better approach to build own model first and then cross-verify with the tutorial figures for a complete understanding.

STEP 1: Writing the decision variable and parameters row-wise so as to ensure that multiplication and addition between variables and parameters turn out to be easy when we formulate the objective function. For all the six positions in the structure, we prepare the excel for ADME property, therapeutic value, toxicity value, and the decision variable line, i.e., choice of ith element in the Nth position. We then provide the value for the parameters and set the value of the cells under decision variables to zero. Figure 1 is the screenshot for further understanding.

STEP 2: Next, we prepare and formulate the objective function with the help of STEP 1 where we prepared the entire input matrix of decision variables and parameters. Therefore, we first prepare the multiplicative operations, i.e., ADME Property * (Therapeutic Value – Toxicity Value) * Decision Variable. We then add all such cells for each of the cells prepared from the input matrix. Please refer Fig. 2a, b for further clarity in this regard.

STEP 3: Now we prepare the constraints in the excel sheet. The first constraint is to ensure that all the values as entered in STEP 2 are greater than or equal to zero. In the absence of this constraint, the excel solver may assume negative values for a particular cell. The next set of constraints (one constraint for each position) is to ensure that only one element is fixed to a position. We show the formula for each constraint in separate screenshots as shown in Fig. 3a–g for the purpose of clarity to the students.

STEP 4: Next we prepare the optimization algorithm by initiating the solver function in excel. Students should first go to the "Data" tab and at the right-hand most corners, EXCEL SOLVER will be present. Students are advised to first click the button. A pop-up screen will appear. Students will just need to select the (A) objective function, (B) maximization or minimization option, (C) select the decision variables, and (D) select the constraints. Please note that in addition to the constraints explained in STEP 3, we have also incorporated the binary constraint for the decision variable. Then, we have to click the options button and then click "Assume Non-Negative" and "Assume Linear Model" to ensure that the optimization model is a linear programming problem and all the decision variables are non-negative. Then, we click solve to get our answer. Refer Fig. 4a, b for further understanding.

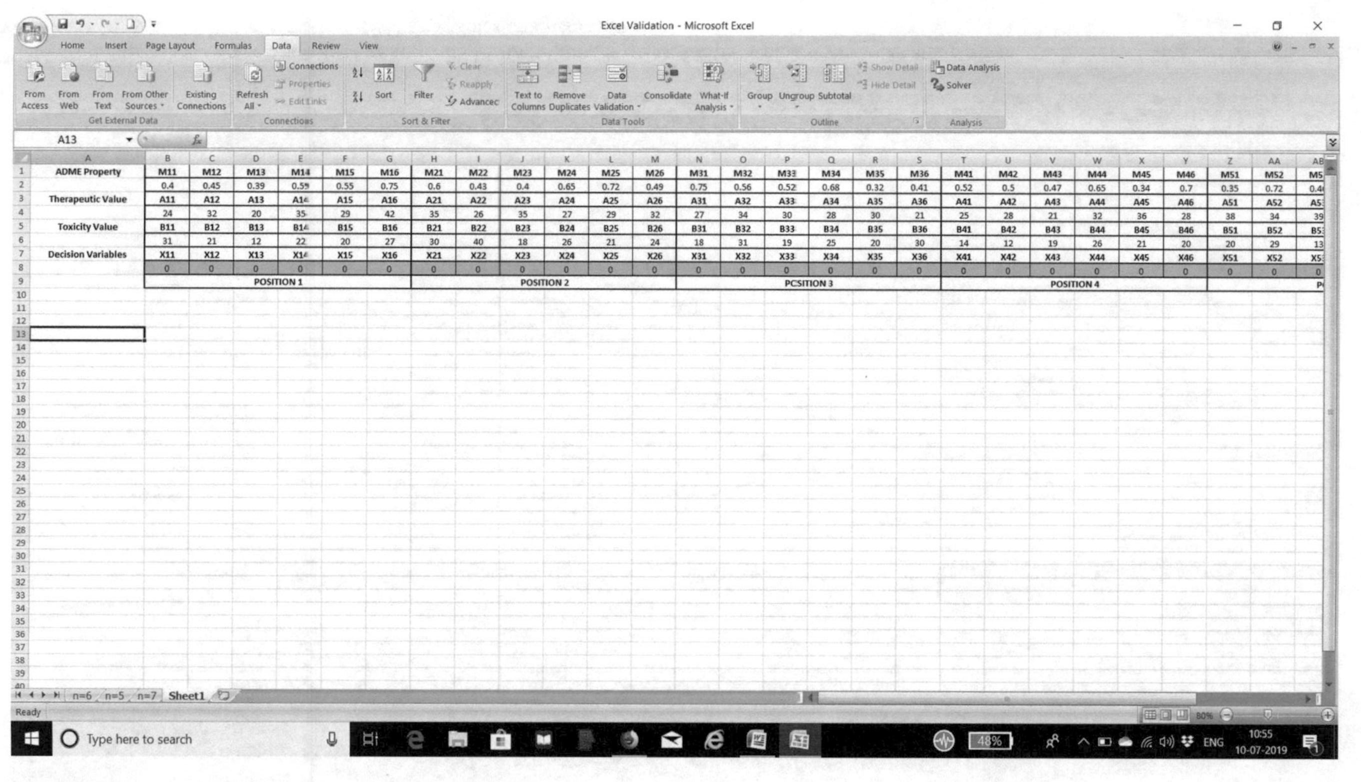

	B	C	D	E	F	G	H	I	J	K	L	M	N	O	P	Q	R	S	T	U	V	W	X	Y	Z	AA	AB
ADME Property	M11	M12	M13	M14	M15	M16	M21	M22	M23	M24	M25	M26	M31	M32	M33	M34	M35	M36	M41	M42	M43	M44	M45	M46	M51	M52	M5
	0.4	0.45	0.39	0.59	0.55	0.75	0.6	0.43	0.4	0.65	0.72	0.49	0.75	0.56	0.52	0.68	0.32	0.41	0.52	0.5	0.47	0.65	0.34	0.7	0.35	0.72	0.4
Therapeutic Value	A11	A12	A13	A14	A15	A16	A21	A22	A23	A24	A25	A26	A31	A32	A33	A34	A35	A36	A41	A42	A43	A44	A45	A46	A51	A52	A5
	24	32	20	35	29	42	35	26	35	27	29	32	27	34	30	28	30	21	25	28	21	32	36	28	38	34	39
Toxicity Value	B11	B12	B13	B14	B15	B16	B21	B22	B23	B24	B25	B26	B31	B32	B33	B34	B35	B36	B41	B42	B43	B44	B45	B46	B51	B52	B5
	31	21	12	22	20	27	30	40	18	26	21	24	18	31	19	25	20	30	14	12	19	26	21	20	20	29	13
Decision Variables	X11	X12	X13	X14	X15	X16	X21	X22	X23	X24	X25	X26	X31	X32	X33	X34	X35	X36	X41	X42	X43	X44	X45	X46	X51	X52	X5
	0	0	0	0	0	0	0	0	0	0	0	0	0	0	0	0	0	0	0	0	0	0	0	0	0	0	0
			POSITION 1						POSITION 2						POSITION 3						POSITION 4						

Fig. 1 Preparing the excel for decision variables and parameters input for solver analysis

(a)

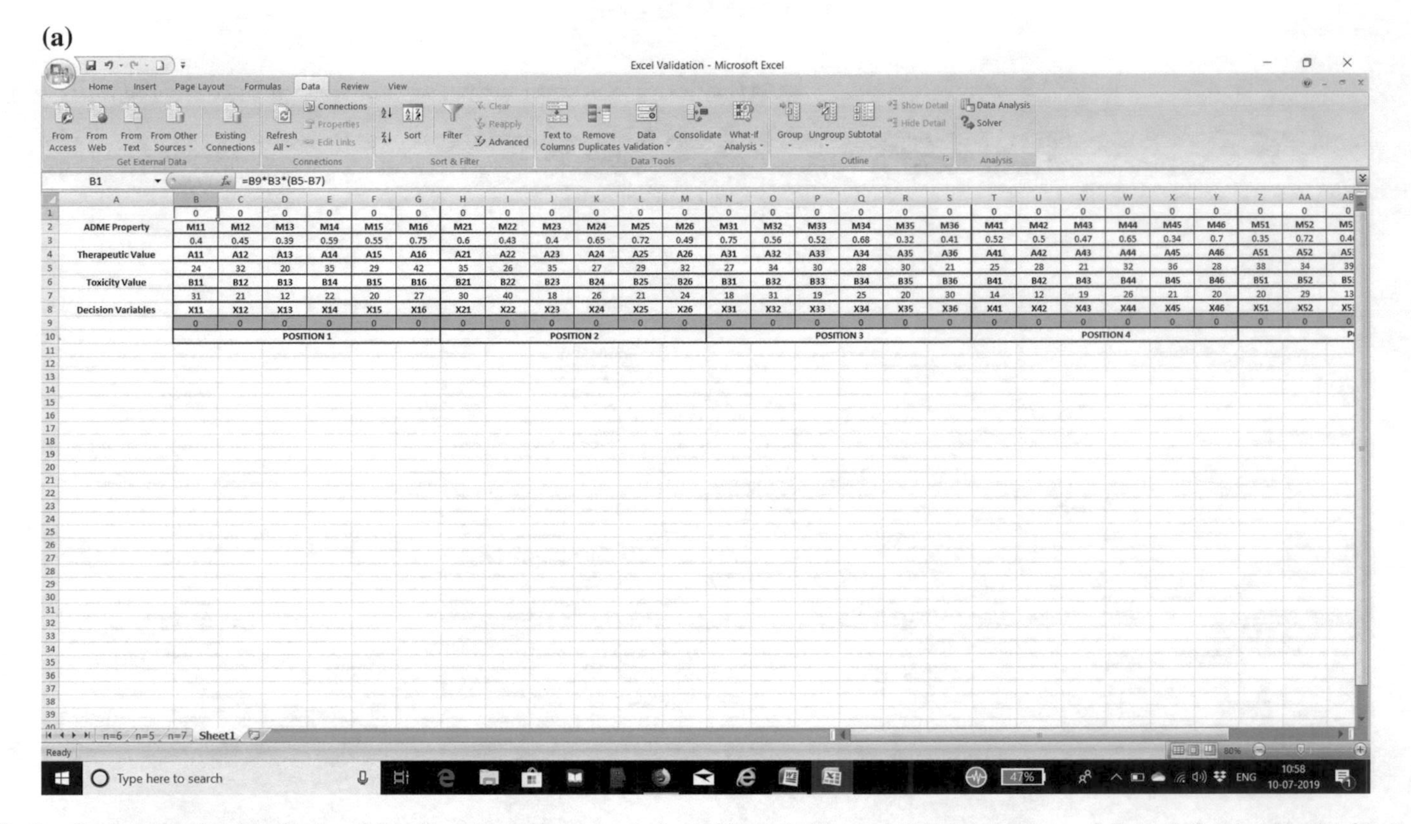

Fig. 2 **a** Formulating the objective function in line with the input matrix formed from decision variables and parameters. **b** Formulating the objective function in line with the input matrix formed from decision variables and parameters

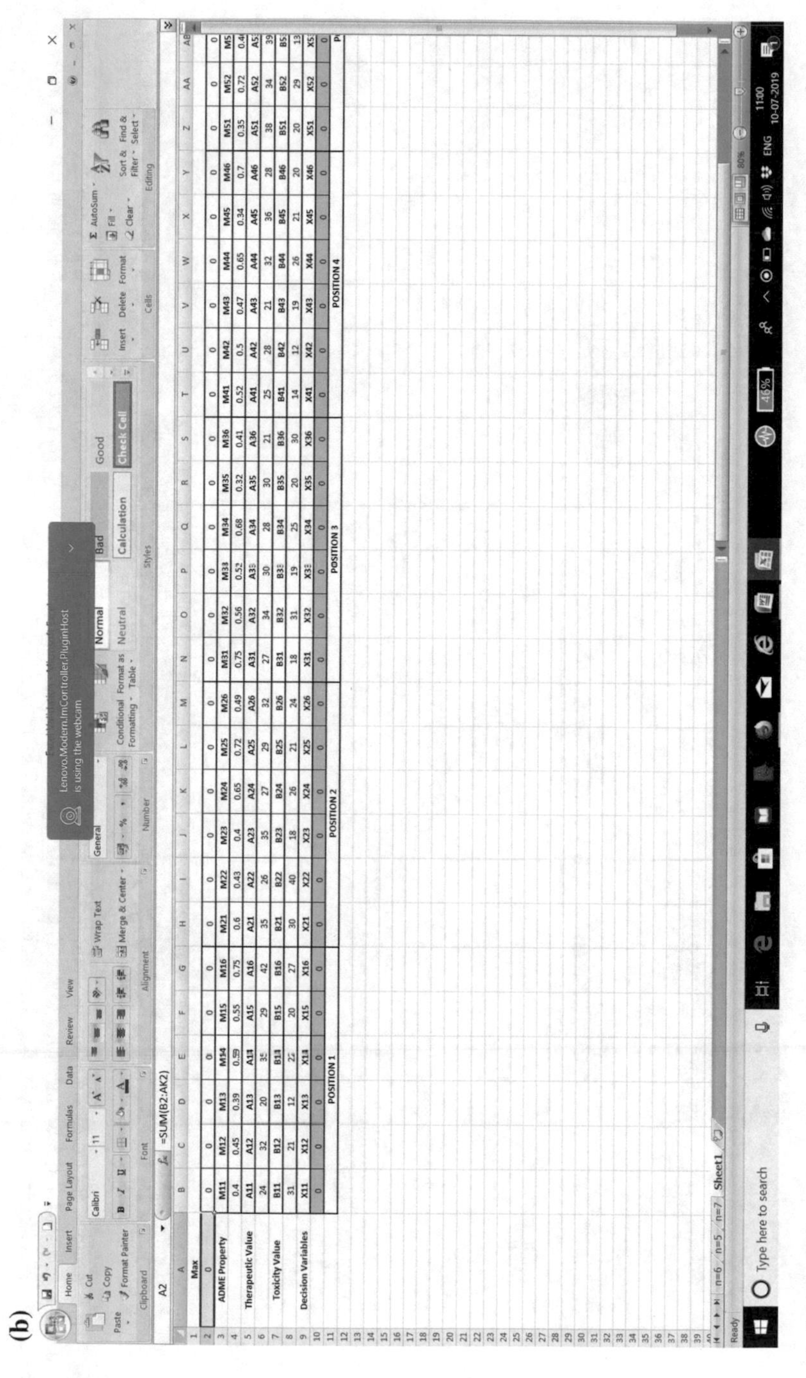

Fig. 2 (continued)

(a)

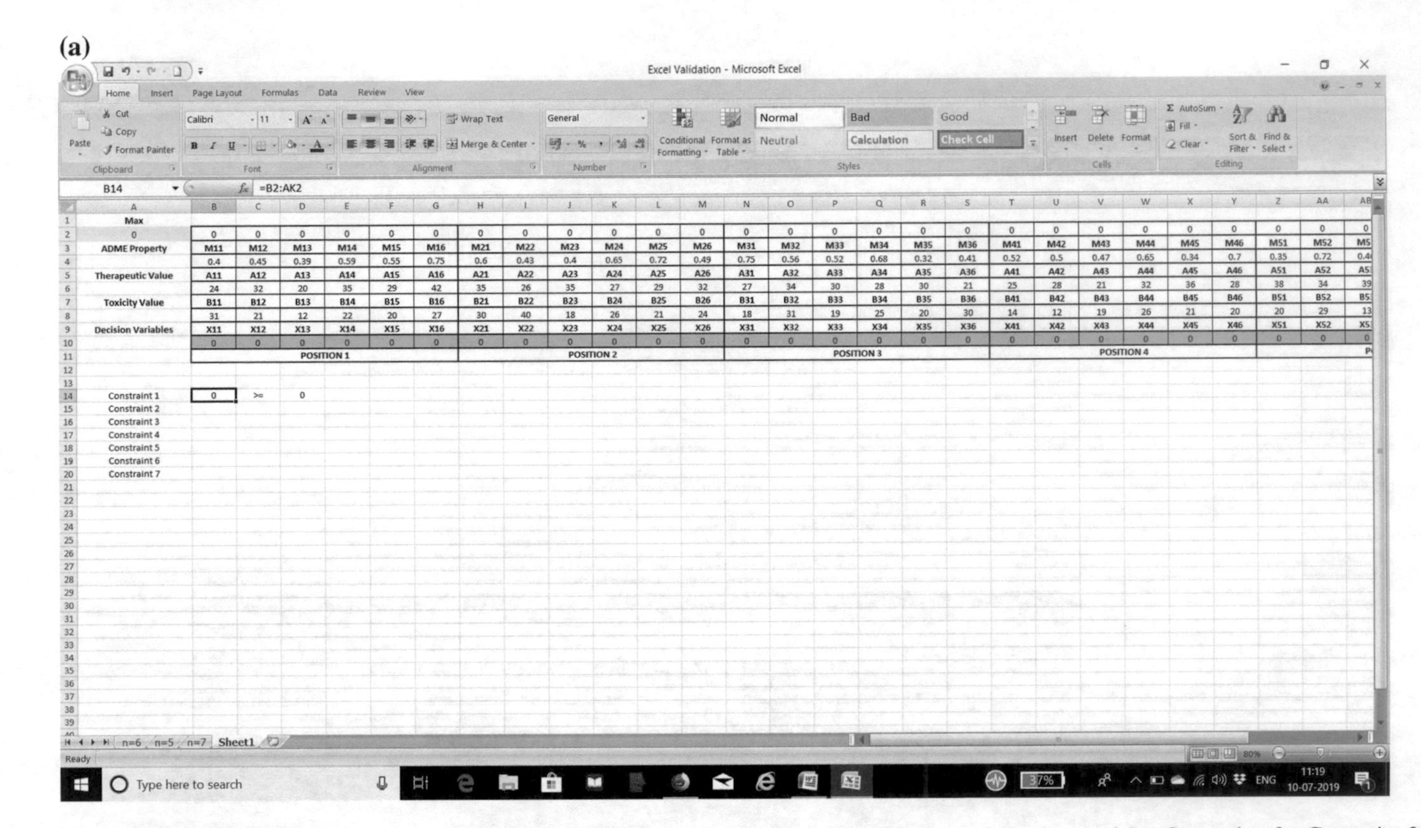

Fig. 3 **a** Screenshot for Constraint 1 in the optimization model. **b** Screenshot for Constraint 2 in the optimization model. **c** Screenshot for Constraint 3 in the optimization model. **d** Screenshot for Constraint 4 in the optimization model. **e** Screenshot for Constraint 5 in the optimization model. **f** Screenshot for Constraint 6 in the optimization model. **g** Screenshot for Constraint 7 in the optimization model

(b)

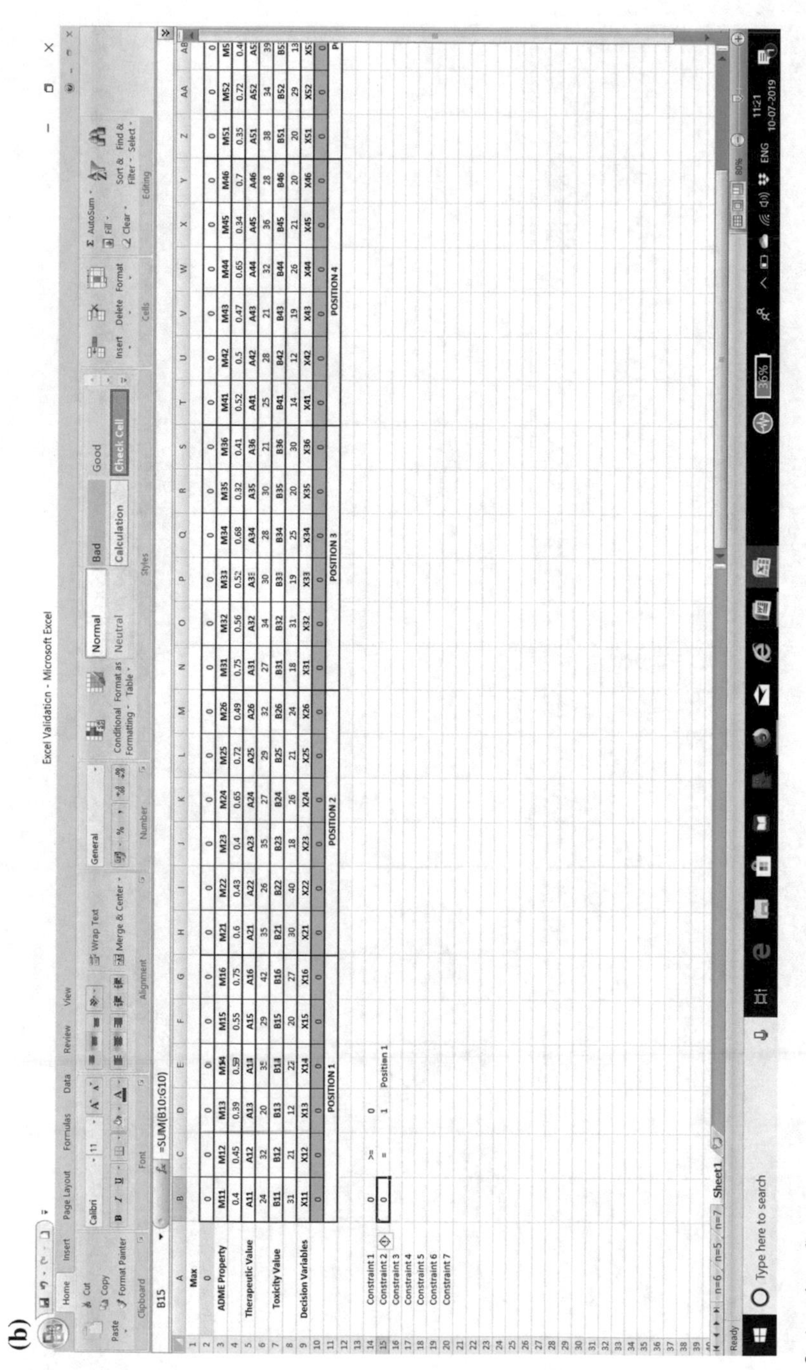

Fig. 3 (continued)

(c)

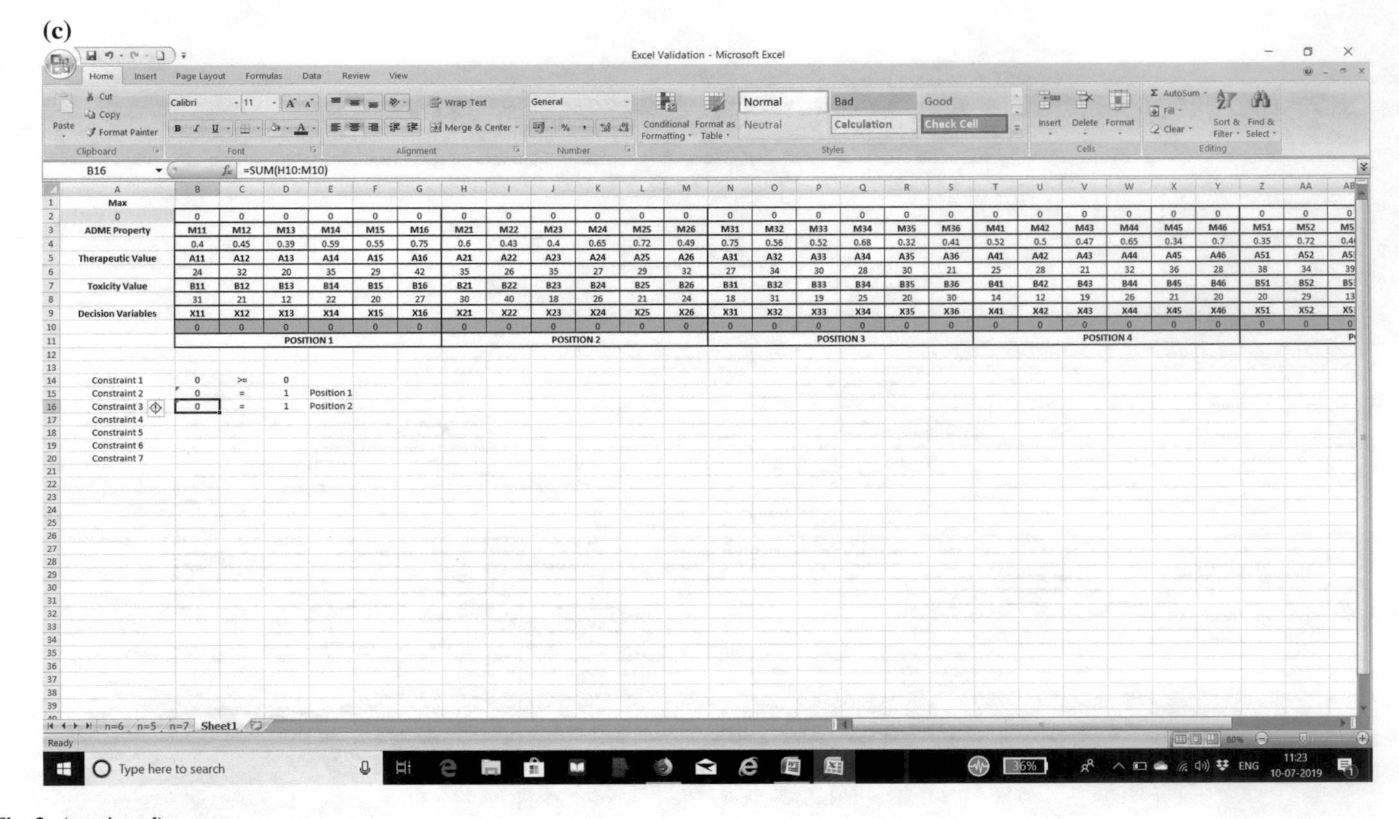

Fig. 3 (continued)

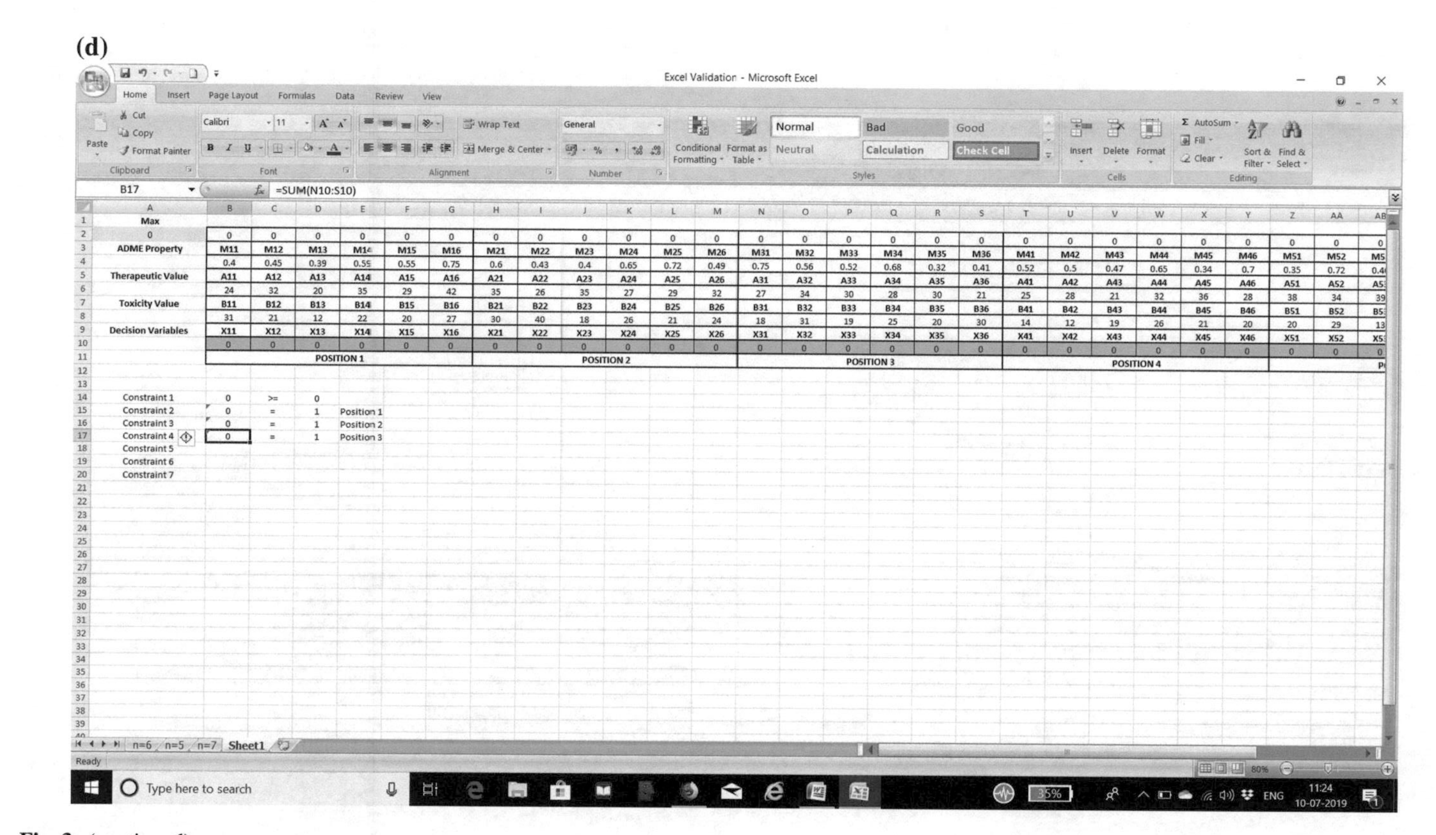

Fig. 3 (continued)

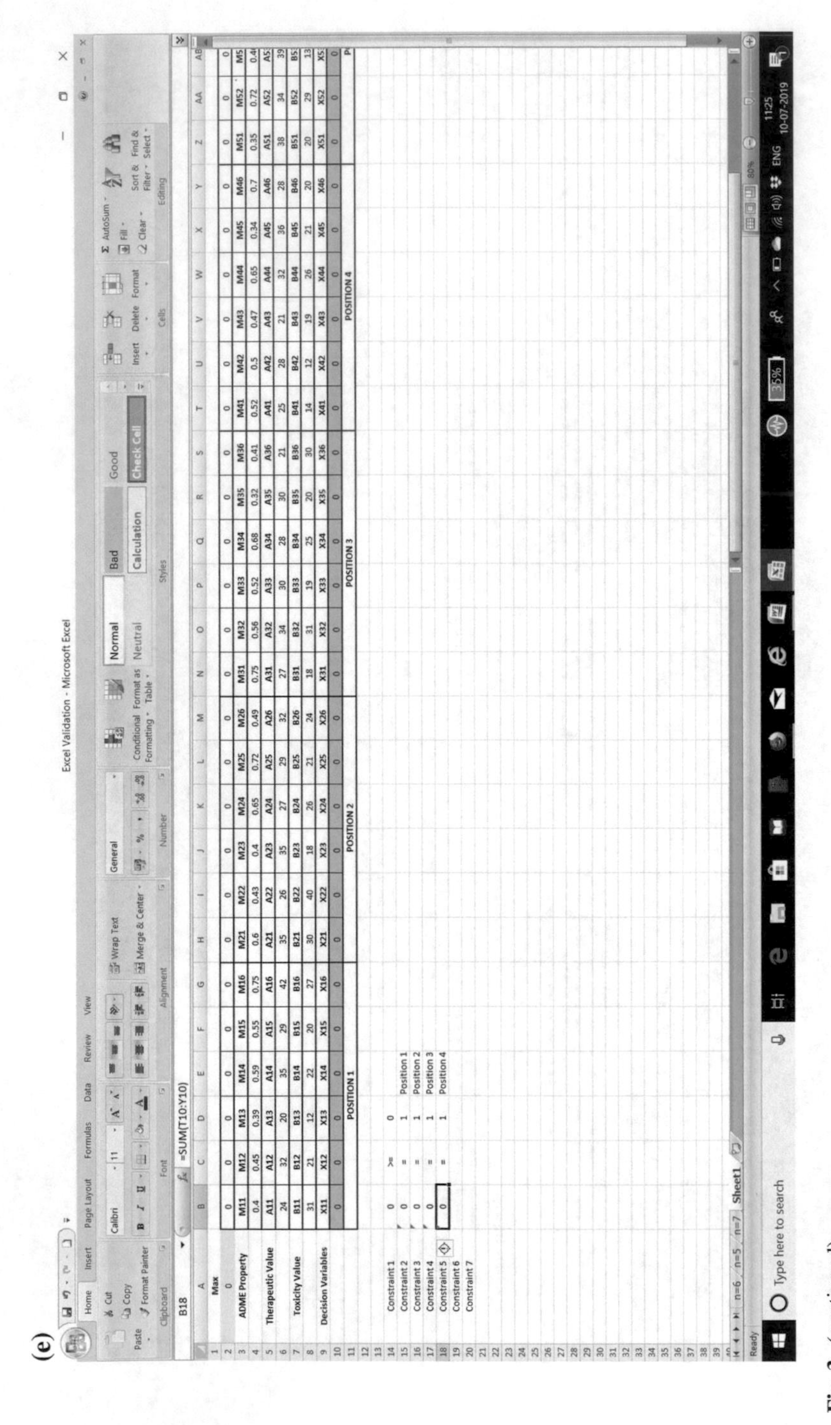

Fig. 3 (continued)

(f)

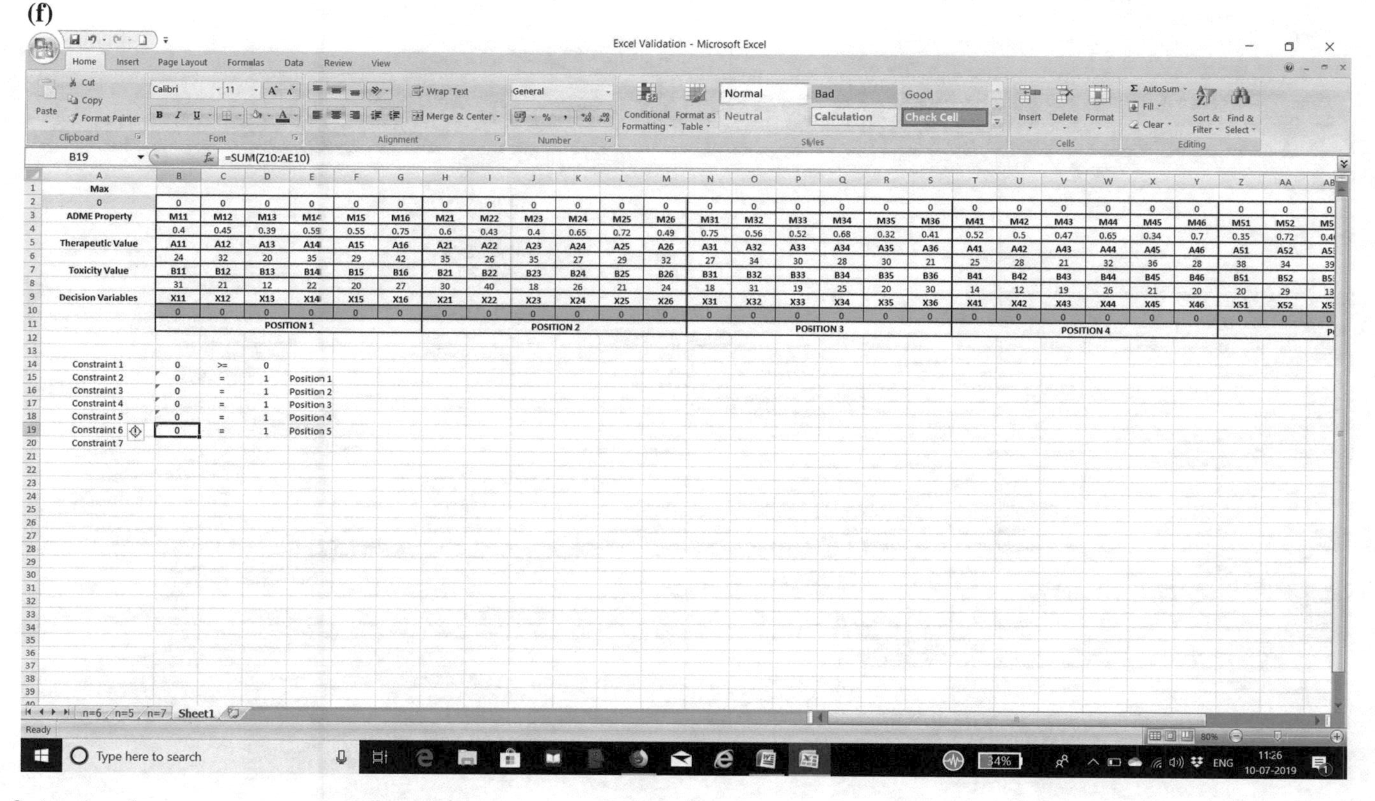

Fig. 3 (continued)

(g)

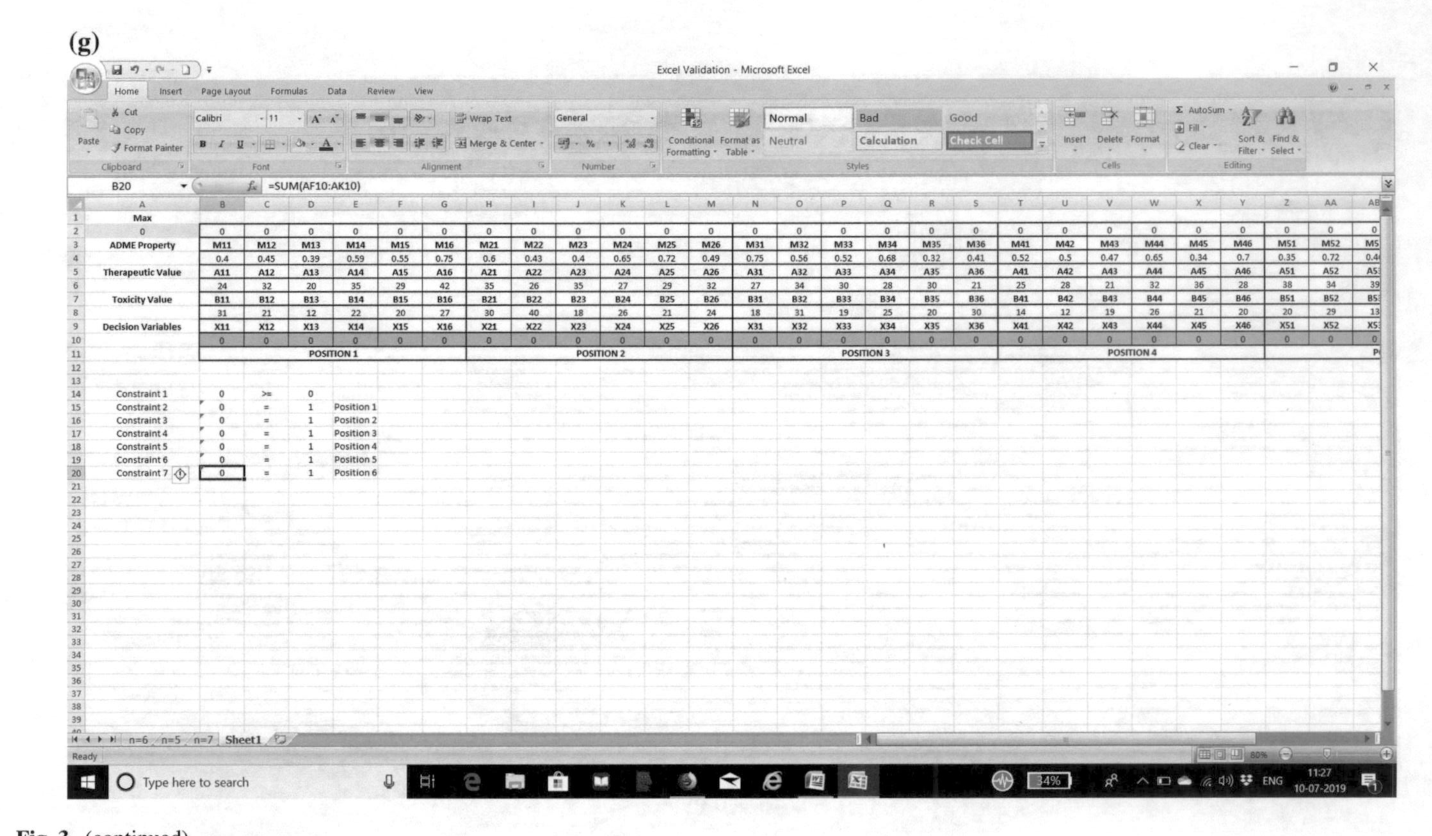

Fig. 3 (continued)

(a)

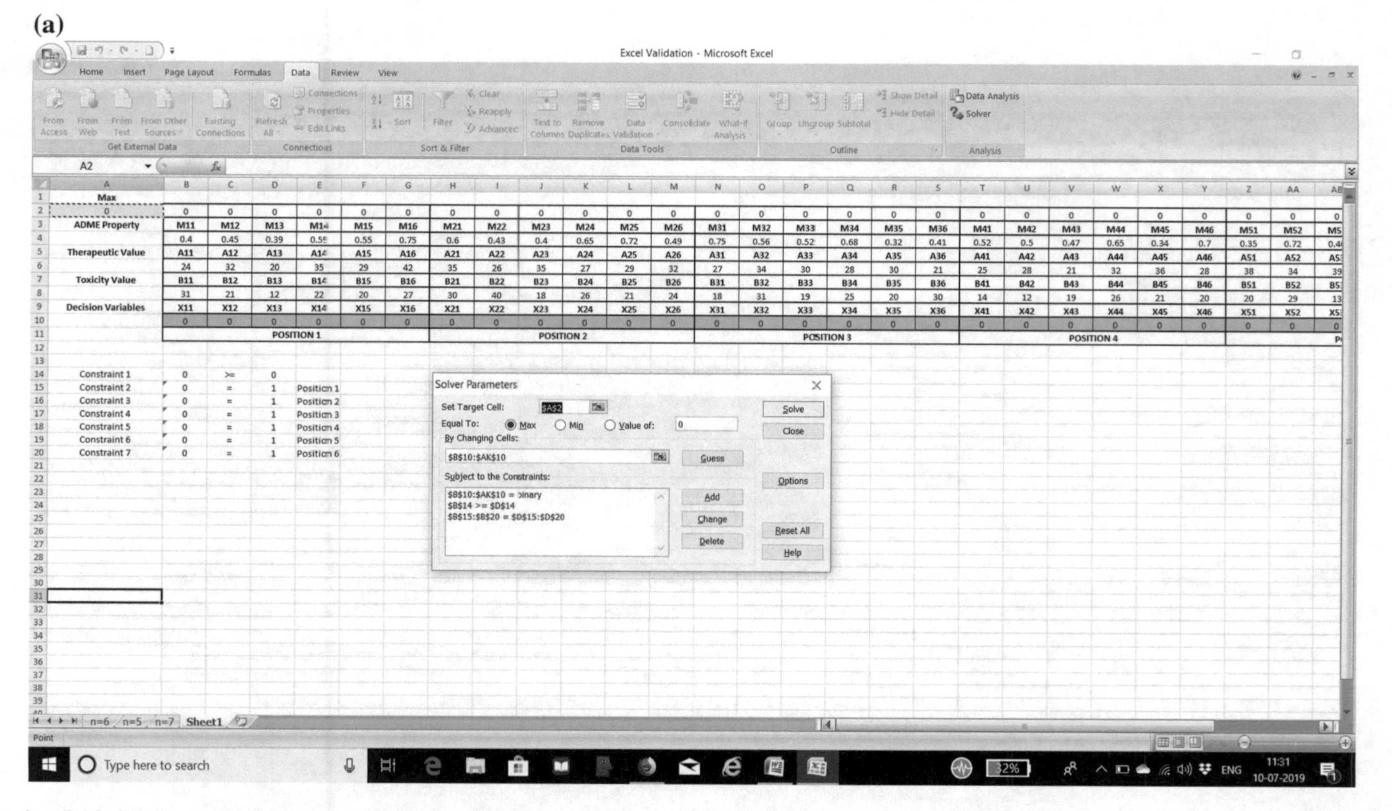

Fig. 4 **a** Initiating the solver function in the Excel and incorporating the constraints, decision variables, and objective function. **b** Incorporating linearity and non-negativity in the optimization model

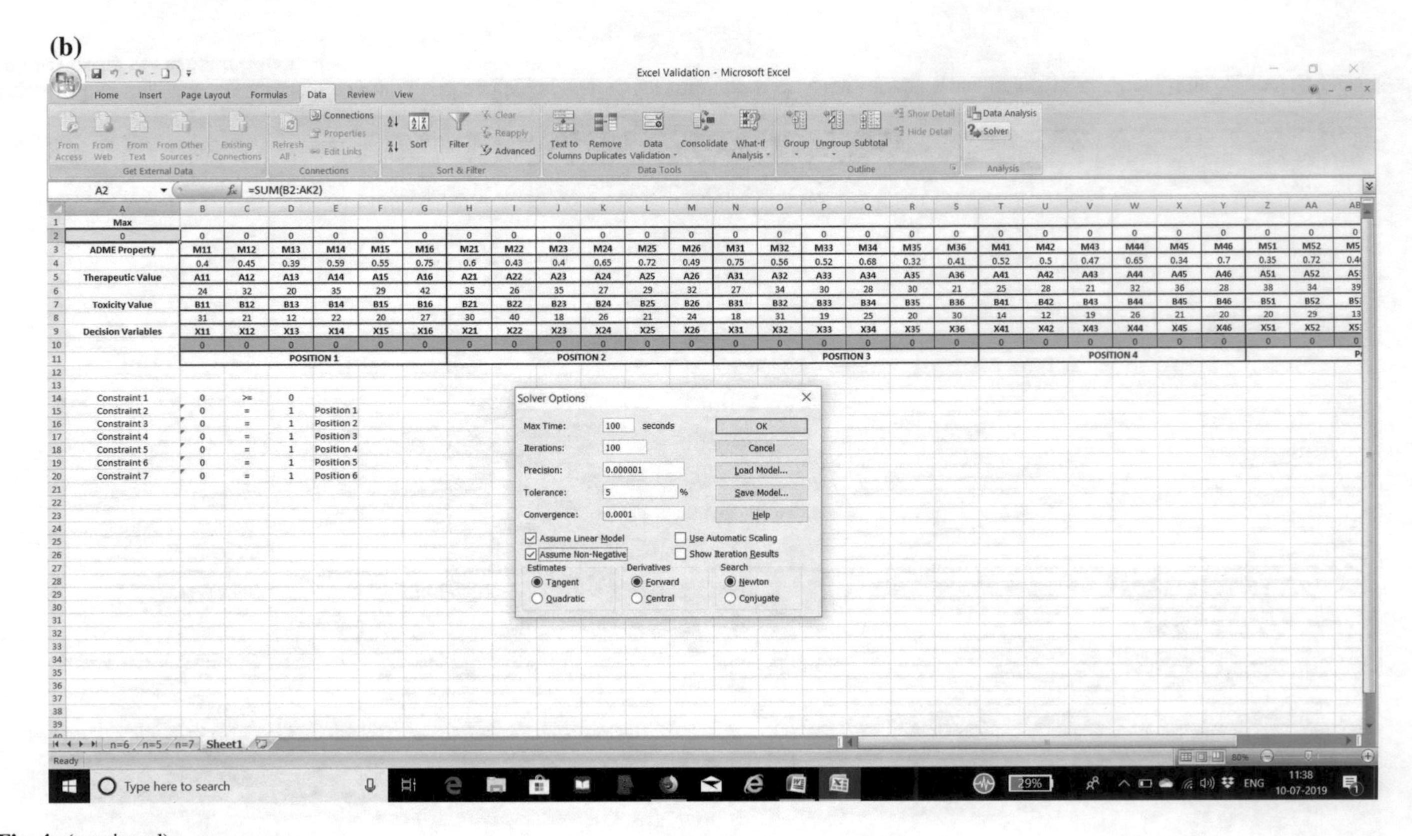

Fig. 4 (continued)

References

1. Burns LR (2014) India' s healthcare industry: innovation in delivery, financing, and manufacturing. Cambridge University Press, Cambridge
2. Shrivastava A (2015) NextGen pharma takes "smart" strides with internet of things
3. Meek T (2018) How IoT is revolutionizing the pharma industry. https://samsungnext.com/whats-next/iot-pharma-biotech/
4. Maroto F (2019) Is the internet of things changing manufacturing? In: Datafloq. https://datafloq.com/read/internet-of-things-changing-manufacturing/1057. Accessed 7 July 2019
5. Sridhar A, Varia H (2016) The healthcare industry could have a lot riding on IoT. Indiatimes
6. Kissick WL (1994) Medicine's dilemmas: infinite needs versus finite resources. Yale University Press
7. Ashburn TT, Thor KB (2004) Drug repositioning: identifying and developing new uses for existing drugs. Nat Rev Drug Discov 3:673–683. https://doi.org/10.1038/nrd1468
8. European Bioinformatics Institute (2018) Train online: drug discovey. https://www.ebi.ac.uk/training/online/course/functional-genomics-i-introduction-and-designing-e/functional-genomics-case-studies/drug-disc. Accessed 13 June 2019
9. Liljefors T, Krogsgaard-Larsen P, Madsen U (2002) Textbook of drug design and discovery. CRC Press
10. Güner FO (2000) Pharmacophore perception, development, and use in drug design, vol 2. Internat'l University Line
11. Cohen CN (1996) Guidebook on molecular modeling in drug design. Elsevier
12. Brown FK (1998) Chemoinformatics: what is it and how does it impact drug discovery. Annu Rep Med Chem 33:375–384
13. Verma J, Khedkar V, Coutinho E (2010) 3D-QSAR in Drug Design—a review. Curr Top Med Chem 10:95–115. https://doi.org/10.2174/156802610790232260
14. Foye WO (2008) Foye's principles of medicinal chemistry. Lippincott Williams & Wilkins
15. Scior T, Medina-Franco J, Do Q-T et al (2009) How to recognize and workaround pitfalls in QSAR studies: a critical review. Curr Med Chem 16:4297–4313. https://doi.org/10.2174/092986709789578213
16. Dudek a Z, Arodz T, Gálvez J (2006) Computational methods in developing quantitative structure-activity relationships (QSAR): a review. Comb Chem High Throughput Screen 9:213–228. https://doi.org/10.2174/138620706776055539
17. Katritzky A, Lobanov V, Karelson M (1995) QSPR: the correlation and quantitative prediction of chemical and physical properties from structure. Chem Soc Rev 24:279–287. https://doi.org/10.1039/cs9952400279
18. Karelson M, Lobanov VS, Katritzky AR (1996) Quantum-chemical descriptors in QSAR/QSPR studies. Chem Rev 96:1027–1043. https://doi.org/10.1021/cr950202r
19. Carlsen L, Kenessov BN, Batyrbekova SY (2008) A QSAR/QSTR study on the environmental health impact by the rocket fuel 1,1-dimethyl hydrazine and its transformation products. Environ Health Insights 1:11–20. https://doi.org/10.1016/j.etap.2009.01.005
20. Cronin MTD, Dearden JC (1995) QSAR in toxicology: 1.-prediction of aquatic toxicity. Quant Struct Relationsh 14:1–7
21. Garg D, Gandhi T, Gopi Mohan C (2008) Exploring QSTR and toxicophore of hERG K+ channel blockers using GFA and HypoGen techniques. J Mol Graph Model 26:966–976. https://doi.org/10.1016/j.jmgm.2007.08.002
22. Das RN, Roy K (2013) Advances in QSPR/QSTR models of ionic liquids for the design of greener solvents of the future. Mol Divers 17:151–196. https://doi.org/10.1007/s11030-012-9413-y
23. Kleandrova VV, Luan F, González-Díaz H et al (2014) Computational tool for risk assessment of nanomaterials: novel QSTR-perturbation model for simultaneous prediction of ecotoxicity and cytotoxicity of uncoated and coated nanoparticles under multiple experimental conditions. Environ Sci Technol 48:14686–14694. https://doi.org/10.1021/es503861x

24. Rücker C, Rücker G, Meringer M (2007) Y-randomization and its variants in QSPR/QSAR. J Chem Inf Model 47:2345–2357
25. Yee LC, Wei YC (2012) Current modeling methods used in QSAR/QSPR. In: Statistical modelling of molecular descriptors in QSAR/QSPR, pp 1–31. https://doi.org/10.3390/ijms10051978
26. Gramatica P (2007) Principles of QSAR models validation: internal and external. QSAR Comb Sci 26:694–701. https://doi.org/10.1002/qsar.200610151
27. Tropsha A, Gramatica P, Gombar VK (2003) The importance of being earnest: validation is the absolute essential for successful application and interpretation of QSPR models. QSAR Comb Sci 22:69–77. https://doi.org/10.1002/qsar.200390007
28. Barchetti U, Bucciero A, De Blasi M et al (2010) RFID, EPC and B2B convergence towards an item-level traceability in the pharmaceutical supply chain. In: Proceedings of 2010 IEEE international conference on RFID-technology and applications. IEEE, pp 194–199
29. Chamekh M, El Asmi S, Hamdi M, Kim TH (2017) Context aware middleware for RFID based pharmaceutical supply chain. In: 2017 13th international wireless communications and mobile computing conference (IWCMC). IEEE, pp 1915–1920
30. Jara AJ, Alcolea AF, Zamora MA, et al (2010) Drugs interaction checker based on IoT. In: 2010 internet things. IEEE, pp 1–8. https://doi.org/10.1109/IOT.2010.5678458
31. Jara AJ, Zamora MA, Skarmeta AF (2014) Drug identification and interaction checker based on IoT to minimize adverse drug reactions and improve drug compliance. Pers Ubiquitous Comput 18:5–17. https://doi.org/10.1007/s00779-012-0622-2
32. Yang G, Xie L, Mäntysalo M et al (2014) A health-IoT platform based on the integration of intelligent packaging, unobtrusive bio-sensor, and intelligent medicine box. IEEE Trans Ind Inform 10:2180–2191. https://doi.org/10.1109/TII.2014.2307795
33. Roy SN, Srivastava SK, Gururajan R (2018) Integrating wearable devices and recommendation system: towards a next generation healthcare service delivery. J Inf Technol 19:4–30

Sudipendra Nath Roy is currently pursuing postdoctoral research in Management Science at the Ivey Business School, Western University, Canada. He had completed doctoral studies in Operations Management and Quantitative Techniques from Indian Institute of Management Indore, India and post-graduate studies in Pharmacoinformatics from National Institute of Pharmaceutical Education & Research Kolkata, India. Sudipendra is passionate about research ideas in the healthcare operations and analytics domain.

Tuhin Sengupta is a Senior Lecturer in the area of Information Technology and Operations Management at Goa Institute of Management. His research interests lie in the domain of supply chain management and social responsibility in operations management. He has published articles in international journals such as Technological Forecasting and Social Change, Production Planning and Control, Computers in Industry, and Journal of Cleaner Production, among others.

Cybersecurity Vulnerabilities in Biomedical Devices: A Hierarchical Layered Framework

F. Badrouchi, A. Aymond, M. Haerinia, S. Badrouchi, D. F. Selvaraj, K. Tavakolian, P. Ranganathan and Sumathy Eswaran

Abstract Any biomedical device requiring power from a source other than the human body or gravity is considered an active device. Currently available active biomedical devices encompass an enormous variety of technologies, ranging from large imaging machines to miniature implantable stimulators. These devices are vulnerable to cybersecurity threats, especially for devices capable of communication with an internet network. An attack exploiting these vulnerabilities can cause a variety of consequences, including data theft, denial-of-service, and serious patient harm. The chapter provides a comprehensive review of cyberattacks on biomedical devices in a hierarchical layered framework (e.g., sensing, communication, and control) with three specific attacks as case studies: (1) MRI unit-based attack, (2) infusion pump-based attack, and (3) implantable medical device attack.

Keywords Cybersecurity · Biomedical devices · Hierarchical layers

1 Introduction

In fall 2013, a team of elite security researchers known as "white hat hackers" was invited to the Mayo Clinic in Minnesota. They were given 40 different medical devices and told to break into them any way they could in an effort to expose vulnerabilities. The team spent one week analyzing the devices and found that every device had backdoor access points making them vulnerable to unauthorized users. The hackers were able to access the devices' control systems via generic default passwords and unsecured operating systems. After gaining access to the system, the

F. Badrouchi · A. Aymond · M. Haerinia · D. F. Selvaraj · K. Tavakolian · P. Ranganathan (✉)
University of North Dakota (UND), Grand Forks, ND, USA
e-mail: Prakash.ranganathan@und.edu

S. Badrouchi
University of Tunis EL Manar (UTM), Tunis, Tunisia

S. Eswaran
Dr. MGR Educational and Research Institute, Chennai, India

P. Raj et al. (eds.), *Internet of Things Use Cases for the Healthcare Industry*,
https://doi.org/10.1007/978-3-030-37526-3_7

hacker can launch a potentially lethal attack, such as causing a medication infusion pump to over administer medication without alerting staff [1].

Any medical device relying on an external power source is known as an active device [2]. Most modern active medical devices utilize some type of processor or computer to execute preprogrammed commands and to communicate with the hospital's network. These computers, particularly their communication channels, pose a security risk due to insufficient communication restriction, encryption, and monitoring. Once a hacker has accessed the device's processor through these insecure channels, he is able to spread the attack throughout the device's control system, actuators, and potentially out through the communication channels to the rest of the hospital network. The insufficient security protocols for these devices, and for the hospital network in general, are due to many factors, including lack of funding for IT specialists in health care, rapid growth of the variety and number of devices sharing a hospital network, and lack of cybersecurity training for the designers of the medical devices [3].

The main focus of this chapter is the cybersecurity threats on active and connected biomedical devices. As cyberphysical systems, biomedical devices are vulnerable to attack vectors such as eavesdropping, spoofing, and jamming. It is important to understand the interaction between sensors, communication, and computing platform of various medical devices in order to gain insights on how these devices are susceptible to cyberthreats.

A hospital network connects various medical technologies used to provide care to patients, including diagnostic, medication delivery, surgical, and life support equipment. Proper cybersecurity must be maintained to protect patient information and insure its confidentiality from unauthorized access and use. A closer partnership and collaboration is required between multiple entities such as hospitals, vendors of medical devices/equipment, and government agencies to mitigate cyberthreats. The United States Food and Drug Administration (FDA) recently started paying more attention to cybersecurity threats. In 2018, the FDA updated the guidance document entitled "Content of Premarket Submissions for Management of Cybersecurity in Medical Devices" which was originally issued in 2014. This document outlines the expectations of new biomedical devices seeking FDA clearance. When comparing the modern cybersecurity demands for insurance companies and financial institutions, the FDA is still behind in making strict regulations controlling connected hospitals and devices [4, 5].

2 Overview of Existing Technologies

Medical devices have many forms and functions in modern health care. Some medical device such as pacemaker is used by an individual, whereas sphygmomanometer or infusion pump is used clinically to assess and treat many people daily. Key security-relevant differences for these device usage scenarios are the amount of personal data stored in the device, sensitivity and quantity of data collected, and type or specificity of therapy delivered. Large clinical facilities have a much greater risk of information theft-type attack for their electronic medical records and billing info but may have fewer security concerns at the device level than do personal users. Hospital medical devices are de-identified, which lessens the risk of a personally targeted attack. However, personal devices and hospital devices are both susceptible to denial-of-service and improper functioning attacks, which will be elaborated upon later in this chapter. The rest of this chapter will primarily focus on personal medical devices; however, the security topics discussed are also relevant to devices used in a commercial setting.

– Connectivity

Connected medical devices optimize the continuous exchange of information between healthcare providers and the devices in contact with the patient [6]. This communication may occur on wired or wireless networks, or using Near-Field Communication (NFC). Wired networks offer benefits of increased speed and reliability compared to wireless networks; however, the wired networks require that equipment be physically connected and thus cannot be transported freely with the patient throughout the hospital. Wired networks may also be more costly due to the custom designing required to fit the system with the existing hospital infrastructure [7]. Some benefits and architectures of medical device connectivity are presented below.

- Reasons for connectivity
  - Connection of multiple sensors and actuators in body.
  - Record data and transmit to practitioner (e.g., Holter monitor, EEG, EKG).
  - Monitor health status and treat (e.g., artificial pancreas, pacemaker).
  - Storage of personal data for device operation (e.g., patient's goal blood sugar level).
- Various connection capabilities of existing devices are ranked by increasing security concerns:
  - Isolated (no external communication from device),
  - Programmable with wand or physical contact by practitioner,
  - Isolated with sensor,
  - Wirelessly connected,
  - In-home data connection (e.g., nightstand data transfer system),
  - Interoperable network (connection of multiple devices),
  - Interoperable network with sensors, and
  - Smartphone-connected devices.

Some examples of connectivity type based on the class of medical devices are presented in Table 1. In addition, the information on some of the working groups/organizations involved in medical device connectivity and the relevant standards are furnished in Tables 2 and 3, respectively.

Table 1 Examples of connectivity type depending on device class

Class of medical device	Examples	Wiring	Connectivity
Implantable devices	Cardiac defibrillator/Pacemaker	Not wired	Wireless body area network (WBAN)
	Cochlear implant	Not wired	Wireless body area network (WBAN)
	Neurostimulator	Not wired	Wireless body area network (WBAN)
Imaging devices	X-ray scan	Not wired	WLAN-based DDR portable radiography
	CT scan	Not wired	WLAN-based DDR portable radiography
	MRI	Wired	Local area network (LAN)
Medication delivery	Infusion pumps	Not wired	WLAN
	Insulin pumps	Not wired	WLAN
	MEMS piezoelectric micropump	Not wired	PAN–WLAN–WPAN

Table 2 Organizations/working groups involved in medical device connectivity

Organization/Working group	Areas of focus
Association for the Advancement of Medical Instrumentation (AAMI)	Initiatives toward decreasing preventable damage to patients and enhance results when the use of complicated health technology is involved in health care [8]
Health Level 7 (HL7)	Standards and framework for exchanging the electronic health records that supports better clinical practice and health service management [9]
CEN/TC 251	Standards for health information and communication technology (ICT) in the European Union [10]
Personal connected health alliance	Supports a patient-centric strategy to health and wellness improvement through private technology and promotes safe clinical-grade data that changes health behaviors [11]
National Institute of Standards and Technology (US)—Health Information Technology	Promotes point-of-care and personal health environments' device communication by developing and advancing software test tools [12]

Table 3 Standards related to medical device connectivity

Standard	Description
Digital imaging and communications in medicine (DICOM)	It describes medical image formats to guarantee that documents are exchanged for clinical use with the required data quality [13]
ISO/IEEE 11073	Standards addressing communication between external computer systems and medical devices and provide comprehensive electronic data capture of information [14]
ISO/TC 215	Enables compatibility and interoperability between autonomous devices, standardization of information and communication technology (ICT) for health sector [15]

3 Active Medical Devices Cyberattacks

Active medical devices rely on alternative source of power, and some examples include Magnetic Resonance Imaging (MRI) scanners, defibrillators, and infusion pumps. These active devices are often connected to a hospital network which allows communication between the diverse devices on the network, including computers, mobile devices, imaging systems, and medication delivery systems. While this network improves the efficiency and continuity of health care, it also creates significant risks due to insufficient monitoring of the network security. Healthcare IT networks are much more vulnerable than other sectors, such as financial services or insurance companies [3]. One reason for the increased cybersecurity risks of hospital networks is the lack of experienced IT professionals employed in the healthcare sector [16].

The motivation behind attacks could be stealing data, causing bodily harm, extortion or threat (e.g., cause diabetic coma by hacking insulin pump), and non-malicious (e.g., caused by unintended commands or interference). The attacks have different types including eavesdropping, denial-of-service, power system disruption, physical damage, artificial sensor readings (to cause incorrect therapeutic output), artificial or unauthorized command, and misuse by authorized programmers. To analyze common active medical devices' cyberattacks, the attack points are identified, a review of biomedical cyberattacks is presented in Table 4, and examples of common biomedical devices and related attacks are studied.

The examples of common biomedical devices and related attacks are presented as follows:

(A) Magnetic Resonance Imaging (MRI)

During the use of an MRI, a patient's physical safety is breached if a metal object in the treatment room is forcefully pulled toward the MRI's very strong magnetic field. Metal objects can be pulled into the MRI with considerable force, thus breaking the MRI and causing a user to be struck, trapped, or otherwise injured by the metal acting as a projectile. This risk is mitigated by placing metal detectors at the entrance to the

Table 4 A review of biomedical cyberattacks

Security property/attack type	Attack examples	References
Authentication (Spoofing)	Impersonate programmer (in order to alter system programming or internal controls only available to device designer/programmers)	[18–28]
	Impersonate controller/user (in order to spoof system controls normally available to a patient, physician, or technician)	[19–25, 29–36]
	Impersonate the medical device	[24, 31–37]
	Impersonate the external device/receiver	[19, 20, 22, 26, 31, 33–39]
	Other attacks not listed above	[40–42]
	Countermeasures to above attacks	[18, 20, 22–24, 30–34, 39, 41–51]
Integrity (Tampering)	Patient data tampering	[19–21, 25, 33–35, 39, 46, 52, 53]
	Malicious inputs: incorrect sensor data	[18, 20–22, 29, 31, 33–35, 37, 49, 52–55]
	Malicious inputs: jamming	[18, 20, 24, 49]
	Malicious inputs: incorrect control commands	[19, 21, 23–25, 34, 38, 44, 49, 55]
	Modify communications: alter output signal	[20, 22, 33, 46, 48, 49, 56]
	Countermeasures	[20, 23, 24, 31, 33, 43–46, 48, 51, 52, 56]
Non-repudiation (Repudiation)	Delete access logs (hide attack history)	[20, 24, 46, 48]
	Repeated access attempts	[20, 24, 33]
	Devices lacking access logs	[20, 24]
	Countermeasures	[19, 20, 23, 24, 33, 44, 48]

(continued)

Table 4 (continued)

Security property/attack type	Attack examples	References
Confidentiality (Information Disclosure)	Disclose medical information (Data theft)	[19–26, 29–33, 37–39, 46, 52, 54]
	Determine type of device or disclose existence of device (for implanted or non-visible devices)	[20, 23, 31, 34, 52, 54]
	Track the device (for implantable or mobile devices)	[20, 30, 31, 34]
	Eavesdropping	[18, 20, 22–26, 30, 31, 33, 34, 38, 39, 44, 46, 48, 55]
	Countermeasures	[18, 20, 24, 26, 31, 33, 45, 46, 48, 52, 54, 57]
Availability (Denial-of-service)	Drain battery (for mobile or implanted devices)	[20, 23, 24, 26, 29–31, 34, 38, 44, 49, 55]
	Interfere with communication capabilities: electronic attack	[18–20, 24, 26, 29–31, 34, 37, 38, 46]
	Interfere with communication capabilities: physical attack (e.g., Physical destruction of antenna or disconnection from wired network)	[18, 24, 30, 37, 54]
	Flood device with data (jamming)	[18, 20, 30, 33, 44]
	Prevent access by authorized personnel (e.g., Prevent access by physician)	[18, 22, 23, 29, 30, 37, 52]
	Countermeasures	[20, 24, 26, 30–32, 43–45, 49, 55, 58]
Authorization (elevation of privileges)	Reprogram the device	[19–21, 23, 24, 29, 34, 37, 38, 46, 54, 55, 59, 60]
	Update/alter therapy of patient	[18–24, 26, 29–31, 33, 34, 44, 54, 61, 62]
	Maliciously change device functioning (e.g., Too much radiation delivery in imaging device or cause device to shock patient)	[18, 19, 21, 22, 24, 26, 29, 31, 34, 44, 46, 54]
	Turn-off device	[20, 29, 44]
	Countermeasures	[20, 23, 24, 26, 45–47, 49, 50]

MRI room to warn staff of metal objects that must be removed before approaching the MRI machine. A physical safety breach could be enhanced by a hacker if he disables the metal detectors at the entrance to the MRI room [16, 17]. Table 5 represents potential MRI cyberattacks.

(B) **Infusion Pump**

An infusion pump delivers liquid medications to the patient's circulation via an intravenous tube. The pump uses an internal motor to deliver the medications at a controlled rate and pressure as set by the pump control system. These systems include alarms to warn staff of potential physical tampering or complications with the medication delivery. The pumps are often wirelessly connected to the hospital network, thus making them vulnerable to a cyberattack via the infusion pump's communication channels. In the event of an attack, the hacker could cause serious harm to patient or even death by altering the medication delivery schedule and pressure or by halting the medication delivery completely. The hacker could also deactivate the system alarms to prevent intervention by care staff [17]. Following the discovery and publication of several infusion pump vulnerabilities, the FDA has launched an infusion pump improvement initiative which aims to reduce the current security risks present in infusion pumps from many manufacturers by implementing stricter regulations which much be satisfied before new pumps may be sold for use in US healthcare systems [63]. Some manufacturers have begun to implement new technology and control architectures into "smart pumps" which satisfy the new FDA criteria [16]. Table 6 shows potential infusion pump cyberattacks.

(C) **Medical Laboratory**

A crucial component of the modern hospital system is a medical laboratory, which processes biological specimens from patients to provide diagnostic data to medical practitioners. The lab's infrastructure is maintained by the Laboratory Automation System (LAS), which regulates equipment such as refrigerators, fume hoods, biological hazard containment systems, ventilation, and other critical safety equipment. Interruptions to this system, as in the event of a hacker attack, could lead to injury of

Table 5 Potential cyberattacks on MRI [17]

Attacker malicious activity	Consequences
Override magnetic field strength limit	Possible patient tissue burns Possibility of damaging the machine
Disable alarms	Unawareness of dangerous conditions by technician
Reboot the machine	Delete configuration settings
Change information of display	Leads to a technician confusion to follow the protocol
Replace patient's files	Wrongly sent diagnosis to a patient

Table 6 Potential cyberattacks on infusion pump [17]

Attacker malicious activity	Consequences
Alter air purge rate or purge process	Syringe line may contain air during therapy
Disable alarms	Unawareness of dangerous conditions by nurse
Reboot the pump	Delete configuration settings
Change information of display	Leads to a nurse confusion to follow the treatment process
Replace patient's files	Wrongly delivered medication to a patient
Falsifying information on the dosage delivered	The equipment shows that the patient received the required dose, however, he did not

the lab employees, loss of patient's specimens, and delivery of incorrect test results to the practitioners [17]. Table 7 depicts potential medical laboratory cyberattacks.

(D) **Heart–Lung Machine**

A heart–lung machine is a device used to maintain an extracorporeal circuit of the patient's blood, called cardiopulmonary bypass. This is necessary during an operation which requires the patient's lungs and heart to be temporarily arrested, such as during a cardiac artery bypass or a lung transplant. While the patient's heart and lungs are nonfunctional, the heart–lung machine draws blood from the body, oxygenates it, and then pumps it back through the patient's circulation. The drug heparin is used to prevent coagulation of the blood as it passes through the machine. Heart–lung machines are critical life support technologies designed for use during difficult and challenging operations. Any alteration to the functioning of the machine poses a significant risk for patient harm or death. If an attacker gains access to the machine through the hospital network, he may cause damage through many different methods. Table 8 explores some possible cyberattacks of the heart–lung machine [17]. Other than studied cases, there are other biomedical devices and systems susceptible to cyberphysical attacks including dialysis machine, medical ventilator, robotic surgical machine, anesthetic machine, active patient monitoring devices, Extracorporeal Membrane Oxygenation (ECMO), medical lasers, Medical Device Data Systems

Table 7 Potential medical laboratory cyberattacks [17]

Attacker malicious activity	Consequences
Block the transfer of information	Critical information are not communicated
Modify test procedures or lab equipment settings	Wrong test results
Corrupt laboratory test results	Makes specialist misdiagnose patient condition and settle on inaccurate treatment choices, recommend an inappropriate medications or direct wrong consideration
Change work orders	Affects patient's treatment

Table 8 Potential heart–lung machine cyberattacks [17]

Attacker malicious activity	Consequences
Alter pump's heparin dosage (excess)	A potential internal bleeding can result from a non-appropriate clot of the blood
Heparin pump shut down	Patient blood clotting possible
Disable alarms	Unawareness of dangerous conditions by technician
Change information of display	Leads to a technician confusion to follow the protocol
Cause random alarms	Leads to a technician confusion to follow the protocol
Reboot the machine	Delete configuration settings

(MDDSs), storage devices for medical images, communications devices for medical images, and Health Electronic Records (HERs).

4 Cyberattack Detection and Prevention

4.1 Medical Device and Hospital Network Cyberattack Anatomy

In order to attack or control a hospital network or medical device, attackers follow an attack procedure composed of five stages [64]:

- Stage 1: Find a target, choose one or more approaches, and then execute attacks, penetrating at least once.
- Stage 2: Gain foothold in a medical device and cautiously seek general information and escalation of privileges. Then begin a lateral movement.
- Stage 3: Continue reconnaissance and identify targets, and move laterally within networks.
- Stage 4: Engage with chosen targets, exfiltrate confidential patient healthcare data and financial records, clean up the artifacts of attack as best as possible, and leave.
- Stage 5: Leave a ransomware tool to run in the network to extort funds directly from the healthcare institution.

Anatomy of medical device and hospital network cyberattack is shown in Fig. 1.

4.2 Tools and Procedures for Detection and Prevention

An effective and efficient cybersecurity plan is necessary for healthcare organizations. According to the Cisco Midyear Cybersecurity Report released in 2016, it takes 100–200 days for an organization to detect possible threats. An effective plan possesses

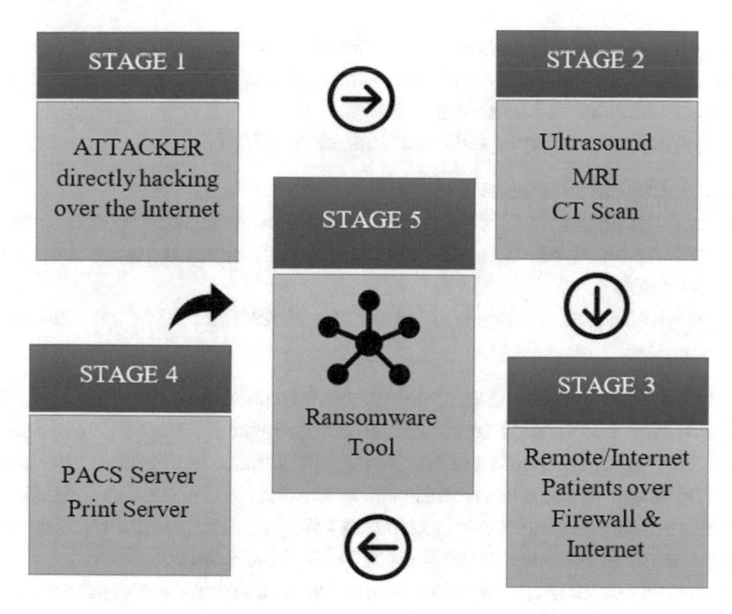

Fig. 1 Medical device and hospital network cyberattack anatomy

strong IT security tools, a strategy to stop emerging threats, and education programs for staff [65]. The robust plan has to secure sensing, control, and communication layers.

The sensing layer of a medical device is responsible for identifying any phenomena in the devices' peripheral and collecting data from the real world. This layer consists of a sensor hub using several transport mechanisms for data flow between sensors and applications [66]. The main attack points for the sensing layer are the sensor's communication with the device and spoofing of the sensor itself to transmit inaccurate sensor information [35, 36, 40, 42, 41, 51]. The sensor link or communication with the device can be secured by encrypting the channel and by maintaining a secure hospital network. Spoofing can be avoided by ensuring proper authentication of the sensor before accepting the data. Many of the novel security approaches for biomedical devices concern body area sensor networks, similar to a local Internet of Things. The main control device on or in the body communicates with several other sensors on the person to establish the network. One current experimental approach to body area network security is to only authenticate sensor nodes within a physical distance from the device to prevent remote attacks. Another method is to use the body's own physiological signals, mainly electrocardiogram (ECG), to generate secure keys.

Wireless connection is the major security concern of the communication layer. Wi-Fi, Bluetooth, and cellular communications may all be victim to eavesdropping, jamming, spoofing, and other remote attacks [38, 20, 33, 18, 24]. Devices should have all unused channels and ports secured to prevent unauthorized access. The network should utilize encryption and firewalls help to secure transmitted data, but these techniques rely on proper maintenance, such as regular password changes and encryption algorithm updates. Many healthcare facilities lack the financial and technical resources to properly maintain such systems, leaving the hospital network and connected devices vulnerable to attack.

Typically, the control layer falls into four categories [23]:

- Access control based on user's identity to get access.
- Access control based on user's role to decide if he is allowed to access or not.
- Access control based on requesting user's set of attributes to decide if he is allowed to access or not.
- Access control based on a risk adaptive model intended to adapt risk-awareness for making decision.

Risks to the control layer involve denial-of-service and reprogramming, which cause the device to stop functioning or to deliver inappropriate therapy. These attacks can be initiated by spoofing, password tracking, or attacks throughout the healthcare network, and result in unauthorized access to the device controls. A large healthcare team can further complicate security issues, as there are many authorized users which may compromise passwords or the network [29, 22–24, 54].

Prevention of control layer attacks can involve more robust encryption and authentication schemes, as well as practice of proper cybersecurity hygiene, such as updating and securing passwords and maintaining an uncompromised hospital network. Maintaining good cybersecurity practices throughout the network prevents attacker access to the device to prevent the opportunity for a control layer attack.

The cyberattack detection tools can be used to identify rogue access points, hidden networks, and stealth port scans. The common cyberattack detection tools for hospitals and healthcare facilities are given in Table 9. To protect against possible security breaches from inside or outside an organization, suspicious activities should be monitored. Table 10 presents the cyberattack indicators and suspicious behaviors [16].

To effectively detect and prevent the cyberattacks in healthcare organizations, some solutions are provided as follows [65, 67, 16]:

- It is important to discover where sensitive data exists, so it can be protected. A reliable way to protect sensitive data is to classify and modify medical database constantly. The sensitive data is usually in the cloud and on-premises. To reduce

Table 9 Cyberattack detection tools

Cyberattack detection tool	Description and function
Wireshark	A network protocol analyzer provides detailed information about the network
Kismet	A wireless network detector
Net Stumbler	A wireless network detector
Snort	A network intrusion detection system for finding attacks and stealth port scans

Table 10 Cyberattack indicators and suspicious behaviors

Suspicious system behaviors	Suspicious user behaviors
• Unplanned reboots • Very slow performance of CPU • Unusual cycles of CPU • Doubtful configurations/software on a server • Connecting information assurance and cybersecurity (BCS) to an unknown IP • Heavy network traffic • Clearing log files • Unwanted patch modifications	• Continuous logins and logouts • Change of software configuration • Increasing account access rights and privileges • Failed login attempts • Account's connection at non-expected time periods • Creating new user accounts • Asking for information regarding the function of the system

the attack surface, sensitive data in non-production environments should be eliminated. Instead, sensitive data can be replaced with realistic, fictional data for test, development, and market research purposes. Data usage activity across a broad range of data stores should be monitored in the cloud and on-premises including databases, big data platforms, SharePoint portals, and file stores.

- Targeting users with excessive access rights and dormant user accounts is an easy way for attackers to access sensitive data. To reduce the risk of data breach, healthcare organization users who have excessive privileges and deactivated dormant user accounts must be identified and monitored. The unusual password activities must be investigated. The password change of communication network or email can be notified by an email. To avoid these types of attacks, a strong password for email and the communication network must be updated at least every 6 months. The unknown emails should be identified. Phishing emails are growing enormously; therefore, the medical and technical staff need to practice safe email protocol and have to be cautious when clicking on online links from unknown sources and opening email attachments.
- Establishment of an intrusion prevention system to detect potential breaches and halt the attack before the target is reached. Installation of a firewall would aid in isolating threats and preventing the spread of attacks between components of a network. Installation of an appropriate antivirus software is required to prevent network users from accidentally downloading malicious software from websites and to filter phishing emails. The cyberattack detection and prevention tools are shown in Fig. 2.

5 A Hierarchical Layered Framework for Biomedical Devices

Biomedical devices are extremely diverse in complexity, connectivity, and implementation environment. Devices vary from an extremely large, stationary MRI machine

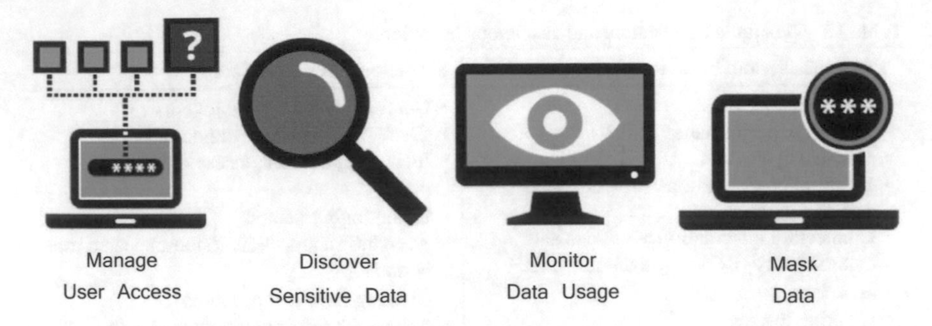

Fig. 2 Cyberattack detection and prevention tools [67]

to a small, implantable stimulator. Previously, in this chapter, cybersecurity topics for biomedical devices have been discussed in general situations to allow the concepts to be applied to as many distinct devices as possible. Three specific examples of biomedical devices are now explored as case studies to further illustrate the cybersecurity concerns of real applications. Three devices considered further are (i) MRI machine, (ii) infusion pump, and (iii) implanted pacemaker. Each of these devices will be examined using a three-layer architecture consisting of sensing, communication, and control layers. The sensing layer includes sensors in communication with the device, which may be internal or external to the device. The communication layer includes the device's communication hardware and software, as well as the networks to which the device is connected. The control layer includes the device hardware and software that handles processing, programming, and device access. The control layer may include cloud processing or other external components.

5.1 Case Study: MRI Unit Cyberattack

MRI units are one of several connected devices that can be attacked by hackers. By gaining access to the MRI unit, hackers can access patient's files and protected information and even change the test procedure and parameters. The attack starts through the communication layer, which is generally the Internet network, and then the hacker can go laterally to gain access to the device's different control layers.

- **Sensing layer attack**:

A hacker can exploit the sensing layer of an MRI unit, for instance, by using metal detectors in the MRI room, a serious physical threat can be created by deactivating these important safety sensors.

- **Communication layer attack**:

The communication is the start point of many attacks on medical devices. The communication layer provides the hacker with access to the system, and from there he

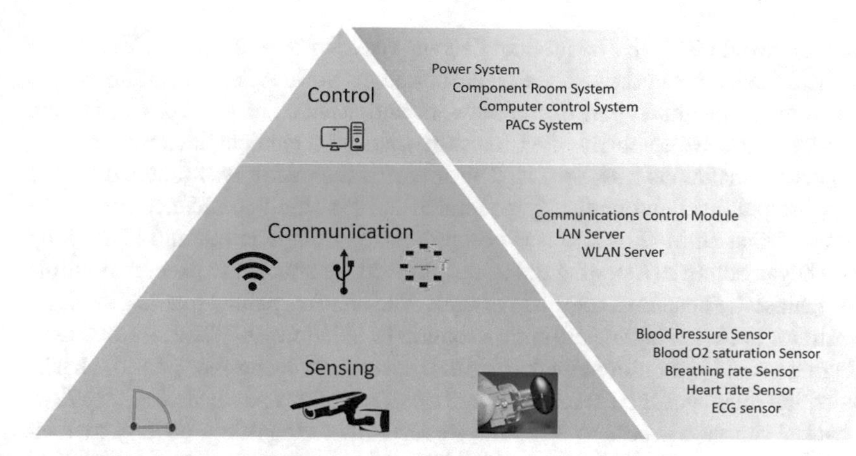

Fig. 3 Three layers in MRI unit

can gain full control of the device. In MRI, one of the communication layer potential attack points is the communication control module. It helps to translate messages between varying wireless communication standards and protocols for retransmission to other devices. The communication system is meant to transmit and/or receive data between physiological sensors, MRI controller, patient monitoring devices, patient entertainment devices, and other computers [68].

- **Control layer**:

The hacker can exploit the computers associated with MRI to change and monitor the operation procedures and parameters as well as MRI system components to cause damage to the equipment. In addition, the attack can reach the Picture Archiving and Communication System (PACS) and gain access to many patients' data.

- **PACS attack**:

The PACS serves to store medical images files such as X-ray, MRI, and CT scan images in Digital Imaging and Communications in Medicine (DICOM) format. It also includes a different type of data, like PDF files, that may be compressed within DICOM files. Hospitals have at least one centralized PACS system connected to all workstations and to the server. If an attacker succeeds to obtain access to the PACS, he can easily spread the malware or gain control to every internal and/or external connected device in the hospital. Figure 3 shows a three-layered framework for an MRI unit.

5.1.1 Attack Overview

In 2015, TRAPX security developed a cybersecurity product and tested it in four US hospitals. The product deploys a shifting minefield of Traps (decoys) and Deception Tokens (lures) that appear identical to the hospital's real IT and IoT assets that no attacker can avoid [69, 70]. The product decoys were deployed inside the VLANs of the medical device networks and the IT corporate network. After several hours, the decoys were an integrated part of the network and acted as medical devices (from a network perspective). Shortly after, malware touched a medical device decoy and tried injecting malicious files into it. The moment the decoy was touched by the attacker, the platform automatically generated the first high-confidence alert. The alert showed that an MRI device was compromised through an internal IT desktop and then began acting as a staging point that allowed the attacker to execute multiple attacks against the hospital's internal network. The attacker gained medical device's administrator access using a well-known exploit of Windows XP. The attacker used this staging point to run more attacks against the network using the "pass the hash" attack, which leverages the PsExec tool and other malicious payloads [64, 71, 72].

A hacker can gain access to a remote server without requiring, usually mandatory, plaintext passwords. This is possible if the attacker uses the underlying NTLM (Microsoft NT Lan Manager) hash of user's password, and this type of attack is commonly called a pass the hash hacking technique. For systems requiring true authentication, this hacking technique is usually unsuccessful; however, the decoy PACS system used as a trap captured the malicious load to allow the success of the attack. By the second day, a malware was discovered in the PACS trap allowed the company to follow the traces of the attack, detect the origin, and collect its details. The origin of the attack was from a device from a totally different segment of the hospital network. The malware learned the PACS location within the network and attempted to access to the PACS trap by performing pass the hash hacking technique. The trap allowed to detect a hidden malware in the hospital network; however, the attack was unsuccessful on the real PACS but the attacker had the impression that the attack was successful [1, 3, 73]. Table 11 presents the threat behaviors in PACS.

Table 11 Threat behaviors in PACS

Type of file	32-bit portable executable application identified as UPX 0.60-3.x
Application used	The application used the Windows graphical user interface (GUI) subsystem
Attack initiation	The malware virus dropped and executed an UPX packed executable in the user temporary directory
Structure of the attack	The malware virus spread via infected local drives, removable drives, emails, and network shares
Attack execution	The file was a DLL. The DLL was injected into the EXPLORER.EXE process, thereby keeping the malware resident in memory. Part of the medical devices had a mapped network share to a central server where medical files were saved (for instance, medical images). The malware attempted to take advantage of this network share and compromised these servers as well, using the same spreading method. In this case, the malware virus used an administrator account that allowed the attacker to access more medical devices from the same vendor. However, the security program alert allowed the security team to mitigate the attack quickly and avoid any further damage

5.2 *Case Study: Infusion Pump Cyberattack*

The components of an infusion pump that are relevant to cybersecurity can be classified into three layers: sensing, communication, and control. If an attacker is able to access one of these layers, he may then be able to spread the attack to the other layers. The components of each layer and some possible attack scenarios are given below.

- **Sensing Layer**

The sensing layer of an infusion pump is primarily composed of internal device sensors which monitor pump function and body-worn sensors to detect the patient's vital signs. To ensure accurate delivery of medication, the pump's flow rate and pressure should be monitored by the internal sensors. The patient vital status is monitored by the body sensors to detect any adverse reactions to the delivered medication. The body-worn sensors may communicate with the device controller via wireless or wired link.

Threats to the sensing layer are loss of sensor function and delivery of incorrect sensor data to the control layer. These attacks may cause the device to deliver inappropriate treatment or to cease treatment altogether. The sensors may be vulnerable to physical or electronic attacks, either of which can modify the sensor data before it is sent to the control layer.

- **Communication Layer**

The communication layer of the infusion pump includes wireless communication with the hospital network and possibly with body-worn sensors. The wireless hospital network allows healthcare providers to communicate with the device to schedule and monitor patient treatment. The hospital network also includes many connected computers, mobile devices, and biomedical devices, forming an Internet of things [74].

The most common attack point for an infusion pump is through the communication layer. The wireless connection is often weakly secured, and the passwords and security that are used may not be adequately updated [74]. Threats to the communication layer include eavesdropping, theft of protected health information, and execution of unauthorized commands.

- **Control Layer**

The device control layer for the infusion pump is an embedded system, onboard firmware and software, and online programming and updates. Loss of function of the infusion pump may occur in a non-attack scenario if a software or firmware update is interrupted or if exposure to harmful conditions (such as a strong MRI magnetic field) causes loss of data on the embedded system.

A common attack point for the control layer is through downloaded updates. If the updates are modified by an attacker, the pump's functioning may be maliciously altered. Inappropriate updates may also cause denial-of-service attacks, such as battery drainage or lockout of authorized personnel [74]. Figure 4 represents three layers

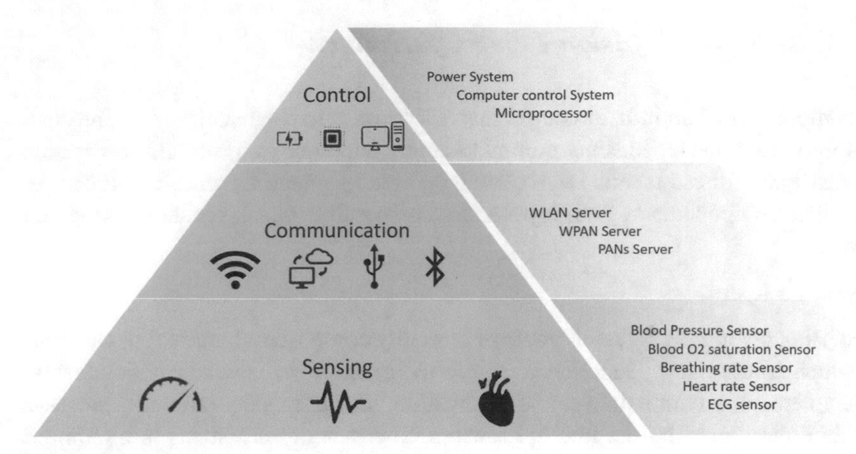

Fig. 4 Three layers in infusion pump

in infusion pump.

- **Attack Overview**

Concern about infusion pump performance and potential malfunction has been growing in recent years, prompting notices by the United States Food and Drug Administration (FDA) to pump manufacturers [63] and the creation of the FDA infusion pump improvement initiative [63]. The lack of continuous monitoring of pump performance after its implementation in the clinical setting is the central issue of the FDA communications. It is likely that some of the malfunctions are due to cyberattacks, but many clinical systems lack the resources to detect such an attack [75]. Because the devices are not adequately monitored by the manufacturer after implementation, their malfunctions may go undetected or undiagnosed [63].

In July 2015, the FDA issued a safety communication, warning healthcare teams that security vulnerabilities had been identified in certain Hospira Symbiq and LifeCare infusion pump models [76]. These vulnerabilities allowed the pump system to be remotely accessed through the hospital's wireless network via the system's communication layer [75]. The attacker could then gain access to the control layer to deliver inappropriate medication dosage or launch a denial-of-service attack [76]. The vulnerabilities in the device were not identified by the manufacturer, but rather by an independent hacker who reported the flaws to the United States Department of Homeland Security (DHS) [77], which then issued a statement about the security vulnerabilities [78]. Although no known attacks were launched on the devices, the affected pump models were pulled from market citing issues unrelated to cybersecurity after the FDA safety communication [76]; however, an unknown number of affected pump models remained in use and were still available from third-party retailers [79]. The DHS Advisory identified several security flaws in the pump devices, including failure to close unused ports (FTP and telnet ports), continued use of a default manufacturer password on port 8443, communication keys stored in plain text on the device, absence of authorization checking on the device, as well as other

Table 12 Cyber threats in infusion pump

Method of attack entry	Attacker gains remote access to the pump via the hospital network, which could be compromised through unsecured emails, etc. Hospira pump shipped with default password that went unchanged in many hospitals
Device vulnerabilities [78]	• Stack-based buffer overflow (can be exploited to execute attack code) • Improper authorization • Insufficient verification of data authenticity (device accepts updates without requiring authentication) • Default hard-coded password • Clear text storage of vital information • Poor key management (private keys and certificates stored on device) • Use of vulnerable software (versions of AppWeb) • Uncontrolled resource consumption (requires manual reboots)
Attack types	Reprogram device, denial-of-service, eavesdrop, track device
Attack outcome	No reported attacks actually occurred. In the event of a real attack, reprogramming the device to inappropriately deliver or withhold medication could lead to patient injury or death. Other attacks include eavesdropping to steal private health information, denial-of-service or jamming to make pump nonfunctional, or tracking the device within the hospital network to track the patient

vulnerabilities [75, 79, 76, 77]. Table 12 presents threat behaviors in infusion pump. Figures 5 and 6 represent network diagram of an MRI unit and an infusion pump, respectively.

5.3 Case Study: Implantable Medical Device Cyberattack

Implantable Medical Devices (IMDs) are used for diagnostic, monitoring, and therapeutic purposes. IMDs should be not only robust and effective but also secure and safe. Since the patient's life is depended on these electronic devices, only the authorized medical personnel should have access to the devices. There are several types of attacks reported by users and hospitals such as theft of protected health information and execution of fraudulent device commands. In this section, control, communication, and sensing layers in IMDs are studied and potential threats in the access schemes are presented to prevent unauthorized access.

The IMD access control schemes are divided into four categories including the access control architecture, the communication channel security keys type, the access control logic, and the access control channel [23].

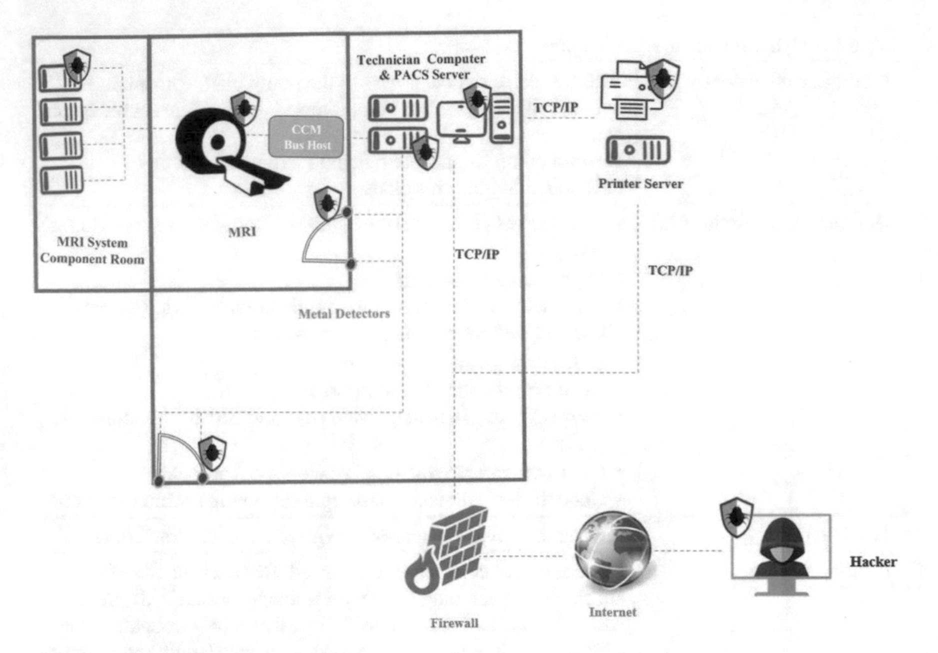

Fig. 5 Network diagram of an MRI unit

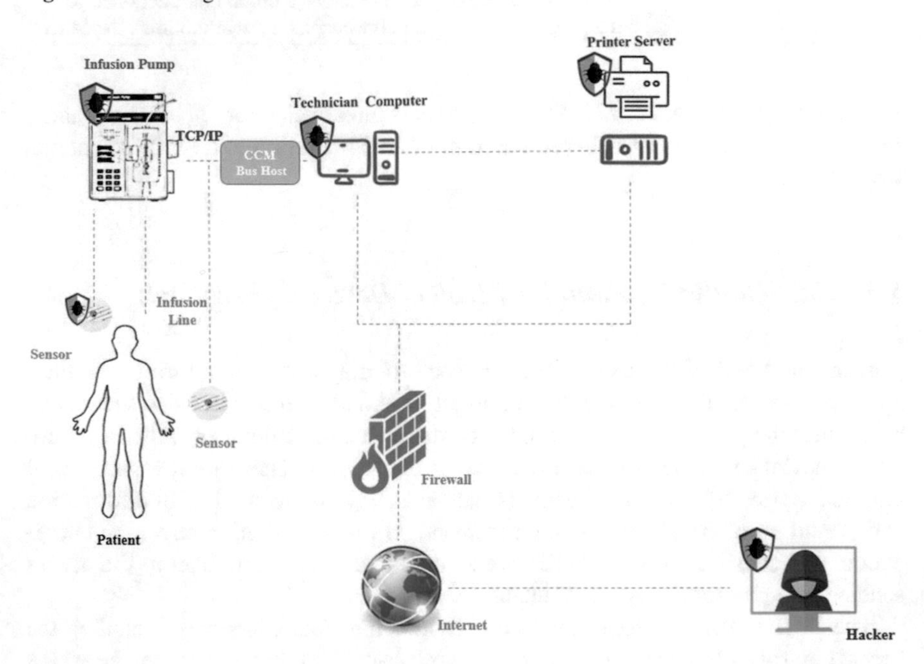

Fig. 6 Network diagram of an infusion pump

- **Control Layer**

Access Control Architecture: The authorized person is able to communicate with IMD directly and indirectly. In the case that user connects to IMD via a proxy device (indirect control), the user is able to specify proxy parameters [23].

Type of Keys: The preloaded permanent keys and the temporary keys generated from a certain source can be used to have direct and indirect access control [23].

Access Control Channel: The access control panel can be managed by ordinary activities such as human muscle motions and sound/video [23].

Access Control Logic: The logic of IMD access control using temporary and permanent keys is different. Access control logic is the key matching for the permanent keys and the access control logic for temporary keys is defined by the properties of the physical channel [26].

- **Communication Layer**

The other layer is communication. It is mandatory to study safety and protection conditions and risks to the Wireless Body Area Network (WBAN) communication structure [52].

The communication design in WBANs system has three levels as follows:

Intra-WBAN communication, the signals measured by sensors will be received by a personnel server (PS) acting as an entrance. The PS sends the collected data to the next level.

Inter-WBAN communication, the second tier is like a bridge between the PS and the user via Access Points (APs) that are accounted as a key component of the communication network.

Beyond-WBAN Communication, in this level, the medical history and specific profile of the patients are accommodated; therefore, a medical environment database is a necessity. It is worth mentioning the personal server in first level can directly connect to the third level of network via General Packet Radio Service (GPRS) or broadband cellular networks.

There are two modes of inter-WBAN communication, infrastructure-based mode communication and ad hoc-based mode communication. The infrastructure-based mode communication is used for most of the WBAN applications and provides better security than ad hoc-based mode communication and also performs like a database server. Although the ad hoc architecture setup is bigger, it promotes motion across much bigger areas [52].

5.3.1 Sensing Layer

The sensors are embedded in sensing layer. The aim of the sensing layer of implantable medical devices is to identify phenomena in human body and obtain data [66]. It is worth mentioning that the locations of sensors are not fixed because the body changes position [52]. Figure 7 depicts three layers in implantable medical devices.

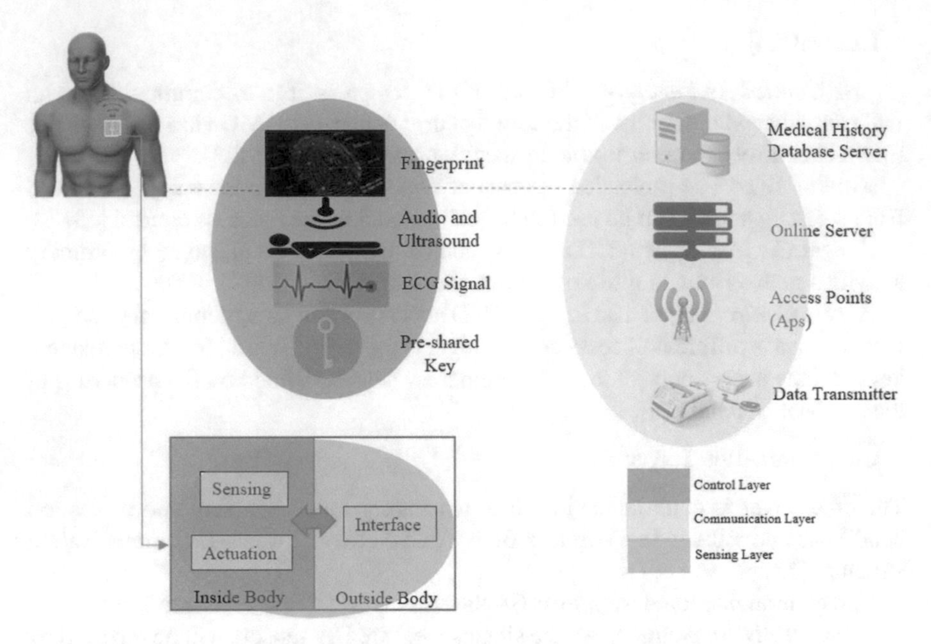

Fig. 7 Control, communication, and sensing layers in IMDs

5.3.2 Attack Overview

A new generation of pacemakers is equipped with wireless technologies to help cardiologists monitor how well the devices are functioning. There is a growing interest in using wireless systems for medical implants for data communication and in charging batteries of medical implants using Wireless Power Transfer (WPT) [80, 81]. Developing medical implants such as the pacemaker with wireless capabilities increases vulnerability to hacking attacks. The hacking attack of pacemakers was reported by the US Food and Drug Administration (FDA) in 2012. According to this report, in some cases the batteries in pacemakers were prematurely drained and in some others the devices were forced to excite the heart at deadly speeds [82]. In this case, the attack occurred in communication layer. To avoid these types of attacks, the patients are required to update their devices' firmware. The update can be done by trained medical staff and there is no need for any invasive surgery. Pacemakers with a remote monitoring unit last longer, have better battery life, have fewer inappropriate shocks and malfunctions, and have improved overall health management [82].

There was another alert issued by FDA regarding safety communication of implantable cardiac devices including Medtronic's Implantable Cardioverter Defibrillators (ICDs) and Cardiac Resynchronization Therapy Defibrillators (CRT-Ds). This FDA communication alerts users to the security vulnerabilities present due to communication between various components of these systems, including the implanted device itself, the home monitoring and data transmission stations, and

Table 13 Potential Implantable Medical Devices (IMDs) cyberattacks

Malicious hacker activity	Consequences
Manipulating access control of an affected product	The attacker is able to inject, modify, and intercept data within the telemetry communication [84]
Connecting to communication protocol	The attacker can change memory in the implanted cardiac device [84]
Having access to external controller unit of IMD	The attacker can reprogram the medical implants [85]
Connecting to medical history database server	The attacker can steal confidential information of the patients
Having access to the sensing layer	The unauthorized personnel are able to monitoring information collected by the sensors and manipulate data from sensors [86]
Controlling power range of transmitter in case that it is used for wireless power transfer (WPT)	The attacker can damage or burn the medical implants

programming devices in the clinic. The manipulation of cardiac device configured by clinic programmers is to be considered an attack in control layer [83].

The Medtronic Conexus Radio Frequency Telemetry Protocol is released by CISA in 2019 [84]. This protocol allows the Medtronic cardiac devices to wirelessly communicate between the implanted device, clinic-based programming and data-display stations, Medtronic-operated programming and update stations, and home data collection stations. Beyond safety features in the current Medtronic's implantable cardiac devices, multiple research teams are developing novel authentication and encryption strategies to improve robustness of medical device cybersecurity. The potential cyberattacks against Implantable Medical Devices (IMDs) are presented in Table 13.

6 Conclusion

A three-layered hierarchical framework categorizing the attack vectors of biomedical devices was discussed. Specifically, how the isolation of sensing, communication, and control layer framework in three medical devices as use cases: MRI unit, infusion pump, and implantable medical devices will help in mitigating the cyberattack vectors was presented. A review of several literatures on possible cyber threats that can occur in biomedical devices was detailed in this chapter. Such a framework will help provide some isolation and lead time to thwart attacks, and enable in implementation of cybersecurity policies in the intrusion detection systems or firewall units in healthcare organizations.

References

1. Robertson J, Reel M (2015) It's way too easy to hack the hospital. Wired. http://www.bloomberg.com/features/2015-hospital-hack/
2. Schich A (2019) Active medical devices. https://www.med-cert.com/en_certification/en_medical-device/
3. TrapX Labs (2015) Anatomy of an attack medjack (Medical Device Hijack), pp 1–39
4. U.S. Food and Drug Administration (2014) Content of Premarket Submissions for Management of Cybersecurity in Medical Devices Guidance for Industry and Food and Drug Administration Staff (Document Issued on: October 2, 2014), FDA Guide, p 6
5. FDA (2014) Content of Premarket Submissions for Management of Cybersecurity in Medical Devices Guidance for Industry and Food and Drug Administration Staff. FDA Guide, p 6
6. Witonsky P (2012) Leveraging EHR investments through medical device connectivity. Healthc Financ Manage 66(8):50–3
7. Brookstone A (2011) Pros and Cons of wireless and local networks. http://www.americanehr.com/blog/2011/08/the-pros-and-cons-of-wireless-and-local-networks/
8. Meldrum SJ (1979) Association for the advancement of medical instrumentation 14th annual meeting. J Med Eng Technol 3(5):259
9. Health Level Seven International (2014) Health Level Seven International: tools & resources. http://www.hl7.org/participate/toolsandresources.cfm
10. CEN/CT, "CEN/TC 251," (2015) European Committee for Standardization. http://cimlaboratory.com/
11. Personal Connected Health Alliance, "Personal Connected Health Alliance," (2018). http://www.pchalliance.org/
12. Brien GO, Brien GO, Edwards S (2017) Securing wireless infusion pumps in healthcare delivery organizations, p 354
13. Rodrigues JJPC, Sendra Compte S, de la Torra Diez I (2016) Digital imaging and communications in medicine. In: e-Health Systems, pp 53–74
14. IEEE 11073-10207-2017—IEEE Health informatics—Point-of-care medical device communication. IEEE Standards Association. https://standards.ieee.org/standard/11073-10207-2017.html
15. ISO, "ISO/TC 215 Health informatics," (1998). https://www.iso.org/committee/54960.html
16. Ayala L (2016) Cybersecurity for hospitals and healthcare facilities
17. Archibold RC (2001) Hospital details failures leading to M.R.I. fatality. The NewYork Times. http://www.nytimes.com/2001/08/22/nyregion/hospital-details-failures-leading-to-mri-fatality.html?src=pm
18. Challa S, Wazid M, Das AK, Khan MK (2018) Authentication protocols for implantable medical devices: taxonomy, analysis and future directions. IEEE Consum Electron Mag 7(1)
19. Wu F, Eagles S (2016) Cybersecurity for medical device manufacturers: ensuring safety and functionality. Biomed Instrum Technol 50(1)
20. Camara C, Peris-Lopez P, Tapiador JE (2015) Security and privacy issues in implantable medical devices: a comprehensive survey. J Biomed Informat 55
21. Klonoff DC (2015) Cybersecurity for connected diabetes devices. J Diabetes Sci Technol 9(5)
22. Zheng G, Zhang G, Yang W, Valli R, Shankaran R, Orgun MA (2018) From WannaCry to WannaDie: security trade-offs and design for implantable medical devices. In: 2017 17th international symposium communication informative technology ISC 2017, vol 2018-Janua, pp 1–5
23. Wu L, Du X, Guizani M, Mohamed A (2017) Access control schemes for implantable medical devices: a survey. IEEE Internet Things J
24. Ellouze N, Rekhis S, Boudriga N, Allouche M (2017) Cardiac implantable medical devices forensics: postmortem analysis of lethal attacks scenarios. Digit Investig
25. Zheng G et al (2019) A critical analysis of ecg-based key distribution for securing wearable and implantable medical devices. IEEE Sens J 19(3):1186–1198

26. Rekhis S, Boudriga N, Ellouze N (2017) Securing implantable medical devices against cyberspace attacks. In: 2017 2nd international conference anti-cyber crimes, ICACC 2017, pp 187–192
27. Pycroft L, Aziz TZ (2018) Security of implantable medical devices with wireless connections: the dangers of cyber-attacks. Expert Rev Med Devices 15(6):403–406
28. Mcdonald KA, Security CI, Clinic M, Wirth A, Architect DH (2018) The intersection of patient safety and medical device cybersecurity
29. Pycroft L et al (2016) Brainjacking: implant security issues in invasive neuromodulation. World Neurosurg 92
30. Altawy R, Youssef AM (2016) Security tradeoffs in cyber physical systems: a case study survey on implantable medical devices. IEEE Access 4
31. Hasan R, Zawoad S, Noor S, Haque MM, Burke D (2016) How secure is the healthcare network from insider attacks? An audit guideline for vulnerability analysis. In: Proceedings—international computer software and applications conference
32. Meng W, Li W, Wang Y, Au MH (2018) Detecting insider attacks in medical cyber–physical networks based on behavioral profiling. Future Generat Comput Syst
33. Kompara M, Hölbl M (2018) Survey on security in intra-body area network communication. Ad Hoc Netw 70
34. Arney D, Venkatasubramanian KK, Sokolsky O, Lee I (2011) Biomedical devices and systems security. In: Proceedings of the annual international conference of the IEEE engineering in medicine and biology society, EMBS
35. Williams PAH, Woodward AJ (2015) Cybersecurity vulnerabilities in medical devices: a complex environment and multifaceted problem. Med Devices Evidence Res 8
36. Ali B, Awad AI (2018) Cyber and physical security vulnerability assessment for IoT-based smart homes. Sensors (Switzerland)
37. Stine I, Rice M, Dunlap S, Pecarina J (2017) A cyber risk scoring system for medical devices. Int J Crit Infrastruct Prot
38. Kramer DB, Fu K (2017) Cybersecurity concerns and medical devices lessons from a pacemaker advisory. JAMA J Am Med Assoc
39. Lee M, Lee K, Shim J, Cho SJ, Choi J (2017) Security threat on wearable services: empirical study using a commercial smartband. In: 2016 IEEE international conference on consumer electronics-Asia, ICCE-Asia 2016
40. Jagannathan S, Sorini A (2016) Self-authentication in medical device software: an approach to include cybersecurity in legacy medical devices. In: ISPCE 2016—proceedings: IEEE symposium on product compliance engineering
41. Pozzobon O, Canzian L, Danieletto M, Chiara AD (2010) Anti-spoofing and open GNSS signal authentication with signal authentication sequences. In: Programme and abstract book—5th ESA workshop on satellite navigation technologies and European workshop on GNSS Signals and signal processing, NAVITEC 2010
42. Salem A, Zaidan D, Swidan A, Saifan R (2016) Analysis of strong password using keystroke dynamics authentication in touch screen devices. In: Proceedings—2016 cybersecurity and cyberforensics conference, CCC 2016
43. Anderson S, Williams T (2018) Cybersecurity and medical devices: are the ISO/IEC 80001-2-2 technical controls up to the challenge? Comput Stand Interfaces
44. Kulac S, Sazli MH, Ilk HG (2018) External relaying based security solutions for wireless implantable medical devices: a review. In: Proceedings of the 2018 11th IFIP wireless and mobile networking conference, WMNC 2018
45. Gao Y, Liu W (2015) A security routing model based on trust for medical sensor networks. In: Proceedings of 2015 IEEE international conference communication software networks, ICCSN 2015, pp 405–408
46. Wazid M, Das AK, Kumar N, Conti M, Vasilakos AV (2018) A novel authentication and key agreement scheme for implantable medical devices deployment. IEEE J Biomed Heal Informat 22(4):1299–1300

47. Das AK, Wazid M, Kumar N, Khan MK, Choo KKR, Park YH (2018) Design of secure and lightweight authentication protocol for wearable devices environment. IEEE J Biomed Heal Informat
48. Challa S et al (2018) An efficient ECC-based provably secure three-factor user authentication and key agreement protocol for wireless healthcare sensor networks. Comput Electr Eng 69:534–554
49. Ellouze N, Rekhis S, Boudriga N, Allouche M (2018) Powerless security for cardiac implantable medical devices: use of wireless identification and sensing platform. J Netw Comput Appl
50. Paliokas I, Tsoniotis N, Votis K, Tzovaras D (2019) A blockchain platform in connected medical-device environments: trustworthy technology to guard against cyberthreats. IEEE Consum Electron Mag 8(4):50–55
51. BSI (2019) Multi-part Document BS EN 419251—security requirements for device for authentication. The British Standards Institution. https://landingpage.bsigroup.com/LandingPage/Series?UPI=BS EN 419251
52. Al-Janabi S, Al-Shourbaji I, Shojafar M, Shamshirband S (2017) Survey of main challenges (security and privacy) in wireless body area networks for healthcare applications. Egypt Informat J 18(2)
53. Kohli S, Exploring cyber security vulnerabilities in the age of IoT. Cyber Security Threats, IGI Global, 1609–1623
54. Xu J, Venkatasubramanian KK, Sfyrla V (2016) A methodology for systematic attack trees generation for interoperable medical devices. In: 10th annual international systems conference, SysCon 2016—Proceedings
55. Mosenia A, Jha NK (2018) OpSecure: a secure unidirectional optical channel for implantable medical devices. IEEE Trans Multi Scale Comput Syst 4(3):410–419
56. Mikson C, Hammargren L, Strunk E (2017) Medical devices and data: protecting patients and their PHI
57. Alabdulatif A, Khalil I, Yi X, Guizani M (2019) Secure edge of things for smart healthcare surveillance framework. IEEE Access
58. Chizari H, Lupu EC (2019) Extracting randomness from the trend of IPI for cryptographic operators in implantable medical devices. IEEE Trans Dependable Secur Comput
59. Gaukstern E, Krishnan S (2018) Cybersecurity threats targeting networked critical medical devices. In: ASEE IL-IN section conference, vol 2
60. Owens B (2016) Stronger rules needed for medical device cybersecurity. Lancet 387(10026):1364
61. Slotwiner D (2019) Editorial commentary: cybersecurity of cardiac implantable electronic devices—role of the clinician. Trends Cardiovasc Med
62. Slotwiner DJ, Deering TF, Fu K, Russo AM, Walsh MN, Van Hare GF (2018) Cybersecurity vulnerabilities of cardiac implantable electronic devices: communication strategies for clinicians. Hear Rhythm
63. FDA (2014) Infusion pumps—infusion pump improvement initiative
64. Trapx B (2018) MEDJACK.4 medical device Hijacking, pp 1–29
65. Sabio R (2017) 5 ways to detect a cyber attack. Huffpost. https://www.huffingtonpost.ca/2017/01/30/detect-cyber-attack_n_13880814.html
66. Sikder AK, Petracca G, Aksu H, Jaeger T, Uluagac AS (2018) A survey on sensor-based threats to
67. Anand K (2016) Healthcare cyber security and compliance guide. Imperva
68. Brown MJ, Herrera B (2013) Method and apparatus for MRI compatible communications. US20140275970A1
69. Tomlinson K (2017) The lurker in your MRI machine wants money, not your life. Archer Energy Solutions LLC. https://archerint.com/the-lurker-in-your-mri-machine-wants-money-not-your-life/
70. TrapX (2019) The most effective solution for advanced breach detection. https://trapx.com/product/
71. Ewaida B (2010) Pass-the-hash attacks: tools and mitigation, p 53
72. Jadeja N, Parmar V (2016) Implementation and mitigation of various tools for pass the hash attack. Proc Comput Sci

73. Perez R (2017) Article 29 Working Party still not happy with Windows 10 privacy controls. Haymarket Media, Inc. http://www.scmagazine.com/home/security-news/privacy-compliance/article-29-working-party-still-not-happy-with-windows-10-privacy-controls/
74. O'Brien G, Edwards S, Littlefield K, McNab N, Wang S, Zheng K (2018) Securing wireless infusion pumps in healthcare delivery organizations
75. CISA (2013) Hospira Symbiq infusion system. Biomed Saf Stand 43(18):144
76. FDA (2017) LifeCare PCA3 and PCA5 infusion pump systems by Hospira: FDA safety communication—security vulnerabilities. https://wayback.archive-it.org/7993/20170112164109/http:/www.fda.gov/Safety/MedWatch/SafetyInformation/SafetyAlertsforHumanMedicalProducts/ucm446828.htm
77. Thomson I (2015) This hospital drug pump can be hacked over a network—and the US FDA is freaking out. Register. https://www.theregister.co.uk/2015/08/01/fda_hospitals_hospira_pump_hacks/
78. CISA (2015) Hospira Plum A+ and Plum A+3 Infusion systems. Biomed Saf Stand 45(8):60–61
79. Stanley N, Coderre M (2016) An introduction to medical device cyber security a European perspective. Healthc Inf Manag Syst Soc
80. Shadid R, Haerinia M, Sayan R, Noghanian S (2018) Hybrid inductive power transfer and wireless antenna system for biomedical implanted devices. Prog Electromagn Res C 88(June):77–88
81. Haerinia M (2018) Modeling and simulation of inductive-based wireless power transmission systems. In: Olfa K (eds) Energy harvesting for wireless sensor networks: technology, components and system design, 1st edn., De Gruyter: Berlin, Germany; Boston, MA, USA, pp 197–220
82. Alpine Security (2019) Most dangerous hacked medical devices. https://www.alpinesecurity.com/blog/most-dangerous-hacked-medical-devices
83. US FDA (2019) Cybersecurity vulnerabilities affecting medtronic implantable cardiac devices, programmers, and home monitors: FDA safety communication
84. Department of Homeland Security (2019) Medtronic conexus radio frequency telemetry protocol
85. P. S. Development (2011) Integrated circuits for implantable medical devices
86. Cichonski J (2019) Security for IOT sensor building management systems case study

Foued Badrouchi is currently a Ph.D. candidate at the University of North Dakota (UND), Grand Forks, North Dakota, USA. He received his B.Sc and M.Sc. degree in Petroleum engineering from Boumerdes University (UMBB), Algeria, in 2015. He is currently an Instructor and Teaching Assistant at the Department of Petroleum Engineering. He is also a Lab Manager and serves as the President of the Society of Petroleum Engineers UND student chapter. He is also named as Technical Advisor for a Petroleum Cybernetics graduate program in Algeria. He is part of a team focusing on kidney transplantation amelioration. His research interest includes Petroleum Engineering, machine learning, biomedical engineering, and kidney transplantation.

Abby Aymond is a Master of Biomedical Engineering student at the University of North Dakota (UND). Her thesis focus is the development of an electronic device to monitor and analyze cardiovascular signals in the user's home environment. She received a Bachelor of Science in electrical engineering with a focus in biomedical engineering from UND.

Mohammad Haerinia received his B.Sc. and M.Sc. degree in Electrical Engineering. Currently, he is researching at the University of North Dakota, ND, the USA in the field of Biomedical Engineering. His research interest includes wireless power transfer (WPT), WPT for medical devices, design of the implantable antenna, and applied electromagnetics. He is a member of IEEE-Eta Kappa Nu (IEEE-HKN), the honor society of IEEE. He serves as a Reviewer for

Institution of Engineering and Technology (IET) Journals (Power Electronics, Electronics Letters and Microwaves, Antennas & Propagation), and also IEEE Journals (Antennas and Wireless Propagation Letters, Antennas and Propagation Magazine).

Samarra Badrouchi is a graduate student at the Medical School of Tunis, Tunisia. She is currently completing her residency in Nephrology at the Internal Medicine and Nephrology Department, Charles Nicolle's Hospital, Tunisia. She worked for one year as an intern in different departments in the hospitals of Tunis and worked one year as a volunteer in the Endocrinology Department in the Tunisian Institute of Nutrition. She succeeded in the national exam of specialization in medicine. She is currently working on her Medical Doctor degree (Ph.D.) and she is the head of a research team focusing on studying and ameliorating the Kidney Transplantation Experience using Machine Learning. Her research interests include dialysis, kidney transplantation, and the use of artificial intelligence in the medical field.

Daisy Flora Selvaraj is currently a postdoctoral research fellow at the University of North Dakota (UND), Grand Forks, North Dakota, USA. She received her B.E degree in Electrical and Electronics Engineering from Bharathidasan University, India, in 1999 and the M.E degree in High Voltage Engineering from Anna University, India, in 2008 and the Ph.D. degree in Electrical engineering from Visvesvaraya Technological University (VTU), Belgaum, India in 2018. From 2013 to 2017, she was a Senior Research Fellow at R&D Management Division of Central Power Research Institute, Bengaluru. Her research interest includes smart grid, data analytics, cyberphysical systems, control algorithms for smart grid, condition monitoring of power apparatus, and machine learning algorithms.

Kouhyar Tavakolian joined the Electrical Engineering department in March 2014. Prior to joining UND, he was a postdoctoral fellow at ECE department at the University of British Columbia, Vancouver, Canada for 2 years. He received his B.Sc. in Biomedical Engineering from Tehran Polytechnic in 2000, M.Sc. degree in Bioelectrical Engineering from Electrical Engineering department at the University of Tehran in 2003, and another M.Sc. degree in Computer Science from University of Northern British Columbia, Canada in 2005. His particular interest is in biological signal and image processing, biomedical instrumentation, and noninvasive cardiology technologies, and he has published more than a hundred journal, conference proceedings, patents, and book chapters in these fields.

Prakash Ranganathan is currently an Assistant Professor of Electrical Engineering and also serving as the Research Director for Data Energy Cyber and Systems (DECS) Laboratory at the University of North Dakota (UND). His research areas include operations research, smart grid, data mining, and cybersecurity. He is a senior IEEE member and member of Research Institute for Autonomous Systems (RIAS), a center for advancing autonomous systems, data, and cybersecurity research. He also plays a leadership role in cyber educational initiatives for the North Dakota University System (NDUS). He is a recipient of the College of Engineering and Mines (CEM)'s Dean's Outstanding Faculty Award; North Dakota Spirit Faculty Achievement Award from UND Alumni Foundation recognizing his significant contribution in teaching, research, and service and a Public Scholar Award from Center for Community Engagement. He earned his Ph.D. in Software Engineering from North Dakota State University (NDSU). He also plays a mentorship role for several native American students and tribal college faculty across the tribal reservations in the State of North Dakota.

Sumathy Eswaran is currently a professor of Computer Science and Dean at Dr. MGR Educational and Research Institute, India. She holds rich experience of 15 years from Industry and 15 years in academics. She has 30+ publications. Her interest is in data management, data sciences, and education management.

Smart Healthcare Use Cases and Applications

A. R. Charulatha and R. Sujatha

Abstract The growth of IoT is tremendous and is making its presence into nearly every space from industries to health care. The healthcare industry is now getting embraced by technological innovations. IoT is making the promise of smart and connected care a reality. Leading technologies such as Big Data, IoT, advanced analytics, and many other technological modernizations have turned the old-style health care into smart health care. Smart health care can be defined as using mobile and electronic technology for efficient diagnosis of the disease, better-quality treatment of the patients, and improved quality of lives. The healthcare industry is rapidly adopting Internet of things technologies in everything from wearable's to patient monitoring, in order to improve precision, endorse efficiency, cut costs, and boost health and augment safety. The newest research conducted by industry experts shows how the market for smart healthcare solutions is growing at a tremendous pace. IoT is an enabler to drive better asset utilization; new revenues achieve improved care for patients and reduced costs. In addition, it has the potential to revolutionize how health care is delivered. The new features offered by distributed analytics and edge intelligence, if successfully applied for time-sensitive healthcare applications, have great potential to accelerate the discovery of early notification of emergency situations to support smart decision-making. Smart health care, which monitors users' living settings and health status using wearable sensing devices and collecting their data over a network under daily life, is expected as a new trend. It is getting more attention along with the increase of demands of preventive care. This chapter gives an overview on the range of applications for the Internet of Things, share examples that illustrate how IoT products and services are being deployed around the globe, by heathcare industry in some areas like image management, visualization, remote health and monitoring, healthcare asset tracking, health monitoring using wearable devices, enhanced drug management, and patient flow analysis. IoT customer case

A. R. Charulatha (✉)
Department of Computer Science, Stella Maris College, University of Madras, Chennai, India
e-mail: latha.arc@gmail.com

R. Sujatha
School of Information Technology & Engineering, Vellore Institute of Technology, Vellore, India
e-mail: r.sujatha@vit.ac.in

P. Raj et al. (eds.), *Internet of Things Use Cases for the Healthcare Industry*,
https://doi.org/10.1007/978-3-030-37526-3_8

studies help to demonstrate the breadth of possibilities for IoT applications in health care.

Keywords Health care · Big data analytics · Distributed analytics · Edge intelligence · Hospital management

1 Introduction

1.1 Health Care

The health of human is primary for the growth of the nation in both technical level and economical level. Normally, health is classified into physical, emotional, mental, social, environmental, and spiritual. Ensuring ill-free pleasant state is called as health and in the process of maintaining and improving the same falls under health care. Health care is the largest sector in any nation and need for the well-being in ultimate need of all the people surviving in the world. A large amount of revenue flow is prevailing along with ample employment opportunities in all various phases. Health care encompasses clinics, devices, and gadgets to address the various issues, insurance sector, drugs, and so on. Digitalization and systemization of traditional healthcare unit made it support all the stakeholders in a big way. The proposed software framework in this chapter is a great step toward health surveillance [1]. The work carried out this challenging particularly for elderly people health by tracking and observing with the help of the multi-agent system and used efficient highly user-friendly interface along with reinforcement technique to strengthen the system [2–4]. Data sharing in health care is a significant and cumbersome process with various stakeholders from patient, hospital, private clinics, insurance, and pharmacies. Work insists on sharing data among cross-organization for providing best and timely service to all involved based on the time frame. Still, policies prevail for exchange of data but perfect designing of the system is required to smooth the process [5]. Data sharing comes with the issue of security. Various technologies used are authentication, encryption, data masking, and access control to tackle cross-organization in the process of sharing data. These have given a preview about laws governed in different places across the globe. Privacy-preserving is challenging due to the hefty data generated in each process [6]. The exponential growth of data made the decision-making process tough and at times impossible. Researchers normally use statistics and economy-related stuff to narrow down. But all this cumulated pave way for data mining and its highly interdisciplinary field that fetched ideas of various disciplines. Various tasks like anomaly detection, classification, clustering, association rule mining, regression, and summarization accumulated the data. Usage of data mining is inevitable and in the healthcare industry, it's widely used along with machine learning concept for faster decision-making [7]. Global healthcare outlook given by Deloitte in shaping the future indicates the need for care outside the walls of the hospital and also mentions it as an increasing trend. This could be aided with the

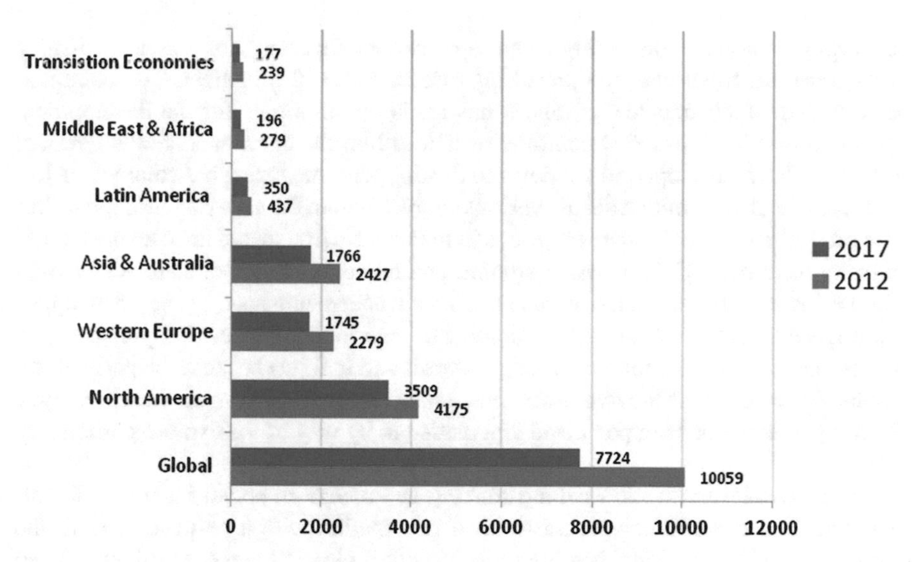

Fig. 1 Healthcare spending in USD Billion

help of virtual health. Digital reality—combination of augmented, mixed, and virtual reality component, IoMT—interconnected all devices with the patient for monitoring and tracking and so on to address the challenges in a medical environment for ensuring treatment at earliest. So many challenges are faced based on demographic and economic policies across the world. In spite of so many hurdles, the spending on a reliable system to serve patient is on a steep increase. Figure 1 illustrates the healthcare spending provided by economic intelligence unit [8].

1.2 IoT

Internet of things (IoT) is one of the main favorable technologies within the modern-day age. The worldview evaluation is taken into consideration by way of utilizing savvy and self-configuring items which could interact with each different by means of the worldwide setup framework. Ultimately, these unified in-built among large quantities of various gadgets talk to IoT as a taxing innovation that empowers plentiful and inescapable computing programs. Hence, the exact range of commercial enterprise IoT applications is developed and deployed in several domain names like transportation, agriculture, energy, health care, food technique business, military, environmental observance, or security police work. Eventually, IoT unites the devices and different gadgets to the Internet; it performs a core function to hold the development of smart facilities. The dynamic matters accumulate diverse varieties of statistics from this present reality circumstance [9]. Sometime later, the extraction of essential information from IoT data can be applied to improve and boost our everyday lifestyles with setting aware applications that may, for example, display substance identified with the prevailing circumstance of the client. The combination of huge facts and IoT advances has made opportunities for the development of administrations for a few complex structures like clever cities. A few big record advances have developed to support the dealing with the extensive volumes of IoT records, which are collected from various sources within the savvy environment. But the progression of IoT and its programs in many exclusive spaces are causing a noteworthy increment of the massive amount and numerous kinds of statistics. Within the period in-between, massive facts and its advancements have opened new application openings for industries and the scholarly world to grow new IoT preparations. Consequently, the combination of large records and IoT, just because the particularly dynamic evolution of the two areas, make new research challenges, which anyway have up to now not been perceived and tended to by way of the explore community [10].

The essential motivation behind making use of IoT in social insurance is collectively and dissects nonstop restorative information with a purpose to limit the constraints of conventional healing remedy, except cloud ranges are utilized to keep and analyze the gathered medicinal facts circulate. Consequently, the assembled data approximately the patient's well-being repute permits the human offering institutions to create typical social coverage programs and advance the contemporary administrations and preparations, for instance, programs for far off observing, nourishment, therapeutic merchandise, scientific gadgets, restorative workplace, or clinical coverage. Consequently, the utility of IoT in human offering area allows discovering the satisfactory health situation and getting a better plan for patients [11].

1.3 Big Data Analytics

The growth of big data is well mentioned by Domo.

According to Domo, world's Internet usage has increased steeply. On comparison of the year 2016 with 2017, the global Internet population has grown 7.5%. Data never sleeps 6.0 that provides the insights of the generated data for every minute. It's predicted that by 2020, each resident on earth will create 1.7 MB of data each second [12].

- The weather channel receives 18,055,555 forecast requests.
- Giphy serves 1,388,889 GIFS.
- Netflix users stream 97,222 h of video.
- Snapchat users share 2,083,333 photos.
- LinkedIn gains 120+ new professionals.
- YouTube users watch 4,333,560 videos.
- Twitter users send 473,400 tweets.
- Texts sent 12,98,611.
- Skype users make 176,220 calls.

- Instagram users post 49,380 photos.
- Americans use 3,138.420 GB of Internet data.
- Spotify streams over 750,000 songs.
- Uber riders take 1,389 trips.
- Venmo processes $68,493 peer-to-peer transactions.
- Google conducts 3,877,140 searches.
- Bitcoin 1.25 new are created.
- Reddit receives 1,944 comments.
- Tumblr users publish 79,740 posts.
- Amazon delivers 1,111 packages.

The above stats show us that huge data is generated via various sectors [13].

Big data is retrieving of hefty data from various sources like web, mobile devices, and other sorts of electronic gadgets. Integrating the data and managing and analyzing the data are a challenging task. The characteristics of data are volume, veracity, velocity, and variety. Best practices are based on goals align big data, use the center of excellence to optimize the transfer of knowledge, and cloud operating makes it still more useful [14].

The ultimate need for big data analytics is that it provides the patient-centric facility, tracking the disease spread at earlier by analyzing data, hospital quality validating and optimize treatment strategy, and so on. Each and every researcher works with a different strategy and brings a versatile framework to ensure optimal usage of data among various stakeholders. Electronic health record acts as the base to serve all sorts of service for taking the decision and achieved by integrating the required algorithm in a tactical manner [15]. IoT is the important counterpart of big data. Sensors produce data at each time stamp and interconnection of various devices makes the framework potential resource for researchers. This chapter shows clearly the combination of IoT with big data in the manufacturing industry and similar happens in the healthcare industry [16].

Big data analytics relying on IoT finds great application in health care like health monitoring system in a real-time and remote fashion, ubiquitous recognizing using inference system, life care, and emergency system, treating the disease at earliest [17]. Research is carried out for analyzing big data with the healthcare wearable devices. Model is designed based on consumer and providers' perspective. Efficiency and privacy risk are taken into consideration in consumer and benefit and cost based on the provider's point of view, respectively. Scope of work is possible by taking into account all perspectives [18].

Gartner provided great insight into big data in various industries, and it illustrates medical and insurance having great hands in Fig. 2 [19].

1.4 Smart Health Care

Smart Health Care

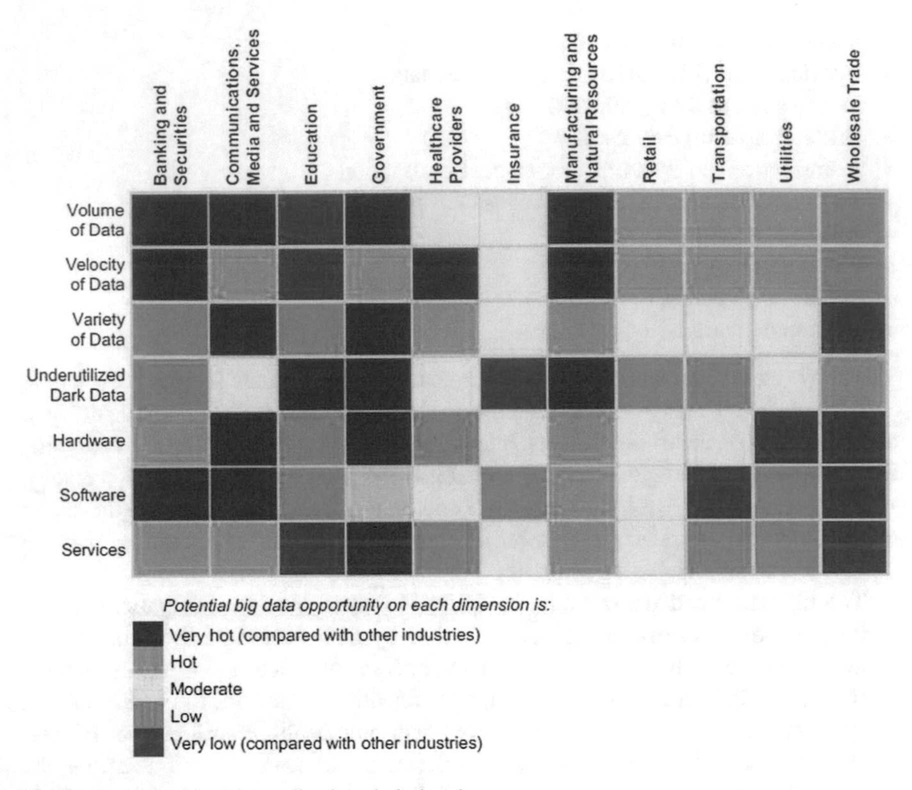

Fig. 2 Gartner—big data applications in industries

A smart cities concept joins hands with electronic health to provide smart health. Fascinating words like e-health, m-health, and s-health are made this era of ICT prudent. Machine learning concept is rocking s-health with its fast algorithms like deep learning, deep forest to make highly accurate decision-making in various places like glaucoma diagnosis, Alzheimer disease analysis, bacterial sepsis diagnose, and cataract treatment. Smart health is a framework comprising data acquisition, the flow of data, and processing of the same with trending algorithms [20]. Google trend illustrated in Fig. 3 shows that e-health, m-health, and s-health are active research terms in recent years. The interest of researchers and the popularity of the terms are

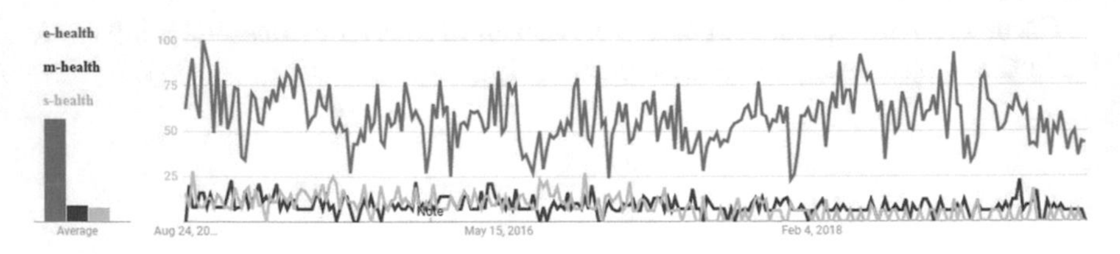

Fig. 3 e-health, m-health, and s-health based on Google trend

competing in nature. Technologies are making door to serve people at a faster phase in health industry [21].

Medical ontology is a great milestone in organizing the related terms under a single umbrella. Preparing ontology is a lengthy process after the number of discussions. Various steps are entity extraction and taxonomy formation, and interactions among concepts are mentioned as relationships and axioms creation. Consistency checking is made finally to ensure no redundancies. Ontology-based system is a great boon to the remote area and in absentee of medical experts to give preliminary guidance based on medical history and semantic of constructed ontology [22–24]. A smart home is an interesting phenomenon, and they have developed a home ontology that helps in providing semantics for the words exchanged via devices interconnected in the home. Knowledge sharing is performed by combining smart home with cloud computing to make the processing faster and accurate. Health monitoring system is optimized by incorporating cloud environment and patients get an immediate response [25].

1.5 Distributed Analytics and Edge Intelligence

In the current era, the data to be handled is large and faster processing is a quiet challenging task. To overcome this, edge along with distributed analytics is utilized. In the distributed analytics process, data is spread across multiple nodes and algorithms run and finally aggregated to get insights. In massive data scenario, a fast solution is possible by working on nodes. Smart farming and smart homework with the help of these technologies [26]. Decentralized way of handling data is the unique feature of edge computing process. The nearby spot is utilized for analyzing the data. Introduction of intelligence in the computing process is the great shift from the traditional way of handling data. Benefits of edge computing are decision-making is faster, communication cost is reduced, and based on requirement load balance is maintained. Characteristics like mobility, autonomy, security, local and WAN network bandwidth, prioritization, peer communication, and self-organization need all sectors resolved by using a tactical manner of intelligence with machine learning algorithms [27]. Slotted way of collecting the data is taken into consideration to make the environment hassle-free and efficient data analysis.

The work was carried out with edge of thing to make it cost-effective in nature [28]. By combining the idea of edge computing work carried out in all sectors and in this work, care is taken to consider the emergency situation of the patient and serving them at the fast phase to ensure safety. Integrated cognitive concept is based on data and resource along with cloud and edge platform based on the situation healthcare function [29].

2 Smart Healthcare Use Cases and Applications

The world population grows at a faster pace and so is the addition of new diseases in people. People of all ages are affected, and the hospitalization costs of health care for these diseases are more. The health monitoring of the common people without hospitalization is made possible with help of technologies like IoT, EoT, and CoT. More advancements and findings in sensing technologies create possibilities to develop wearable devices to monitor health and human behavior. These transformations through these technologies are a boon to elderly people in particular. The innovation of sensing technologies facilitates to develop smarter systems to monitor human behaviors regularly. In recent years, the mobile and wearable technologies which are developed to collect data from human based on their activities and vital signs have increased. Wrist wearables, accelerometer, pedometer as well as sensors which are used to calculate heart rate and those devices that provide important data are commonly available in market. Also, people use devices which monitor their sleep and stress levels to help people on the regulation of their activities [30].

The IoT concept in healthcare domain involves tracking, authentication, automatic data collection, and sensing. The medical condition data about a person is confidential, and data should not be exposed to unauthorized party. If there is no proper security mechanism, then data can be mishandled by malicious user leading to the doctor prescribing wrong medicines or giving bad treatments to their patient. For example, changes to a blood test result may exacerbate the patient's condition because of accepting a mismatched blood during blood transferring process [31].

2.1 Healthcare Monitoring

A typical healthcare architecture of wearable devices is shown in Fig. 4. Many researches are undertaken in identifying various sensors and algorithms to extract data from these wearables in an efficient way.

Md. Zia Uddin, in his work, proposes a sensor-based wearable system for foreseeing the activity by means of recurrent neural network on device like PC or laptop. Multiple wearable healthcare sensors supply the input data of the system with help of sensors like electrocardiography, magnetometer, etc. An recurrent neural network is trained based on the features, which is then used for predicting the activities [32].

Sun, Zang et al. proposed a study on emerging technology identity recognition with respect to gait pattern of an individual. Elderly patients tend to share their wearable devices with other family members or friends of their age. To access these wearable devices, it would be difficult for them to remember passwords. Also, the data present in these wearable devices should be secured. To protect the data as well as making it easily accessible by elderly, a gait-based identity recognition method used for the access control of aged people wearable healthcare devices is introduced. This lessens the problem that occurs because of gait fluctuation within a person and

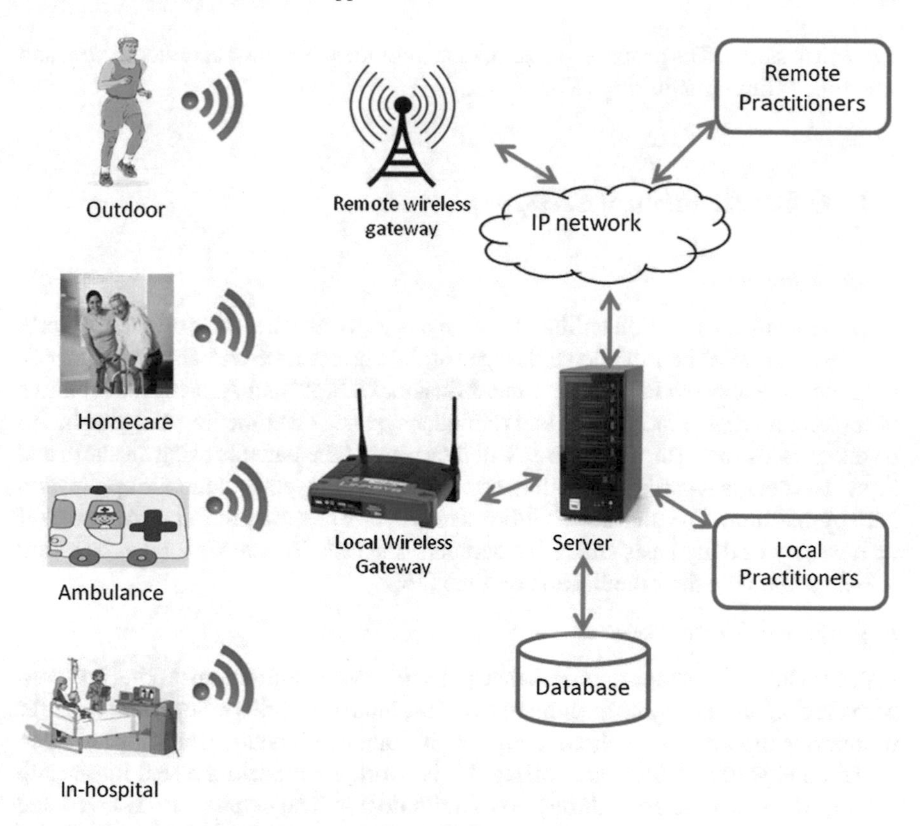

Fig. 4 Typical architecture of wearable devices in health care

provides a considerable access control recognition rate improvement more than 95% when compared to existing methods [33].

Romare et al. suggested that intensive care unit patient's conditions can change at a rapid rate, necessitating a quick and correct response from staff in charge of the unit to save life. For making proper decision on treatment to be offered to these patients, vital signs are important. Smart glasses are a relatively new platform for applications that works by touch or voice and can display text, images, take pictures, and transfer these data using Wi-Fi or Bluetooth to communicate, which thereby possibly improves observation and safety of patients in intensive care [34].

Zouka and Hosni aim at combining artificial technology in a healthcare monitoring system. This actually facilitates the system to work as an independent smart healthcare model which decides the treatment priority by itself depending on the collected health parameters from the sensors. The researcher proposes a model containing a trust environment which is in charge for collecting the physiological data from the patient's body. The collected data is communicated through mobile communication to IoT hub where the raw data using logic-based algorithm gets converted into linguistic form. The fuzzy-based algorithm is skilled in inference system to get the patient status. The proposed system, then, provides reliable, accurate, secure, and real-time patient monitoring [35].

2.2 Other Healthcare Sectors

Drug management

To prevent any dysfunction or illness, patients have to take medicine on time. Elderly people often miss their medicine dosages at the correct time and also forget which medicine they have to take at that time. Minaam, D. S. A. and Abd-ELfattah build a pillbox for medicine monitoring and reminder system. The time the medicine has to be taken needs to be set. The pillbox will then remind the patients using an alarm and light. The details regarding the pill to be taken are displayed by a mobile application held by the client. The traditional pillbox needs to be stacked by the client or caretaker on a weekly or daily basis which is a cumbersome task. This model comes as an aid to elders to intake their medication on time [36].

Employee health management

Kati and Otto proposed an approach that will handle various problems taking into concern the characteristics and the limitations of the industry workers. Several devices for monitoring the workplace, discovering a varied range of biodata, which are analyzed based on objective details, are collected. The worker's biodata are sent to e-health server, which will be gone through by family doctor. The details are reviewed and suggestions are given based on the details collected over a period of time. This helps the industry to have a concern on their employees and also increase the employee's performance by taking care of his health issues at the correct moment [37].

Patient Identity management

Benjamin et al. proposed an algorithm to collect consistent patient's health data in a uniform and well-timed manner which is the prime factor in making healthcare decisions. Cloud infrastructure is proposed to maintain a consolidated view of data appropriate to patient for hospital management and doctors, an essential requirement for facilitating performance management of care processes. Cloud computing technologies help healthcare providers to communicate information, improve association, and reduce cost on computing infrastructure [38].

Remote health monitoring

Majeed et al. developed "CogSense" an IoT device system that uses conventional sensors to enable instantaneous concern for patients, and professional response with the caretakers and doctors in a combined framework. This researcher captures a person's emotions and approximate physiological changes using voice recorder and camera to identify the emotions of the person and to predict the physiological changes such as heartbeat and blood pressure [39].

2.3 Wearable Devices

Wearable devices have been life-changing for those with chronic disease like diabetes, pain, and heart ailments. Companies produce various wearable devices likc fitness trackers, smartwatches, etc., as illustrated in Fig. 5.

In a survey conducted in 2017, 45% of the smartwatches are used for activity tracking (Fig. 6) which is one way of monitoring health.

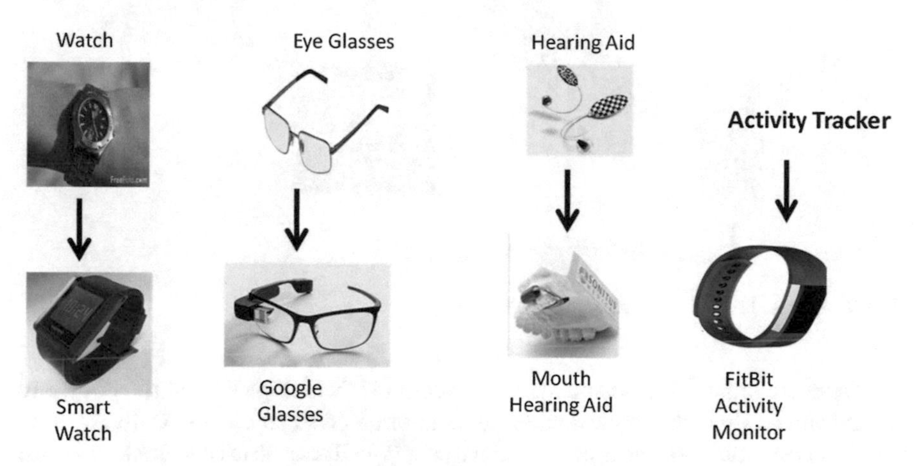

Fig. 5 Innovation of health monitoring wearable devices

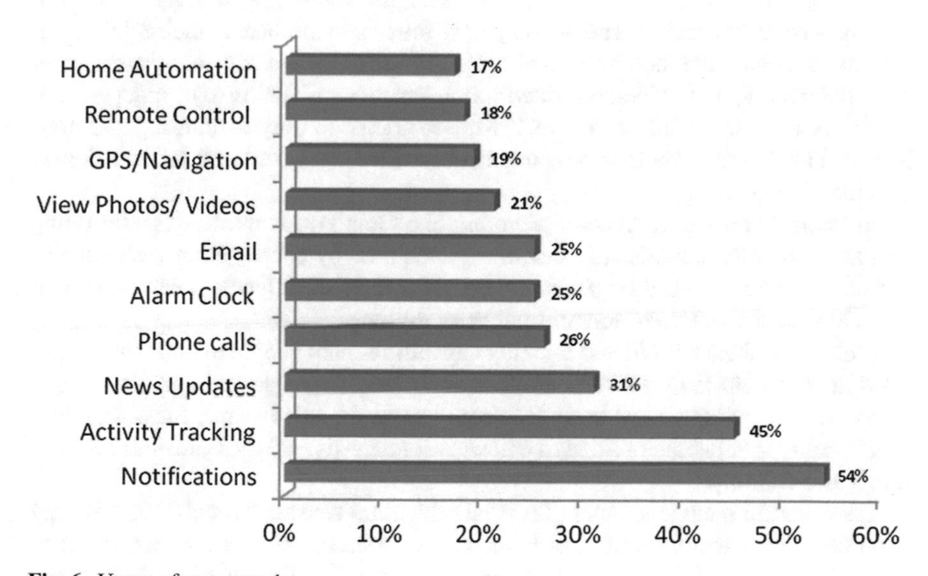

Fig. 6 Usage of smartwatches

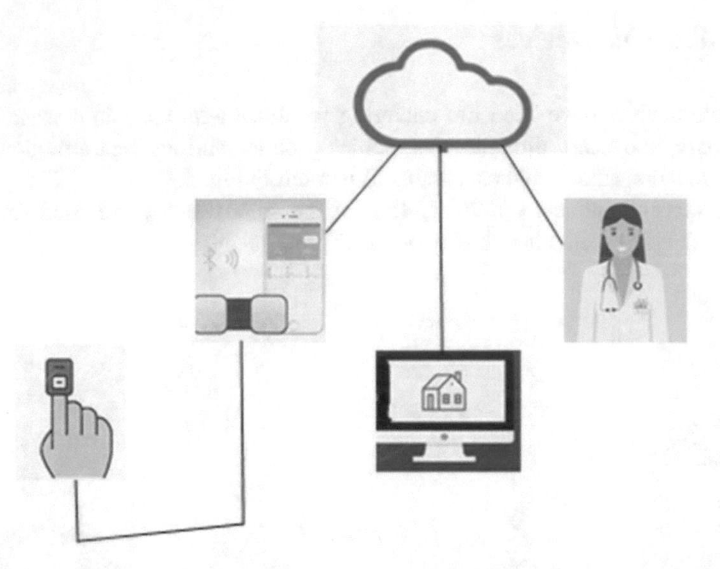

Fig. 7 Remote health monitoring through wearable

There are smart glucose monitors (Dexcom G5) which placed on the body and linked wirelessly with mobile devices to monitor blood sugar continuously. An electrical nerve stimulation wearable to relieve pain (Quell) can be used to track activities and sleep patterns to adjust pain-management intensity, as well as provide proper sleep and practical relief throughout the night for patients with severe pain. For elderly persons to monitor whether they have fallen and intimate to their relations or caretakers a vital-sign monitor wearable UnaliWear's Kanega with an accelerometer and GPS tracking is a voice-controlled watch which helps elderly to be independent.

The benefits of wearable devices are not restricted to only monitoring and notification but also for remote treatment and preventive care. A typical process flow is specified in Fig. 7.

In terms of remote treatment, wearable like OmniPod is used as insulin pump that automatically administers exact dosage required by coordinating with glucose monitor. LifeVest is used by patients who are at the risk of having heart attacks; it gives electrical shock to restore normal heart rhythms.

Many wearables with fitness tracking capabilities help people to maintain proper lifestyle and help them to keep track of their health and defend against chronic diseases. Also, these wearable devices come in an attractive shape, form, and ease functionality that people of all ages can wear it modestly and these devices are very much user-friendly.

Triboelectric nanogenerators (TENGs) which are sensors for extracting energy from the mechanical vibrations of humans have been the area of interest for many research groups working in nanotechnology worldwide. This extraction of energy from vibrations is done through medical devices and small systems which are

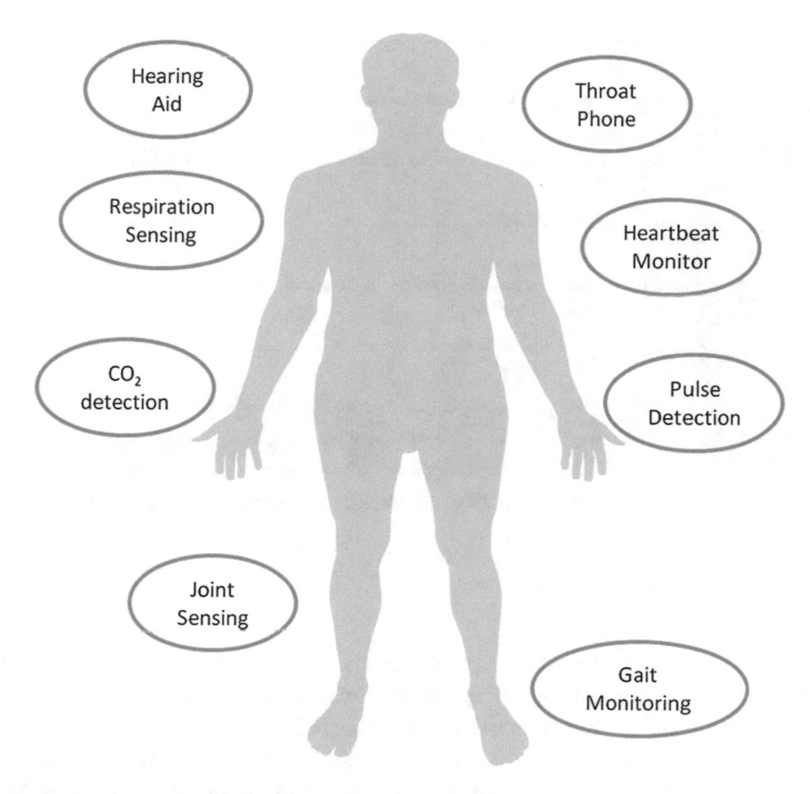

Fig. 8 Typical application of TNEGs in health monitoring

implanted in human body. Few of the TENG sensors which can be implanted in human body are shown in Fig. 8.

The review covers in-depth textile and non-textile TENGs as self-powered health monitors. Textile-based TENGs have advantages like fine air permeability, flexibility, and huge production, which make them very appropriate for wearable applications. Textile-based sensors are self-powered and used to monitor sleep and respiration, whereas non-textile sensors are generally placed on the skin or on outfits. Most non-textile sensors which are self-powered have the capability of multiple sensing abilities, while few have single sensing ability. Examining and supervising motion like joint, biceps, and abdominal respiration plays a major role in postoperative rehabilitation, particularly in the area of sports and fitness management. Heartbeat and pulse when compared to biceps have small amplitudes; thus, it requires the sensors to have high-pressure sensitivity and less detection limits to obtain the heartbeats and pulses information. These TENG sensors have also been useful to monitor voice and work as hearing aids which will be an important application in vocal rehabilitation. TENGs are also used to detect chemicals related to health care [40].

Though wearables are existing in market for longer period, the development of mobile technologies and the awareness on fitness and sport activities has led to gain

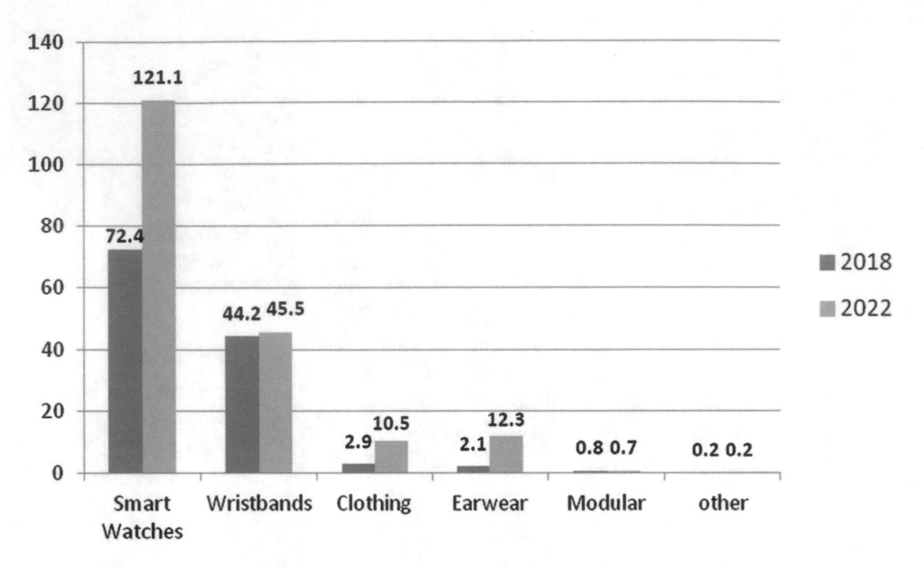

Fig. 9 Wrist wearable market share

a huge market share of wearable devices. Out of a wide range of wearable devices, smartwatches and wrist/fit bands appear to have major market share. Estimations indicate that by 2022 wrist wearables will attain 121 million sold units as shown in Fig. 9 [41]. In addition to their compact size and comfy use, wrist wearables also include sensors for providing constant data with regard to vital signs like heart rate, temperature, and environmental variables related to movements that can be used for a variety of purpose. Similarly, other wearable sensors, such as tattoos, outfits worn, or diapers, have a good market share.

3 Smart Home

It's latest in the IoT market to provide the comfortable life to elderly people. The population of elderly people is on an increasing level. Due to the lifestyle change, independence is required in all ways. It's time to ensure that elderly people are out of risk in all ways. To face this task, a number of sensors and devices are on the market. The main challenge in this group is a health issue. Constant monitoring and helping them with required assistance is on great demand. In these initial stages, home automation is the process involved remote control of lights, entertainment system, and other appliances. But recent days, it's incorporated with elderly care and research on progress with robotics for this purpose [42]. Great leap to this robotics-based work on the previous is the privacy deduction scheme and purely to handle attackers. Lot of work was carried out on using supervised and unsupervised algorithms for monitoring the activities happening inside the home. In this privacy-based system,

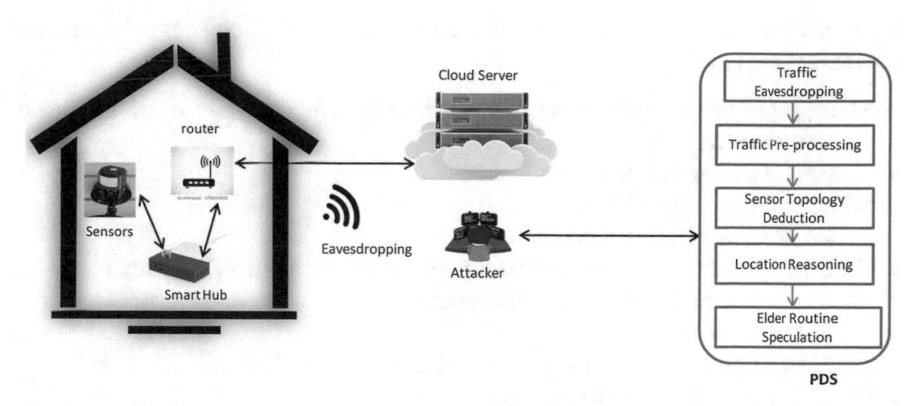

Fig. 10 PDS workflow

concern is with aiding privacy for elderly people and multiple sensors used for this purpose in his case study. He has made clear flow of task like shown in Fig. 10 [43, 44].

4 Benefits and Challenges of IoT in Health Care

Benefits

Joyia et al. explained that IoT has lots of benefits in the field of healthcare monitoring especially for aged people and those with chronic diseases. These devices are used in monitoring and as preventive care. Some of the benefits are listed below:

- Convenient lifestyle.
- Health care is economical.
- Survival rate of patient is improved.
- Disease management is instantaneous.
- Life's quality is improved.
- End user (patients) experience is enhanced.
- Patient care is better.
- Reduction in cost.

Major variation in patient's health will make an automatic alert to their caretakers, lifesavers, and different parties, thereby saving lives and time.

Challenges

The author lists some important challenges that need to be taken care in the healthcare domain of IoT. A huge growth and change in IoT and Internet communication field has also undergone a major change, contributing particularly in the healthcare sector. This has led way to reduce the gap between doctors, healthcare services provided by them, and patients enabling ease to use, accuracy, and flexibility. Some of the major challenges are listed below:

- Managing device diversity scale, unstructured, growing, and diverse data at exponential rate;
- Flexibility and evolution of applications;
- Maintaining privacy of data;
- Expertise in medical field is required;
- Hardware-related issues like network performance or memory capacity has to be monitored, while data is shared and stored;
- Security challenges;
- Understanding the working of the wearable devices; and
- Power consumption needs to be less.

These are the challenges that need to be addressed in the field of medical care [45].

4.1 Privacy and Security

Data privacy is essential in the IoT-based health cloud. Healthcare cloud applications are planned and developed based on the different ways of acquiring data from IoT devices. Confidential information of patients are collected from smart devices, summarized through smartphones and uploaded to the healthcare cloud, or transmitted back to smartphones from the cloud. This patient information could also be passed on to third parties. Such information could indicate patients' preferences, behaviors, and habits. Therefore, all agencies who are working in collecting, storing, and communicating patient's information should protect the privacy and secrecy of patient information and avoid compliance and legal suits. Only encrypted details of patients should be shared in cloud.

Authorizing credentials to applications and patient's confidential information is the prime challenge. Cryptographic protocols in health cloud should be implemented and deployed correctly. There is a chance of security breach when the healthcare professionals bring personal devices to have access to medical applications and services.

Vulnerabilities caused in devices and deploying firmware patches is a challenge that causes a dilemma in cloud which maintains the patient data. Many smart applications are vulnerable to code injection attacks, thereby giving provision to attacker to take complete control of the program and memory.

Data packets which are lost during transmission flow through the networks which have to be identified and diagnosed in well-organized manner. Health networks need to be secured, and data loss has to be minimized [46].

5 Conclusion

With the growing population, increase in medical expenditure and new diseases more focus is given to the healthcare sector. With efficient monitoring, most sudden abnormalities in health or chronic diseases can be detected at right time and can be prevented too. These health monitoring tools/wearable devices help patients especially elders to have a check on their health and also help doctors to attend patients remotely, thereby attending immediately on emergency situations. These devices ease the diagnosis work with reference to the data collected from the patient [47].

The IoT also can be implemented in clinical care where critical care patients or patients hospitalized and whose physiological status needs to be monitored continuously can be done using IoT-driven smart devices. This noninvasive monitoring involves sensors to collect complete physiological data of the patients and makes use of gateways and cloud to store, analyze, and transmit the information to caretakers for further necessary analysis and assessment of the patient's health [48]. With proper adherence to privacy policies and an efficient security measures in data handling, the IoT in healthcare sector is definitely a boon to patients and doctors.

References

1. Macedo AA, Pollettini JT, Baranauskas JA, Chaves JCA (2016) A Health Surveillance Software Framework to deliver information on preventive healthcare strategies. J Biomed Inform 62:159–170
2. Shakshuki EM, Reid M, Sheltami TR (2015) An adaptive user interface in healthcare. Procedia Comput Sci 56:49–58
3. Alnanih R, Ormandjieva O (2016) Mapping hci principles to design quality of mobile user interfaces in healthcare applications. Procedia Comput Sci 94:75–82
4. Shakshuki EM, Reid M, Sheltami TR (2015) Dynamic healthcare interface for patients. Procedia Comput Sci 63:356–365
5. Azarm-Daigle M, Kuziemsky C, Peyton L (2015) A review of cross organizational healthcare data sharing. Procedia Comput Sci 63:425–432
6. Abouelmehdi K, Beni-Hssane A, Khaloufi H, Saadi M (2017) Big data security and privacy in healthcare: a review. Procedia Comput Sci 113:73–80
7. Jothi N, Husain W (2015) Data mining in healthcare–a review. Procedia Comput Sci 72:306–313
8. https://www2.deloitte.com/global/en/pages/life-sciences-and-healthcare/articles/global-health-care-sector-outlook.html
9. Manogaran G, Thota C, Lopez D, Vijayakumar V, Abbas KM, Sundarsekar R (2017) Big data knowledge system in healthcare. In: Internet of things and big data technologies for next generation healthcare. Springer, Cham, pp 133–157
10. Kitchin R (2017) Big data—hype or revolution. In: The SAGE handbook of social media research methods, pp 27–39
11. Da Xu L, He W, Li S (2014) Internet of things in industries: a survey. IEEE Trans Industr Inf 10(4):2233–2243
12. https://www.domo.com/assets/downloads/18_domo_data-never-sleeps-6+verticals.pdf. Accessed 18 Feb 2019
13. https://blog.capterra.com/15-important-education-statistics-and-facts-you-should-know/. Accessed 18 Feb 2019

14. Kaur P, Sharma M, Mittal M (2018) Big data and machine learning based secure healthcare framework. Procedia Comput Sci 132:1049–1059
15. Archenaa J, Anita EM (2015) A survey of big data analytics in healthcare and government. Procedia Comput Sci 50:408–413
16. Mourtzis D, Vlachou E, Milas N (2016) Industrial Big Data as a result of IoT adoption in manufacturing. Procedia Cirp 55:290–295
17. Saheb T, Izadi L (2019) Paradigm of IoT big data analytics in healthcare industry: a review of scientific literature and mapping of research trends. Telemat Inform
18. Wu J, Li H, Liu L, Zheng H (2017) Adoption of big data and analytics in mobile healthcare market: an economic perspective. Electron Commer Res Appl 22:24–41
19. http://bigdata.black/business/communications/big-data-applications-in-industries/. Accessed 17 Aug 2019
20. Rayan Z, Alfonse M, Salem ABM (2019) Machine learning approaches in smart health. Procedia Comput Sci 154:361–368
21. Zeshan F, Mohamad R (2012) Medical ontology in the dynamic healthcare environment. Procedia Comput Sci 10:340–348
22. Verhaak PF, Meijer SA, Visser AP, Wolters G (2006) Persistent presentation of medically unexplained symptoms in general practice. Fam Pract 23(4):414–420
23. Mostefai S, Bouras A, Batouche M (2005) Effective collaboration in product development via a common sharable ontology. Int J Comput Intell 2(4):206–212
24. Walsh SH (2004) The clinician's perspective on electronic health records and how they can affect patient care. BMJ 328(7449):1184–1187
25. Puustjärvi J, Puustjärvi L (2015) The role of smart data in smart home: health monitoring case. Procedia Comput Sci 69:143–151
26. Rahman H, Rahmani R (2018) Enabling distributed intelligence assisted future internet of things controller (fitc). Appl Comput Inform 14(1):73–87
27. https://www.iec.ch/whitepaper/pdf/IEC_WP_Edge_Intelligence.pdf
28. Alam MGR, Munir MS, Uddin MZ, Alam MS, Dang TN, Hong CS (2019) Edge-of-things computing framework for cost-effective provisioning of healthcare data. J Parallel Distrib Comput 123:54–60
29. Chen M, Li W, Hao Y, Qian Y, Humar I (2018) Edge cognitive computing based smart healthcare system. Futur Gener Comput Syst 86:403–411
30. De Arriba-Pérez F, Caeiro-Rodríguez M, Santos-Gago J (2016) Collection and processing of data from wrist wearable devices in heterogeneous and multiple-user scenarios. Sensors 16(9):1538. https://doi.org/10.3390/s16091538
31. Nawir M, Amir A, Yaakob N, Lynn OB (2016) Internet of Things (IoT): taxonomy of security attacks. In: 2016 3rd international conference on electronic design (ICED). IEEE, pp 321–326
32. Uddin MZ (2019) A wearable sensor-based activity prediction system to facilitate edge computing in smart healthcare system. J Parallel Distrib Comput 123:46–53
33. Sun F, Zang W, Gravina R, Fortino G, Li Y (2020) Gait-based identification for elderly users in wearable healthcare systems. Inf Fusion 53:134–144
34. Romare C, Hass U, Skär L (2018) Healthcare professionals' views of smart glasses in intensive care: a qualitative study. Intensive Crit Care Nurs 45:66–71
35. El Zouka HA, Hosni MM (2019) Secure IoT communications for smart healthcare monitoring system. Internet of Things
36. Minaam DSA, Abd-ELfattah M (2018) Smart drugs: improving healthcare using smart pill box for medicine reminder and monitoring system. Futur Comput Inform J 3(2):443–456
37. Kaare KK, Otto T (2015) Smart health care monitoring technologies to improve employee performance in manufacturing. Procedia Eng 100:826–833
38. Eze B, Kuziemsky C, Peyton L (2017) A patient identity matching service for cloud-based performance management of community healthcare. Procedia Comput Sci 113:287–294
39. Al-Majeed SS, Al-Mejibli IS, Karam J (2015) Home telehealth by internet of things (IoT). In: 2015 IEEE 28th Canadian conference on electrical and computer engineering (CCECE). IEEE, pp 609–613

40. Yi F, Zhang Z, Kang Z, Liao Q, Zhang Y (2019) Recent advances in triboelectric nanogenerator-based health monitoring. Adv Funct Mater 1808849
41. Richter F, The predicted wearables boom is all about the wrist. https://www.statista.com/chart/3370/wearable-device-forecast/. Accessed 20 Sept 2018
42. Ramoly N, Bouzeghoub A, Finance B (2018) A framework for service robots in smart home: an efficient solution for domestic healthcare. IRBM 39(6):413–420
43. Lee MC, Lin JC, Owe O (2019) PDS: deduce elder privacy from smart homes. Internet of Things 100072
44. Burrows A, Coyle D, Gooberman-Hill R (2018) Privacy, boundaries and smart homes for health: an ethnographic study. Health Place 50:112–118
45. Joyia GJ, Liaqat RM, Farooq A, Rehman S (2017) Internet of Medical Things (IOMT): applications, benefits and future challenges in healthcare domain. J Commun 12(4):240–247
46. Alasmari S, Anwar M (2016) Security & privacy challenges in IoT-based health cloud. In: 2016 international conference on computational science and computational intelligence (CSCI). IEEE, pp 198–201
47. Yang Z, Zhou Q, Lei L, Zheng K, Xiang W (2016) An IoT-cloud based wearable ECG monitoring system for smart healthcare. J Med Syst 40(12):286
48. Gelogo YE, Hwang HJ, Kim HK (2015) Internet of things (IoT) framework for u-healthcare system. Int J Smart Home 9(11):323–330
49. Valerio L, Conti M, Passarella A (2018) Energy efficient distributed analytics at the edge of the network for IoT environments. Pervasive Mob Comput 51:27–42
50. Sazonov E (ed) (2014) Wearable sensors: fundamentals, implementation and applications. Elsevier

A. R. Charulatha obtained her M. Sc. degree in Computer Science from Anna University in 2002 and later her M. Phil. in 2003. She has a teaching experience of 12 years and is currently serving as Assistant Professor in Stella Maris College, Chennai. She has attended various seminars, conferences, and workshops. She has published articles and papers in various journals. Her areas of interests include networks, data mining, automata theory, and database management system. She is currently pursuing her research in the field of networks.

R. Sujatha completed the Ph.D. degree in Vellore Institute of Technology, in 2017 in the area of data mining. She received her M.E. degree in computer science from Anna University in 2009 with university ninth rank and done Master of Financial Management from Pondicherry University in 2005. She received her B.E. degree in Computer Science from Madras University, in 2001. She has 15 years of teaching experience and has been serving as an Associate Professor in School of Information Technology and Engineering in Vellore Institute of Technology, Vellore. She organized and attended a number of workshops and faculty development programs. She actively involves her in growth of institute by contributing in various committees in both academic and administrative levels. She gives technical talks in colleges for symposium and various sessions. She acts as advisory, editorial member, and technical committee member in conferences conducted in other educational institutions and in-house too. She has published a book titled software project management for the college students and also has published research articles and papers in reputed journals. She used to guide projects for undergraduate and postgraduate students. She currently guides doctoral students. She is interested to explore different places and visit the same to know about the culture and people of various areas. She is interested in learning upcoming things and gets herself acquainted with student's level. Her areas of research interest include data mining, machine learning, image processing, and management of information systems.

IoT Use Cases and Applications

G. Priya, M. Lawanya Shri, E. GangaDevi and Jyotir Moy Chatterjee

Abstract IoT in health care is wireless communication system of applications and devices which connects health providers and patients to detect, observe, track, and store medical information and statistics. In this chapter, various case studies of smart healthcare system have been discussed. A model which would monitor aspects of a human body such as his pulse rate and temperature are described. Smart IOT-enabled healthcare wearable device is used to aid paralyzed person for daily chores using machine learning to get better in understanding the patient gestures over time. Health monitoring system pill box and a pulse rate sensor is discussed for Alzheimer's patients. The system is based on Arduino-Uno microcontroller and uses accelerometer and pulse sensor to get data from the patient.

Keywords Internet of things · Healthcare system · Arduino-microcontroller · Machine learning

1 Introduction

The Internet of things plays an significant role in the healthcare industry. Healthcare industry is improved in terms of increasing efficiency, low costs, and having more focus on patients care. We have discussed a model which is helpful to the elderly people and the patient who need constant health inspection. His data can be accessed

G. Priya
School of Computer Science and Engineering, Vellore Institute of Technology, Vellore, India
e-mail: gpriya.raj@gmail.com

M. Lawanya Shri (✉)
School of Information Technology and Engineering, Vellore Institute of Technology, Vellore, India
e-mail: lawanyaraj@gmail.com

E. GangaDevi
Loyola College, Chennai, Tamil Nadu, India
e-mail: smgangadevi@yahoo.co.in

J. M. Chatterjee
Lord Buddha Education Foundation, Kathmandu, Nepal
e-mail: jyotirchatterjee@gmail.com

P. Raj et al. (eds.), *Internet of Things Use Cases for the Healthcare Industry*,
https://doi.org/10.1007/978-3-030-37526-3_9

by his/her doctor, and immediate actions can then be taken. The data which are obtained from sensors are uploaded in the cloud, and they can be accessed by anyone. The data collected from sensor can be accessed from smartphone app which shows us the whole information of the user's body. In the next case study, the data that is transmitted over low power 433 MHz transmitter to local computer which further performs the data processing and store onto the cloud. Some hospitals and NGOs are coming forward to serve paralytic patients whose whole or partial body disabled by the paralysis attack. Those people are unable to deliver their requirements as they are unable to speak well nor do they deliver via sign language. In such scenario, the proposed structure helps disabled people in presenting a message on the LCD by simple gesture of any portion of his body. This system helps the patient to send message via GSM whatever he wants to send in SMS when there is no one to take care of him. In the third analysis, medicine dispenser is implemented. Generally, every person forgets to take their pill at once or more than once, but for patients who are on a multifaceted pill administration, not taking prescribed medicines at the right dosage and at the exact time can have main consequences, predominantly if they are elderly people. To our pillbox, we have attached a buzzer that will buzz every time a patient has to take a medicine. We have also included a pulse sensor which will detect the heart rate of the patient and indicate the agitation state of the patient. The results will be displayed using an LCD.

2 Pulse Rate Monitoring System

IOT is nothing but transforming or converting information of data from the physical world into the digital world for making it possible to analyze data to operate tasks [1]. Since our objective is based on health care, the proposed system should be able to manage huge volume of patient's medical data. The need for health care is growing nowadays to improvise admittance to health precaution, raise quality, and reduce cost. In IoT, devices collect and share data directly with others and the cloud is to assemble record and study new data streams quicker and more precisely.

The base for integrating all the things that are all the physical objects such as sensor-based networks is accomplished by using radio radio-frequency identification (RFID), NFC, and other wireless technologies [2]. The Internet-oriented vision provides connection between devices and Internet that described as smart objects. The data collected from sensors is analyzed and interpreted by semantic-oriented vision. When building a device related to health care, three main categories to be considered are tracking of objects, identification, and automatic sensing. The IoT adopts a notable part in a wide scope of public assurance applications, from overseeing chronic diseases toward one side to anticipating malady at the other side.

2.1 Clinical Care

The physical status of hospitalized patients needs continual observation by utilizing IoT-driven and noninvasive checking. This organization uses sensors to collect wide-ranging physical data and uses the cloud to store the data and then send the inspected data remotely to parent for helping investigation [3]. It exchanges the method toward having a comfort proficient stopped by common interims to plaid the patient's imperative symbols, rather than specifying a nonstop computerized sequence of data. At the same time, it improves the environment of care through steady attention and reducing the cost of care by providing the necessity for a parental figure to efficiently take part in data collecting and examination.

2.2 Remote Checking

There are persons universally all over the world whose well-being may suffer in light of the information that they don't have organized admittance to viable health checking [4]. These provisions can be used to safely understanding health information from a variety of sensors, apply difficult designs to separate the data, and then share it over remote availability with restorative professionals who can create suitable healthy proposals. Wearable healthcare systems contain pulse sensors, pulse oximetry sensors, respiratory rate sensors, blood pressure, and body temperature sensors.

Technologies that enable the IoT in health care possible are as follows:

1. Low-power operation,
2. Integrated precision—Analog capabilities, and
3. GUI.

We have built a framework that will plan a calendar which is properly planned for the entire worker in light of their heartbeat rate and the quantity of hours they spent working. The principle intention is the representative to client proportion which is a disturbing number. To counter this worry, this framework is going to be built. It includes fields such as defence, security, finance, banking, etc. Before we start, we have to ensure about the worker part we are thinking about. The high representative to client proportion pushes the worker past their well-being limits. These situations prompt individuals sitting and working for extended periods or extra timework [5]. It influences them socially by diminishing their available time. In this proposed method, we have built a heartbeat checker by using Arduino board, temperature sensor, pulse rate generator, and some wires (Fig. 1).

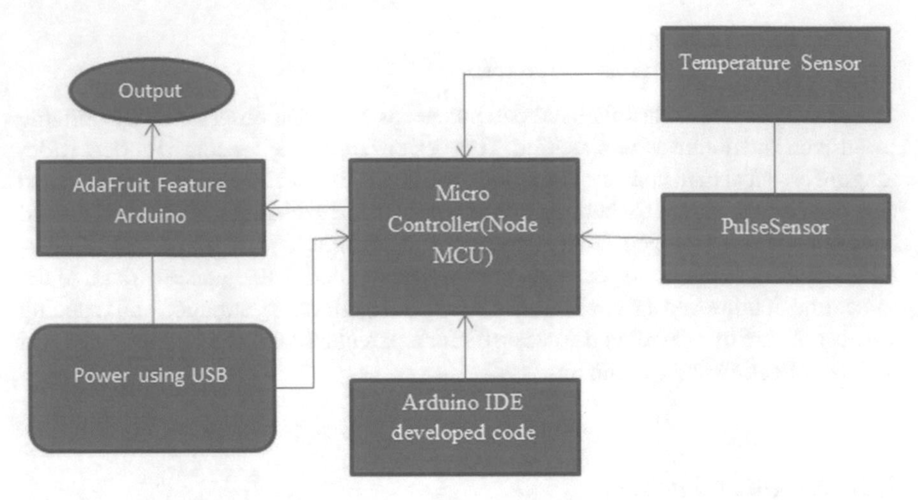

Fig. 1 Architecture of microcontroller

3 Hardware Components

Working With Node MCU:

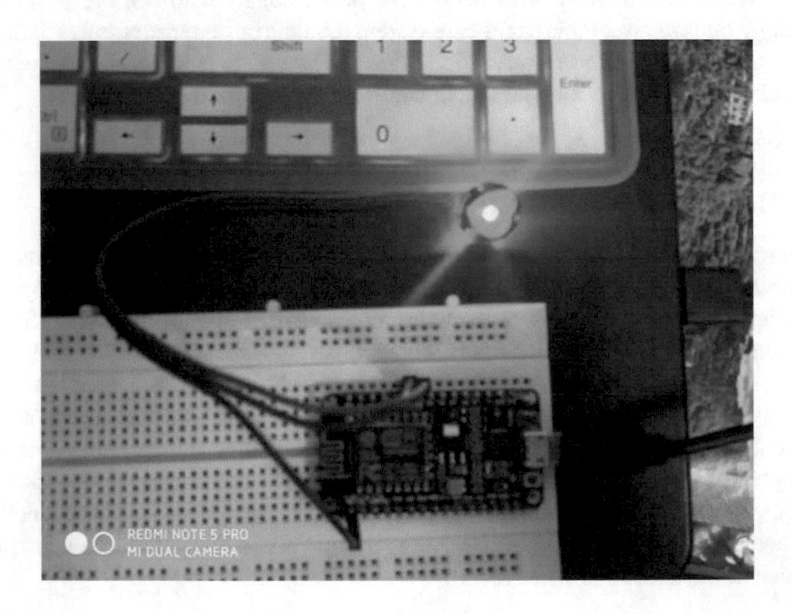

Trying with Arduino UNO:

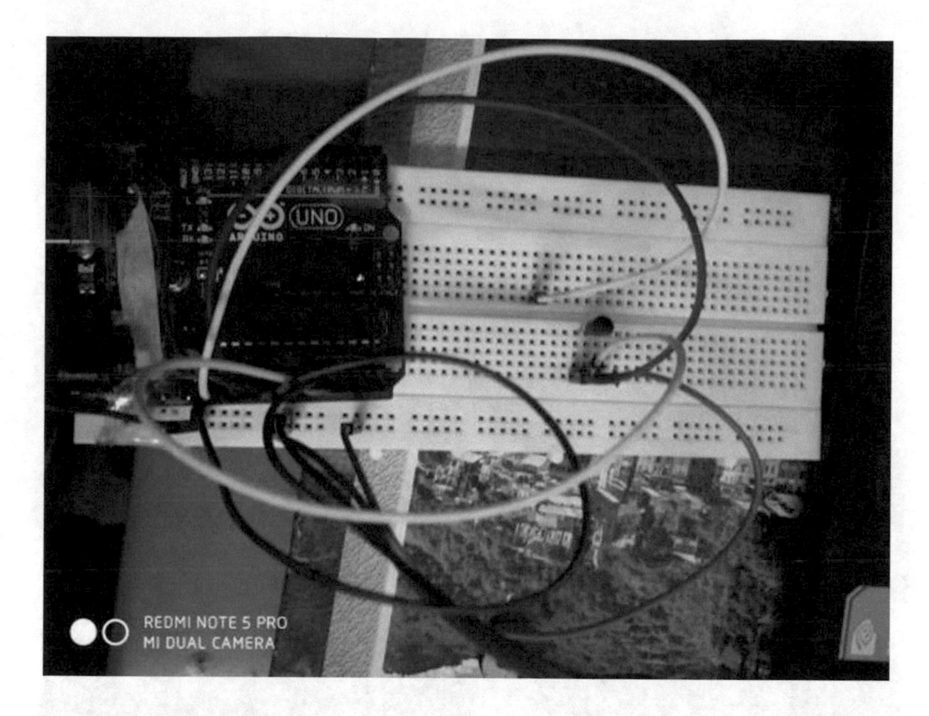

Output Screens

Verifying code:

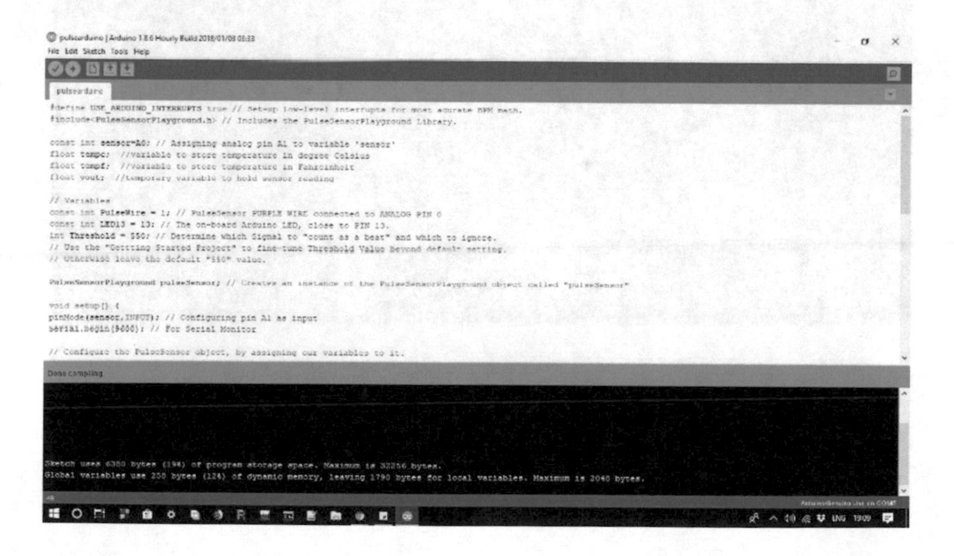

Uploading code to NodeMCU/Wi-Fi module Successfully:

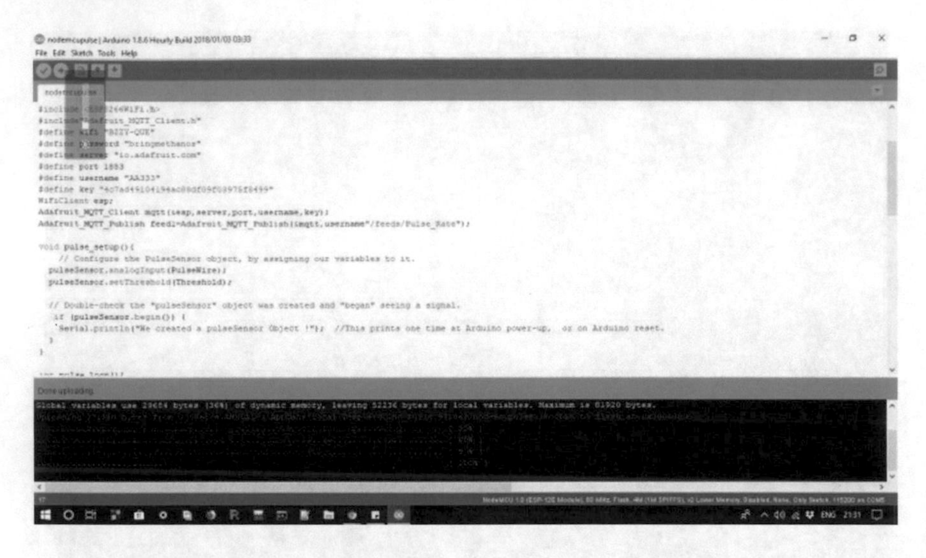

Open Source (AdaFruit compiling): Through Wi-Fi Module:

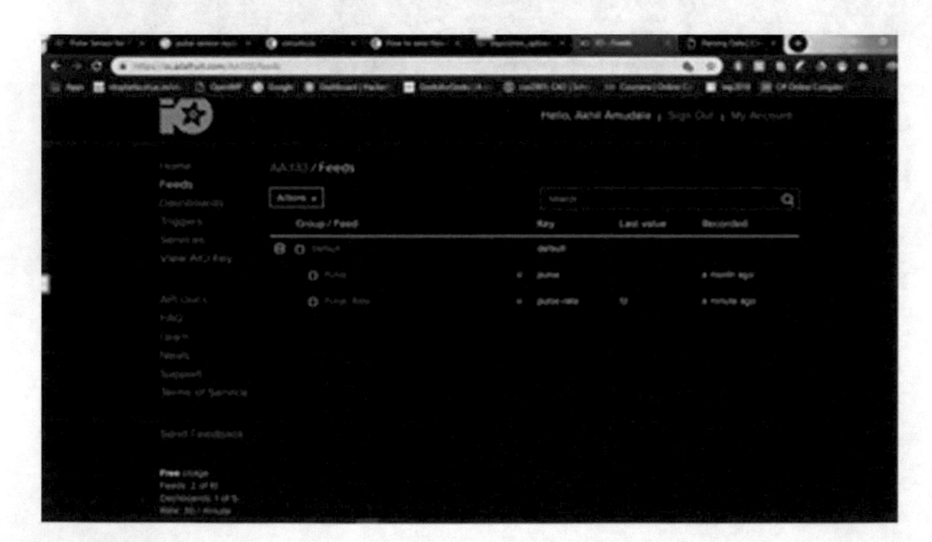

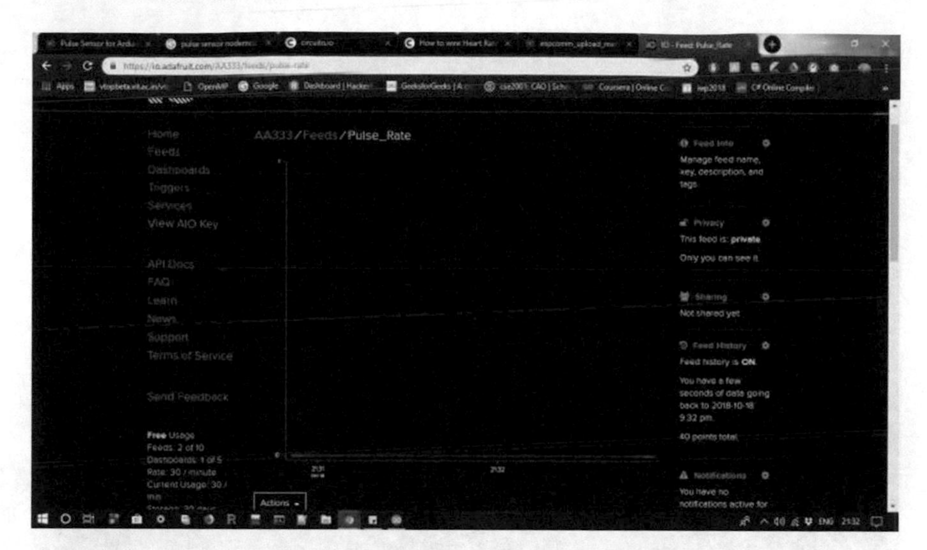

Analytics part:

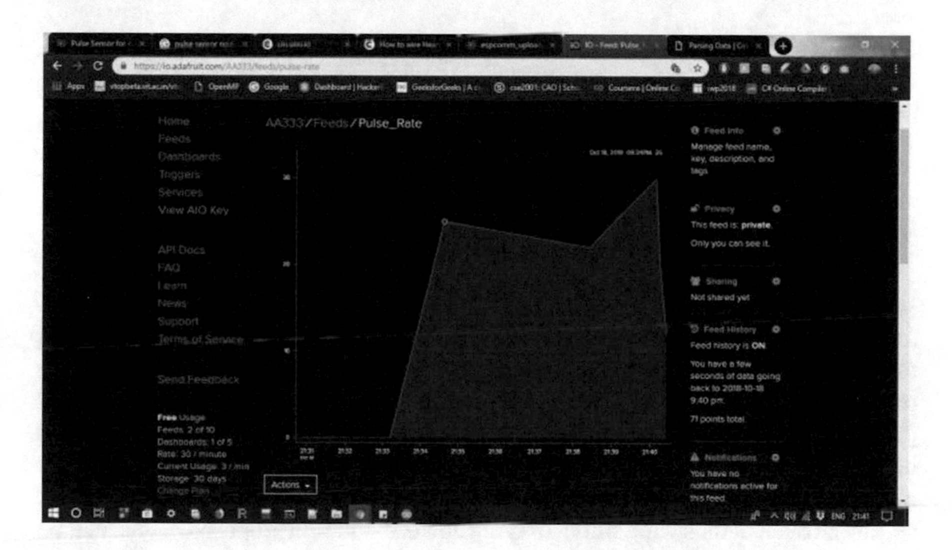

Values:

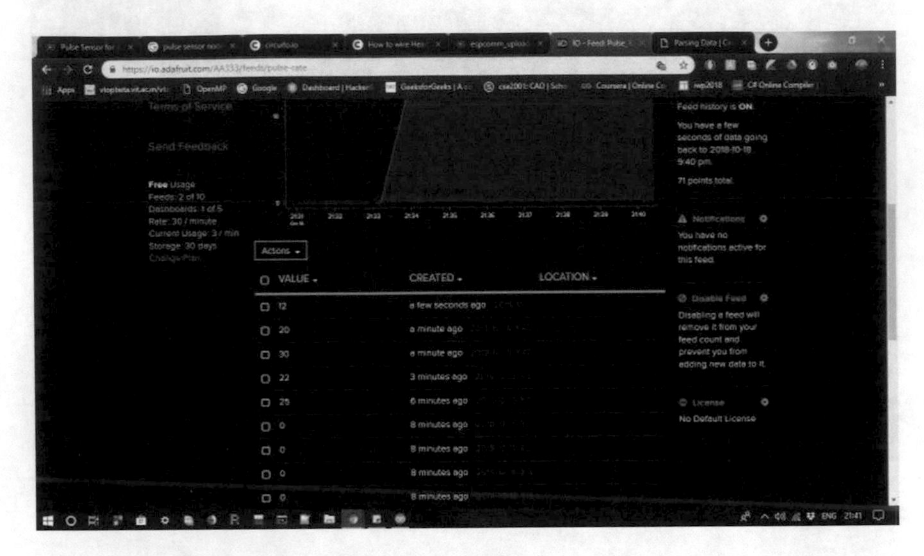

NodeMCU uses a Wi-Fi module which is an advantage over Arduino since it makes easier for user to understand and process but still we can use better pulse sensors so that it would read input values so quickly and can work efficiently.

4 Smart Glove for Paralyzed Patients

In our body, if a muscle loses its function, it causes paralysis. This is due to the information which is sent our brain and muscle goes wrong. The sudden happening of paralysis can be partial or to a greatest extent. It can occur on one or both halves of our body. It can also take place in one region of our body, or it can be generalized [6]. This makes it difficult for the person with paralysis to perform daily tasks such as turning on lights, asking for help, etc. Another problem is that a paralyzed person is more prone to diseases related to the heart, since they restrict their daily movements and spend most of their time sitting or lying down. A solution proposed in this method is a smart device similar to a glove that the person can use and with simple gestures with the hands performs a variety of functions.

The glove will be a Arduino-based IOT device mounted with the accelerometer and a pulse beat sensor. The communication would be done through 433 MHz trans-receiver module. The transceiver is composed of a transmitter and a receiver in a one unit as a pair. It also suggested to wireless communication devices like handphones, two-way radios, cordless telephone sets, and mobile two-way radios [7]. An RF transmitter unit is a minute size PCB efficient to transfer radio wave and balance radio wave to carry bits of data. RF transmitter modules offer data to the transmitted phase, when it is worked with a microcontroller. These transmitters are used to control

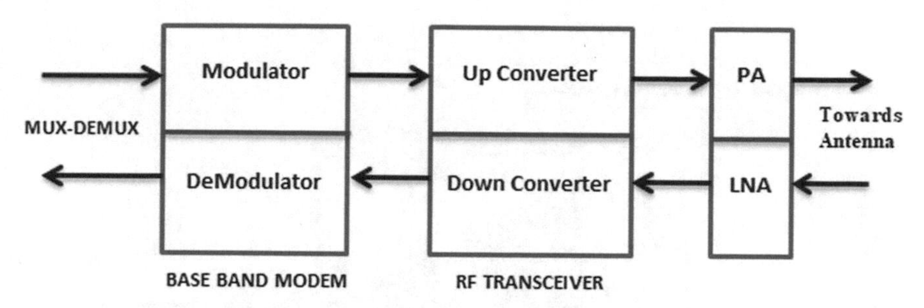

Fig. 2 Block diagram for trans-receiver module

the requirements to order the maximum acceptable transmitter power output, band edge, and the requirements of harmonics.

An RF receiver unit holds the modulated RF signal to demodulate them. There two different types of RF receiver modules are superregenerative receivers and superheterodyne receivers. In general, superregenerative modules are very low-cost one. The projects which cost low will use a series of amplifiers to remove the data modulated by a carrier wave. The given modules vary and they are inaccurate due to their frequency operation with the voltage and temperature of the power supply [8]. The main advantage of heterodyne super receiver modules is a high efficiency compared to the superregenerative. They offer high stability and precision in a wide range of temperatures and voltages. This stability arises from a stable glass design which in turn leads to a relatively more expensive product (Fig. 2).

The equipped accelerometer is ADXL330 which uses a lot of less power and is a three-axis accelerometer. It continuously monitors the movement and sends the data over the Arduino for transmission. The heart pulse sensor is connected to Arduino as analog input. The main technique of working with the heartbeat sensor is photoplethysmograph [9]. With the help of this principle, the variation in the volume of blood in an organ is calculated by the changes in the intensity of the light which passes through that organ (Fig. 3).

The data sent over the transmission is a string enclosed within two parentheses, and extra bit of string is attached at the end. This is due to accommodate the loss last strings sent over transmission as the 433 MHz cannot support high speed, e.g., "[25,2,8,62]LOSS". On the receiver side, the string is parsed and if the data is highly corroded it is discarded. On the practical basis, the trans-receiver can support up to 3000 bits/s which is enough to send the sensor data. The recognized movement can be uploaded to cloud for further data analytics or be used to call specific functions from the receiving computer to perform operations which helps the paralyzed person [10].

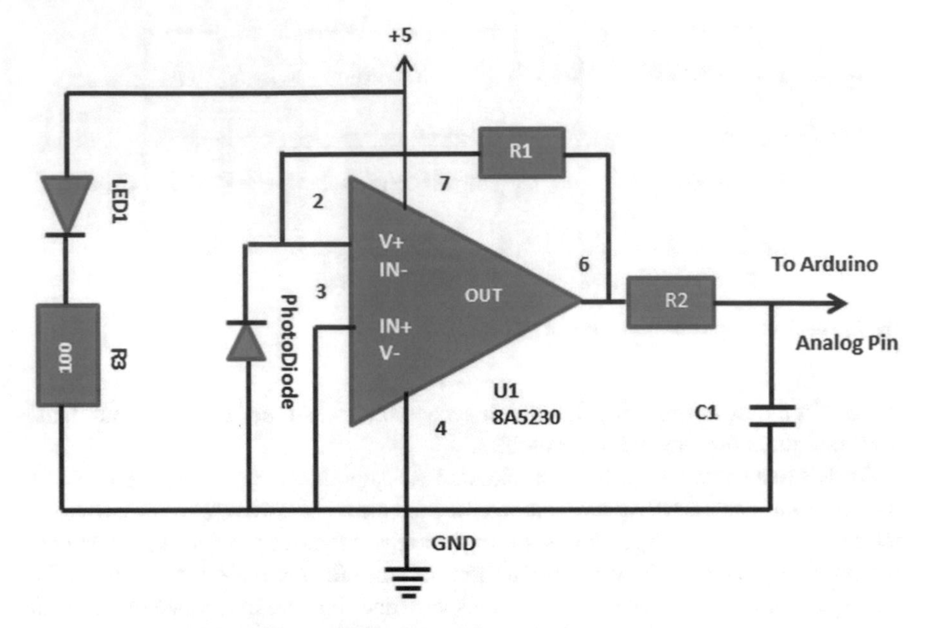

Fig. 3 Schematic of heartbeat sensor

4.1 Machine Learning on the Incoming Data

After the three-axis data and the heartbeat sensor data are received, the ML is performed to recognize the gesture. The model we use is K-nearest neighbor. A good classification algorithm which is simple and robust is KNN algorithm. And because of this, the algorithm can give highly good results. KNN algorithm can also be used for regression problems also. Instead of voting from the nearest, this methodology will be used for averages of nearest neighbors, which is the main difference here [11]. At first, the glove is trained over a gesture where the patient repeats a particular movement and all the data are recorded. This gives a specific pattern of values for each axis. After the training, the system is ready to perform whenever the movement is applied.

4.2 Data Analytics Over Collected Data

After sufficient data about patient is collected, we can perform data analytics to get hidden information such as what requirements he desire at a particular point of day. These data can be uploaded to cloud for further processing. Also, cloud will enable remote monitoring of the data through web or mobile app. Data was able to travel within the range of several feet which makes the 433 MHz trans-receiver perfect for home applications. It is better than other alternatives such as Bluetooth and Wi-Fi Shield as it is a low cost for small data transmission and is extremely power efficient. The range can be improved using an antenna.

However, for continuous large data transmission, other alternatives such as Bluetooth and 2.4 GHZ transmitter may be used. The machine learning model is efficient to recognize the simple gestures like horizontal/vertical waves [12]. However, for complex gesture, it was not accurate because the accelerometer was not sufficient. For this, we need gyroscope and bend sensors. But this would increase the cost of the plan.

5 Automatic Medicine Dispenser

With the development of Internet of things in various fields, we came up with its application in the healthcare domain. This is specifically designed for those on a complex and vulnerable medicine regime where missing even a single medicine becomes a huge risk in their life [13]. The medicine dispenser has also been proved to be useful where patients don't have a caretaker. It is affordable and easy to use. In our proposed method, we have programmed our medicine dispenser according to the regime of user [14]. An alarm has been set up to make the user to remember to take which medicine at what time. The sensor is attached to the medicine cap, whose opening denotes that the patient has taken his medicine and the signal is sent to the Arduino accordingly [15].

If the patient fails to take his medicine, a GSM module attached will send a message to the user that he hasn't taken his medicine. If he still ails to take the medicine, then the message will be sent to his doctor notifying this. The best part of our work is we can have multiple medicine reminders [16]. As a part of innovation, we will be storing his data in a database and uploading it to "ThinkCloud". From here, the user will be able to see how many times he took his medicine in a given month.

5.1 Smart Automatic Medication Dispenser

This was made for those who take medicine without help and aimed for avoiding the consumption of wrong medicine at the wrong time. The components needed for design of reminder to smart medication are raspberry pi zero W (core type-ARM1176JZF-S) interface with LCD16×4, buzzer, led, alarm module (DS3231), multiple pill container, and a stepper motor [17]. At the starting point, switch on the kit and the device will be asked to set the time for alarm and likewise set for the next alarm by allowing the pill into pillbox and close it. As the user sets the time for alarm, the sound is made by the buzzer and also makes the LED blink which is present in the pillbox separately. With the help of using raspberry pi zero W, the interfacing is very easy and simple. The software and the language used for programming are PyCharm and python, respectively.

5.2 Automated Drug Dispensing Systems

This chapter focuses on issues such as the continuous occurrence of errors, wastage of medication, and the inappropriate use of nursing time because of the multiple-dose drug distribution systems which were accepted throughout the world before the unit-of-use packages or unit-dose systems were introduced in early 1960s [18]. These systems replaced multidose systems in which nurses had the greater responsibility for the entire system of medication, which gathers the administering of hundreds of doses of medicine along with paperwork, inventory control, and dose preparation. On the other hand, unit-dose systems facilitate the nurses with separately packaged and labeled doses at eight or more hour intervals that are ready to administer according to the routine schedule determined by the nurse narrated by [19]. Building on this success, Johns Hopkins Hospital further introduced an automated feature into this existing unit-dose system by making the whole technique, from physician prescription entry to hourly dose administration, computer-assisted [20].

5.3 Construction of a Smart Medication Dispenser with High Degree of Scalability and Remote Manageability

This method proposes a smart medication dispenser which is of a high degree of remote manageability. The hardware architecture which aims for scalability is designed for a dispenser in order to gain an extensible hardware architecture and to focus for remote manageability, an agent program was also installed. The working of the dispenser is, when the real-time clock attains the predetermined medication time and the user tends to press the dispense button at that duration, the predetermined medication is dispensed from the medication dispensing tray (MDT) [21]. In the proposed dispenser, the medication allotted for each patient is maintained in an MDT. One smart medication dispenser consists of only one MDT. With respect to this aspect, the dispenser can be extended to add more and more MDTs which will support multiple users to use one dispenser. The final observation of implementation and verification proved that the proposed dispenser operated in a normal way and it performs the management operations from the medication monitoring server.

5.4 Design of Automatic Medication Dispenser

This paper importantly focused on providing medication to aged persons on time. This automatic medication dispenser is architectured especially for users who cannot afford professional supervision at all times. The population of adults and elders can benefit from this design of device as it neglects expensive in-home medical care. The major objective of this design was to keep the device simple and cost–benefit. It relieved the user of the error-prone tasks of doing wrong medicine at wrong time. The important parts of this medication dispenser were a microcontroller interfaced with a keypad, an LED for displaying, a controller, an alarm system, a multiple pill container, and a dispenser. The user is asked to press a button to get the pill and to reset the alarm button. The second alarm was installed to indicate the optimal availability of the pills stored in the container to intimate the user to refill the dispenser with the required quantity of pills. First, we will connect and complete the setup and the circuit. Real-time clock will be running and as soon as it reaches a current time, we'll code the Arduino to send the output to the LCD display and the buzzer. The LCD display will display the time slot of the medicine and buzzer will keep on buzzing.

6 Architecture

Now if the person or user takes the pills, i.e., by opening the lid, the IR sensor attached to the lid which will detect that the lid is opened and hence will send the output to Arduino which will stop the buzzer from buzzing, and this action performed will be sent into the log that the person has taken his medicine successfully. In case the person forgets to take the medicine (Lid is not opened), the buzzer will automatically get stopped after that time and will be put on for snooze. If a person once again misses the medicine, the output will be sent to GSM module which in turn will send a message to the person reminding him that he has missed a pill. And if once again the person misses the pill as a last chance, a message will be sent to family members or to the hospital. We will be uploading all the data about the patient whether he has taken his medicine or not in a database and will upload it to the cloud. At the end of the month, the patient will be able to analyze how many days did he/she consume is medicine (Fig. 4).

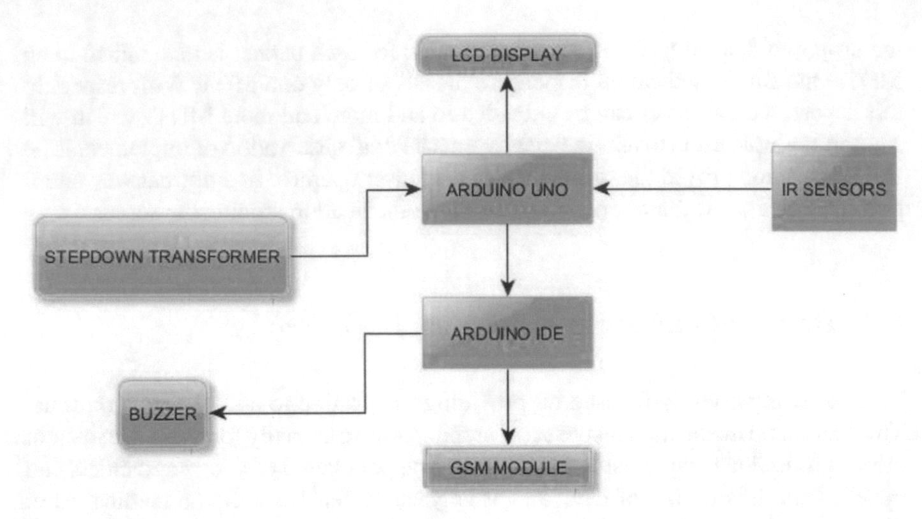

Fig. 4 Architecture

7 Conclusion

In the first case study to monitor the pulse rate, we can implement NodeMCU with a Wi-Fi module used in various workspaces like IT industries and can come up with various solutions so that we can use manpower correctly. The cloud or open source is also user-friendly to operate and shows direct graphical analysis which is an easier way to understand. In the next case study of smart glove for paralyzed patients, few attempts have been made to activate Smart Gloves as tools for hearing problems and speech disabilities. Most of these devices use any one of the following requirements: CMOS cameras, leaf switch-based gloves, copper plate-based gloves, and flex sensor-based gloves, with no innovation presented. In the same order, the different components of each device are common in most cases like microcontrollers, flex sensors, accelerometers, and communication modules. In the scientific literature, four gloves were found and they were compared by analyzing their advantages and disadvantages to make a comfort solution for the end users. The first glove which is developed has the capability to recognize gestures in order to translate them into speech or messages. In certain cases, the main disadvantage of this method is its bend sensors that have limited sensing capacity, which limits its usability. The second glove produced by has the ability to convert language into voice; nonetheless, it uses flex sensors which don't allow a high degree of sensitivity due that they can't bend more than 90°. It also uses sign language as its main tool which is not a universal language. A third glove which can interpret sign language using a wireless function and a screen to display its results has also been presented but it lacks the functionality to translate into voice. Finally, a glove that can translate sign language into audible language has also been designed but a has a limit capacity of storing just 30 gesture.

In the third case study, the proposed work enables the user in a significant way to maintain the health-related issues efficiently by taking medicines on due time. This device is a great relief in a time of competition where under the pressure of work and other liabilities one might forget to take his medicines on the prescribed timing. Making the health a lower priority, hence, the device is a greatly useful one in times like today.

References

1. Sermakani V (2014) Transforming healthcare through internet of things. In: Project management practitioners' conference
2. Kulkarni A, Sathe S (2014) Healthcare applications of the internet of things: a review. Int J Comput Sci Inf Technol 5(5):6229–6232
3. Niewolny D (2013) How the internet of things is revolutionizing healthcare. White paper, pp 1–8
4. Baker SB, Xiang W, Atkinson I (2017) Internet of things for smart healthcare: technologies, challenges, and opportunities. IEEE Access 5:26521–26544
5. Kodali RK, Swamy G, Lakshmi B (2015) An implementation of IoT for healthcare. In: 2015 IEEE recent advances in intelligent computational systems (RAICS). IEEE, pp 411–416
6. Chouhan T, Panse A, Voona AK, Sameer SM (2014) Smart glove with gesture recognition ability for the hearing and speech impaired
7. Rafael V, Glaugo AP (2015) Towards a battery-free wireless smart glove for rehabilitation application based on RFID
8. Soliman M, Abiodu T, Hamouda T, Zhou J, Lung C-H (2013) Smart home: integrating internet of things with web services and cloud computing
9. Enciso-Quispe L, Delgado J. Internet of things based on Arduino technology for people with disabilities
10. Taneja S (2016) Improved KNN algorithm
11. Chouhan T, Panse A, Voona AK, Saamer SM (1989) Smart glove with gesture recognition ability for the hearing and speech impaired. In: Young M (ed) 2014 IEEE global humanitarian technology conference-South Asia satellite (GHTC-SAS). IEEE (2014). The Technical Writer's Handbook. University Science, Mill Valley, CA
12. McCall C (2010) A system that implements automatic medication management and passive remote monitoring to enable independent living of healthcare patients. Doctoral dissertation, University of Central Florida, Orlando, Florida
13. Tsai PH, Chen TY, Yu CR, Shih CS, Liu JW (2011) Smart medication dispenser: design, architecture and implementation. IEEE Syst J 5(1):99–110
14. Balka E, Nutland K (2004) Automated drug dispensing systems: literature review
15. Pak J, Park K (2012) Construction of a smart medication dispenser with high degree of scalability and remote manageability. BioMed Res Int
16. Mukund S, Srinath NK (2012) Design of automatic medication dispenser
17. Sinnemäki J, Sihvo S, Isojärvi J, Blom M, Airaksinen M, Mäntylä A (2013) Automated dose dispensing service for primary healthcare patients: a systematic review. Syst Rev 2(1):1
18. Fang KY, Maeder AJ, Bjering H (2016) Current trends in electronic medication reminders for self care. Stud Health Technol Inform 231:31–41
19. Shojania KG, Duncan BW, McDonald KM, Wachter RM, Markowitz AJ (2001) Making health care safer: a critical analysis of patient safety practices. Evid Rep Technol Assess (Summ) 43(1):668
20. Stillwell K, Stillwell K Jr (2002) Automatic pill dispenser. U.S. Patent 6,427,865
21. Daneshvar Y (1994) Automatic pill dispenser. U.S. Patent 5,372,276

Dr. G. Priya is an Associate Professor in School of Computer Science and Engineering, Vellore Institute of Technology, Vellore. She completed her B.E. in Computer Science and Engineering under Madras University, M. Tech. in Computer Science and Engineering, and Ph.D. in VIT. She published more than 30+ research papers in reputed journals. Her area of interest is trust management, cloud computing, IoT, and deep learning.

Dr. M. Lawanya Shri is working as Associate Professor in School of Information Technology and Engineering at VIT, Vellore. She has 13 years of experience in teaching to UG and PG students. She has published nearly 37 research papers in international journals and 12 conference proceedings. She has co-authored one book: "Computer Architecture for Beginners" and four book chapters. Her research work mainly focusses on cloud computing, web services, Internet of things, blockchain technology, and machine learning.

Ms. E. GangaDevi is working as an Assistant Professor at Loyola College, Chennai since 2016. She is having 8+ years of teaching experiences from different colleges like Vellore Institute of Technology, Vellore, Stella Maris College, Chennai, and B. N. Bandodkar college, Thane, Mumbai. She has published 10 research papers in various journals and 2 book chapters. One of her papers is awarded as a Best paper in International Conference. She has published a book on Data Base Management Systems. She has cleared State Level Eligibility Test during 2016. She is pursuing her Ph.D. from Dr. MGR Educational and Research Institute, Chennai.

Jyotir Moy Chatterjee is currently working as an Assistant Professor (IT) at Lord Buddha Education Foundation (Asia Pacific University of Technology & Innovation), Kathmandu, Nepal. Prior to this, he worked as an Assistant Professor (CSE) at GD Rungta College of Engineering & Technology (CSVTU), Bhilai, India. He has completed M. Tech in Computer Science and Engineering from Kalinga Institute of Industrial Technology, Bhubaneswar, India and B. Tech in Computer Science and Engineering from Dr. MGR Educational & Research Institute, Chennai, India. He has 36 international publications, 2 authored books, 2 edited volume books, and 2 book chapters into my account. His research interests include cloud computing, big data, privacy preservation, data mining, Internet of things, machine learning, and blockchain technology. He is member of various professional societies and international conferences.

Internet of Things for Ambient-Assisted Living—An Overview

A. Vijayalakshmi and Deepa V. Jose

Abstract The traditional family setup that ensures safety and caring for the elderly has changed due to the change in work culture and societal setup. Caring for the bed-ridden with chronic diseases consumes time and money which can be beyond imagination. Ambient-assisted living (AAL) is a boon as it provides an improved quality by monitoring daily routines to provide immediate healthcare services as and when required. Internet of things (IoT) plays a great role in developing technologies for ambient-assisted living. The adoption of this technology has given enormous improvement in the medical and healthcare domain, especially in diagnostic, prevention and patient care activities ensuring utmost comfort. This smart technology has opened up a wide world of possibilities in healthcare which is quite obvious by the massive usage of IoT devices in diagnostic medical equipment and wearable healthcare devices.

Keywords Internet of things · IoT · Sensors · Ambient-assisted living · Elderly care · Palliative care · Medical devices · Pressure ulcer

1 Introduction

Ambient-assisted living (AAL) is an emerging multidisciplinary field which aims to improve the quality in all aspects of our life. This is a concept which includes various products and services enabled with high-end technology which is quite economical and user-friendly. AAL builds a comfortable ecosystem by using various sensors, computing/mobile devices and applications for individual health monitoring. IoT technologies have already proved to be an effective healthcare aid for the elderly and the bedridden with chronic diseases. The wide acceptance of this technology helps in offering better service on time for the needy and relieves the mental stress of the

A. Vijayalakshmi (✉) · D. V. Jose
Department of Computer Science, CHRIST (Deemed to be University), Bangalore, India
e-mail: vijayalakshmi.nair@christuniversity.in

D. V. Jose
e-mail: deepa.v.jose@christuniversity.in

P. Raj et al. (eds.), *Internet of Things Use Cases for the Healthcare Industry*,
https://doi.org/10.1007/978-3-030-37526-3_10

caretakers as continuous monitoring and timely notification will be provided to them by such applications.

2 Internet of Things—An Overview

The word "internet" means a number of applications and rules which are built on computers that are sophisticated and interconnected with each other, which serve people all around the world for communication and connectivity. Now the focus has shifted from the internet to internet of things which reveals two important terms "internet" and "things". The integration of these two terms converges the realm of things into human-made virtual environment which eventually creates internet of things (IoT) phenomena [1]. "Things" refer to any smart devices, sensors, human beings or other objects which are capable of connecting to the internet anywhere without any time constraints. These objects need to be able to communicate with the entities and hence implying that they need to be accessible at any time in any place [1], that is, connectivity at any place and any time is the most important factor in an IoT application. This can be achieved with various types of sensing and computing devices and its communication protocols. Before the emergence of IoT, radio frequency identification was the main sensing technology. As the technology advances, there have been new trends such as wireless sensor networks (WSNs) and Bluetooth devices which helped in the emergence of IoT field.

IoT is widely accepted as it facilitates the interconnection between "things" through the internet. It is a multidisciplinary field which is a combination of data sensing and aggregation techniques, optimization of technologies, data analysis and decision making, artificial intelligence, network and communications and so on. It is quite evident through various applications that the IoT is used not only for just interconnecting various devices but to make important insights and act accordingly which was only in our imaginations a decade ago. These smart devices act as a replacement for humans in many time-consuming, risky and tiring tasks. The whole crux of this technology lies in the ability of these smart devices to identify, communicate and interact among themselves and with everything within its network [2, 3].

All IoT objects possess the characteristics of existence, sense of self, connectivity, interactivity, dynamicity and environmental awareness. With these features, IoT is enabled to offer multitude of services in various fields, including agriculture, monitoring, surveillance and rescue applications, weather forecasting, automating home and personalized healthcare, energy conservation, supply chain, inventory management and control and so on [4]. A comprehensive summary of the same is depicted in Fig. 1 [5].

Because of its distributed nature, huge numbers, heterogeneity and resource constraints, developing security mechanisms for IoT is a daunting task as it creates weak links that malicious entities can easily exploit. A model of IoT with the various components, the IoT devices, gateways, interconnections through internet, cloud storage and the users is represented in Fig. 2.

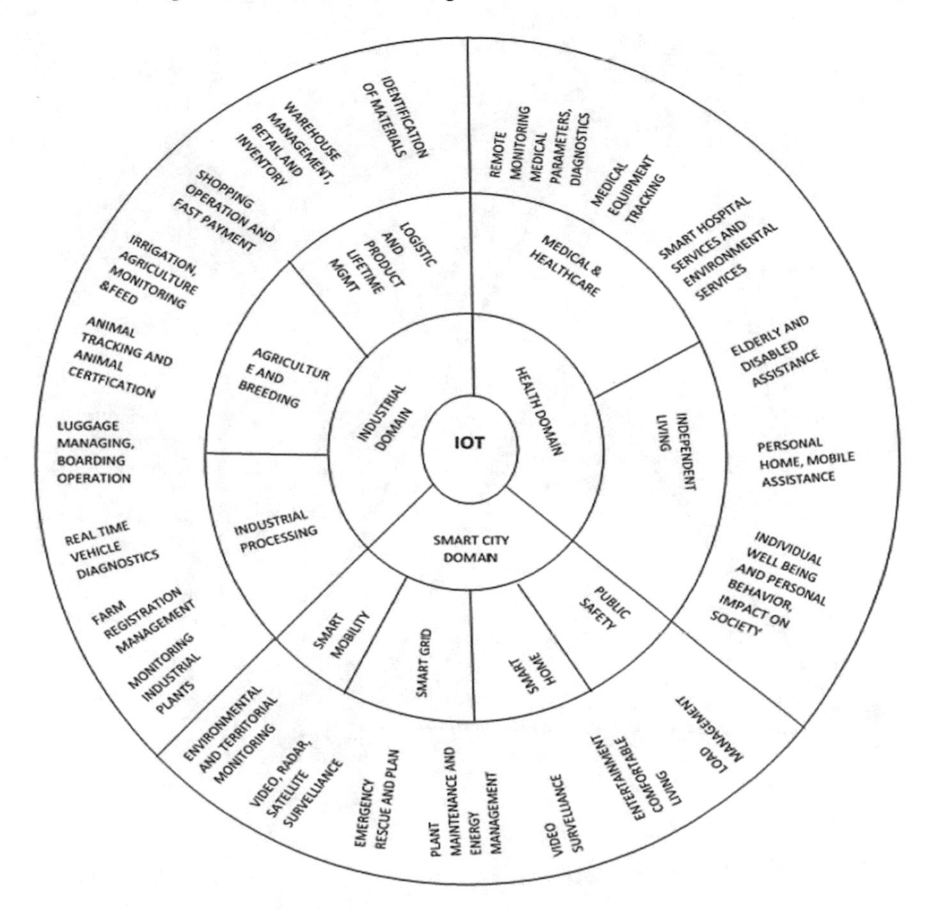

Fig. 1 Overview of IoT applications

2.1 Architecture and Components of IoT

There does not exist any point of reference architecture for IoT as of today. The IoT architecture is usually application-dependent. It is also very essential to have an understanding of the difference between cyber physical systems (CPS) and an IoT application which are used quite synonymously. Lot of research is happening in this area and many architecture models have been proposed [6] in which three- and five-layer architectures are used by majority of applications. Figure 3a, b diagrammatically represents the same. The three-layer architecture has the application network and perception layers. The perception layer or the physical layer is responsible for sensing. The main function of this layer is sensing environment parameters. The interconnections and communications to and from the devices are done by the networking layer, while the application layer provides user-friendly interfaces suiting to the user requirements.

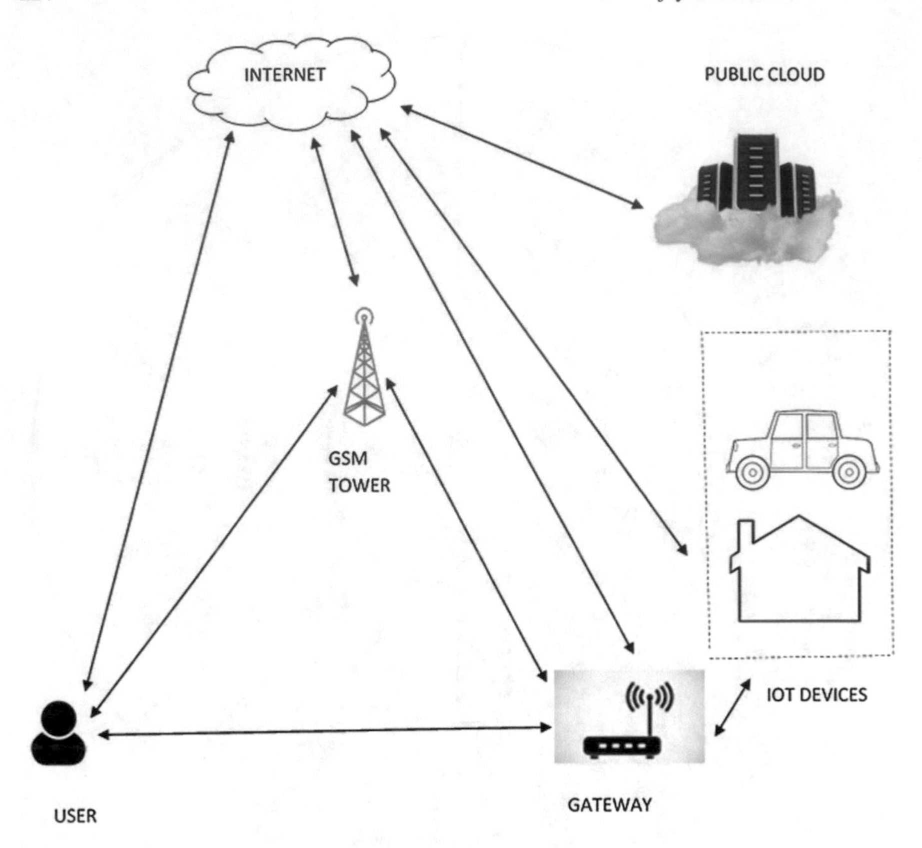

Fig. 2 A model of IoT

The data transfer from the physical to various upper layers happens via various networks. The processing of the data accumulated from the transport layer is the responsibility of the processing layer which employs many technologies for storing and processing data along with providing services to the layers below. The business layer is concerned with the management of the IoT system as a whole including the security and integrity aspects. Any architecture of IoT demonstrates the major functionalities of sensing, processing and networking. IoT devices are a combination of hardware and software, like sensors, actuators Wi-Fi, Bluetooth, Zigbee, and so on. The data processing layer processes the data, analyzes it and take appropriate decisions. For a normal user the direct point of interaction is through the application which is designed for specific applications [7, 8].

To build an IoT application, different IoT frameworks are available which provide guidelines, standards and protocols required for implementation. Some common examples are Eclipse SmartHome, ThingsSpeak, ThingWorx, IoTivity, OpenHAB, Node-RED, AllJoyn, DigitalSTROM, WebNMS, IPSO Alliance, Thread, Open Mobile Alliance, Light Weight Machine to Machine Framework, ThingSquare, AXCIOMA, Xively, The Thing System, IoT ToolKit, ZERYNTH and Cayenne. The

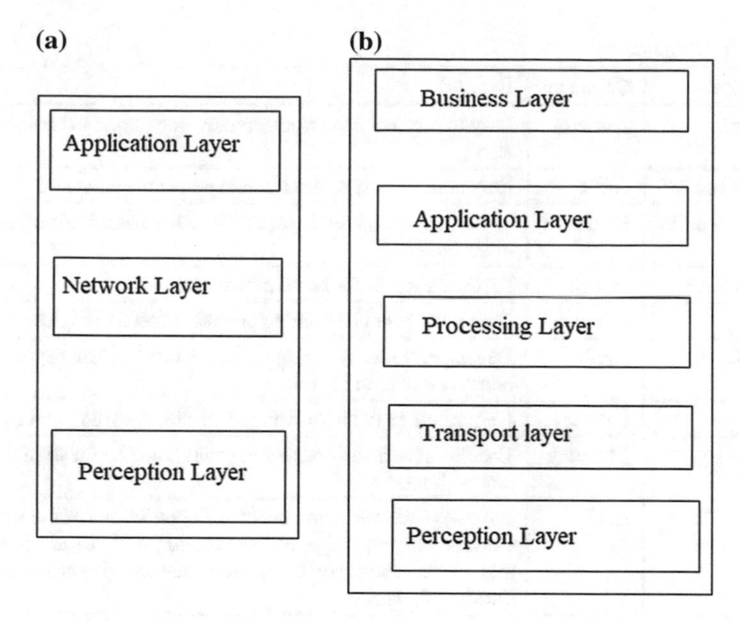

Fig. 3 **a** Three-layer architecture **b** Five-layer architecture

acceptability of these frameworks is dependent on the features it provides especially related to security and privacy aspects. Each of these frameworks has its own features and limitations. The selection of the framework is also dependent on the application requirements. A summary of the various commonly used IoT frameworks mentioning the features of each is mentioned in Table 1 [9].

2.2 *Features and Challenges in IoT*

IoT differs from the traditional networking applications in varied facets. Majority of the IoT devices have resource constraints especially related to size, power and processing capabilities. As these devices are designed mainly for monitoring and surveillance applications, constraints are there in incorporating additional facilities as it will not benefit the used intended. The main features of IoT are depicted in Fig. 4 [9], which differentiate it from the traditional network. Each feature can be a hitch and a boon at various scenarios.

The major challenges that are faced by IoT applications include security, connectivity, reliability and interoperability [10]. Besides that, there are various attacks and threats related to IoT. As IoT is an IP-based network, it is also vulnerable to various attacks. Besides that, IoT lacks a standardized architecture and is prone to various attacks in different layers. Each layer has a number of threats and risks associated to it and the severity of the same depends on the application also. The concept map

Table 1 IoT frameworks

Framework	Company	Features
AWS IoT	Amazon	Easy to connect and ensures secure interaction in offline mode also
ARM Mbed IoT	ARM	Easy connectivity and automatic power management
Azure IoT Suite	Microsoft	Vast range of support irrespective of hardware and software diversity
Brillo/Weave	Google	Specific support for home automation
Calvin	Ericsson	Uses flow-based computing paradigm methodologies
HomeKit	Apple	Developed for easy configuration, control and management of home automation devices
Kura	Eclipse	Kura offers easy interaction IoT devices and the public internet
SmartThings	Samsung	Enable user-friendly access of smart home application through smart phones
Watson	IBM	Provides dynamic configuring and connections of the smart devices with any range, enables the consumer to add devices and connect the newly configurable device without need to enroll with database

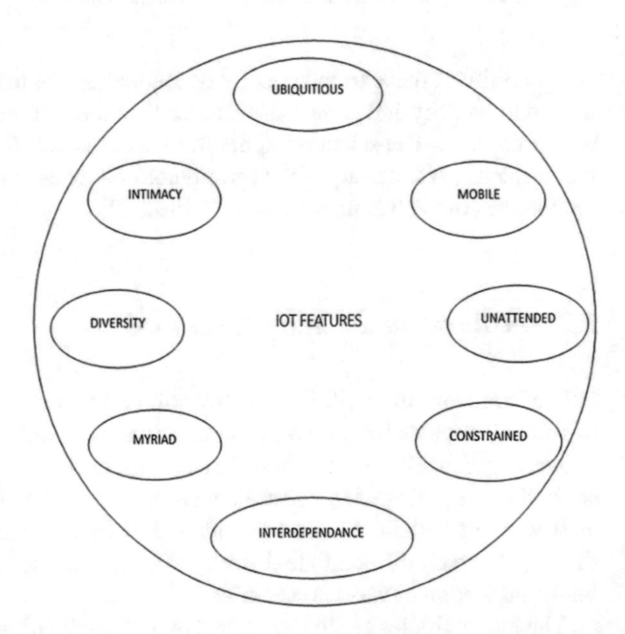

Fig. 4 Overview of IoT features

represented in Fig. 5 helps to gain an understanding of the current state-of-the-art, features, applications, architecture, advantages and limitations of the IoT.

In any IoT application, devices and internet are unavoidable. An edge IoT gadget faces attacks from the internet on one hand and through associated gadgets on the other. An intruder can easily infuse devices into the system. These dangers require

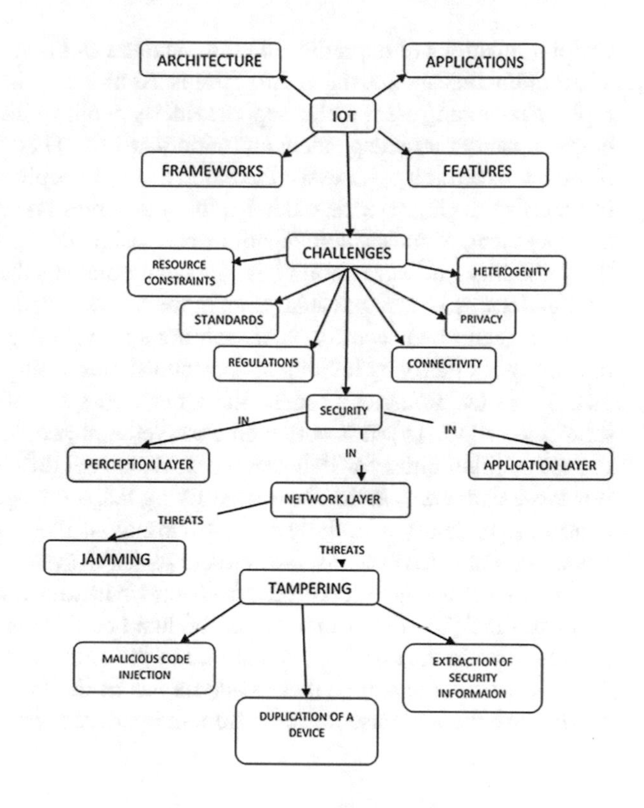

Fig. 5 Concept map

Table 2 Security issues in various layers of IoT architecture

Layer	Security issues
Perception	Device-level threats, denial of service, jamming, tampering
Network	Confidentiality, integrity, compatibility, security, privacy
Application	Software vulnerabilities, authentication, identity and access permission issues, recovery and data security

a complex security design, which needs to consider quite certain imperatives and prerequisites of the IoT. Considering all the features of IoT and how it acts as a challenge is explained mentioning the possible threats to be taken care of. A brief mention of all the threats based on various layers is given in Table 2 [10].

3 Overview of Ambient-Assisted Living

The population of elderly are growing and it is very well noted that majority of them have a desire to live their old-age life at home without bothering their relatives or the caretakers [11]. With advancement in technology, effective support for the elderly in various situations of unpredictable falls, sudden sickness and so on can be provided with continuous monitoring alarm systems. Ambient-assisted living is one of the most rapidly expanding areas which support elderly people with embedded equipment that helps in having an independent and monitored life [12]. The concept of AAL is to imbibe the technology to assist the elderly or the people with unusual requirements in their day-to-day activities. It helps them to achieve independence or autonomy to a great extent. Since such applications are designed with utmost security concerns, the reliability and acceptability is increasing and resulted in wide usage of AAL applications. It is very advantageous in the current world by having greater benefit on their health and security. AAL solutions provide a greater contribution toward the safety of elderly by helping in continuous monitoring of their daily activity [13, 14]. These technologies promise the elderly to stay safe and independent within their houses [11, 15]. It is very well observed that people these days prefer moving to metropolitan cities for living or work, making it difficult to take care of elderly. For these situations, ambient-assisted living helps the aged to live in their comfort zone independently especially in an environment like home [16]. Considering the advantages of AAL systems, the demand for these systems is increasing as health of a person at home can be monitored from anywhere and assistance can be given at any point of time [16, 17]. Moreover, individual health monitoring is most commonly followed due to the massive population and the understanding of systems in medical field. However, the con of these systems lies in the fact that they are yet not fit to accomplish the immense power of human interaction and activities.

3.1 Architecture of AAL

Figure 6 presents the architecture of an ambient-assisted living. The entire architecture can be divided into three layers. Daily routine and issues related to health of an elderly at home can be monitored using data collected from wired, wireless and wearable devices. For this purpose hardware devices are mounted at home. Hardware devices like sensors collect data from the environment and are transferred to a gateway which can communicate with the framework so that monitoring and controlling of all the connected devices could be carried out from the installed location.

Local subsystem consists of devices that are installed at home of an elderly which communicates with the core subsystem via a local area network or wireless network. Local subsystem controls the physical devices and collects the result to transfer them to core subsystem. This is a combination of hardware and software gateway.

Nomadic subsystems are worn by the caregiver. It enables the outdoor activities in places not covered by the local subsystem.

Core subsystem is a software component that is in charge of controlling the system and functions of the data store. Core subsystems can be installed on a local server or in the cloud server.

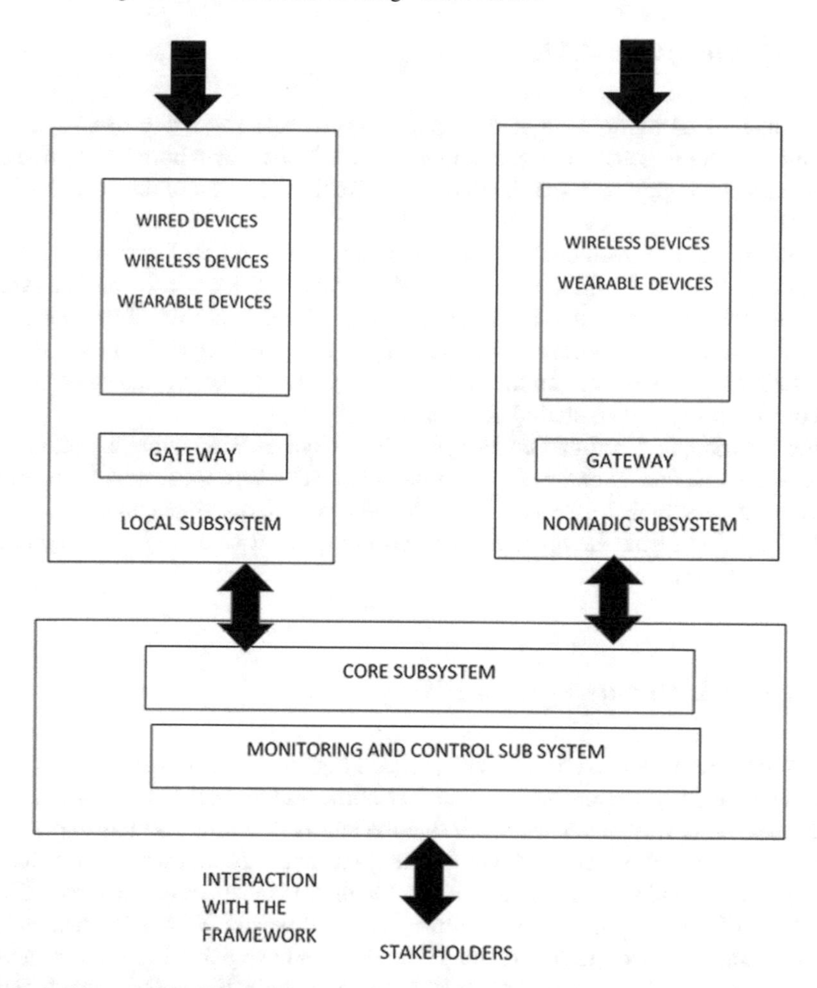

Fig. 6 Architecture of ambient-assisted living

The data collected from the sensors are transferred through communication channels, namely wireless or mobile network, to the gateways. The objectives of the gateways are to collect data from sensors mounted at home.

Monitoring control system includes all those equipment and software components used by caretakers and the staff. The function of this module is controlling, data management and presentation of data to the end-user [18].

3.2 Challenges in AAL

Ambient-assisted living promoted various ways to help the living of people who are aged assisting them to live securely and freely in their own home. Nevertheless, there exist few important issues in ambient-assisted living. Few of the challenges are discussed here.

Dynamic service availability: One of the most important challenge with AAL is service availability. As there are no formal caretakers, there will be an increase in need of social resources and social connections. The availability of these services is very dynamic and handling this dynamicity is a big challenge. There should be a way to institute a structure so that various devices can be connected to each other and mechanically called, started or stopped.

Service mapping: Another challenge with ambient-assisted living is establishing a technique that can automatically map the services that are requested. Some of the service mapping tools that could be developed can overcome this challenge.

Willingness: There should be massive encouragement given to people to participate in AAL system [19].

4 IoT in Ambient-Assisted Living

The population of elderly in this era is much higher when compared to the birth rate. When elderly person prefer to stay at home and are not able to take care of themselves, it is very much necessary that the family or a caretaker has to pay extra attention to them. The costs of the caretakers are increasing and it is necessary that the family has to spend a good financial amount to the caretakers or to the nurses. These can lead to financial pressure in families with aged people. Wearable technologies are a potential solution to this issue. These devices have helped in monitoring the daily activities of elderly at home as well as assisting them. Figure 7 depicts different types of IoT devices for elderly. IoT-enabled devices can be categorized as wearable and non-wearable. At present, advances in wearable and sensor technology help in designing devices that play an important role in monitoring and assisting elderly people.

As most of the elderly suffer from problems and issues related to age, the health-related issues and their symptoms can be monitored continuously that will help in taking effective precautions. Pressure ulcer formation is a serious problem among elderly and bedridden patients that needs utmost care. IoT-enabled devices that help in preventing formation of pressure ulcers in elderly are explained here.

At present, devices like smart watch, smart phone and smart clothing are some of the major wearable technologies assisting elderly at home for conveying health information. Smart phones are ubiquitously carried by everyone every day. Smart watches, on the other hand, can be considered as a networked computer with inbuilt sensors that can capture the physical signals as they are in touch with the skin.

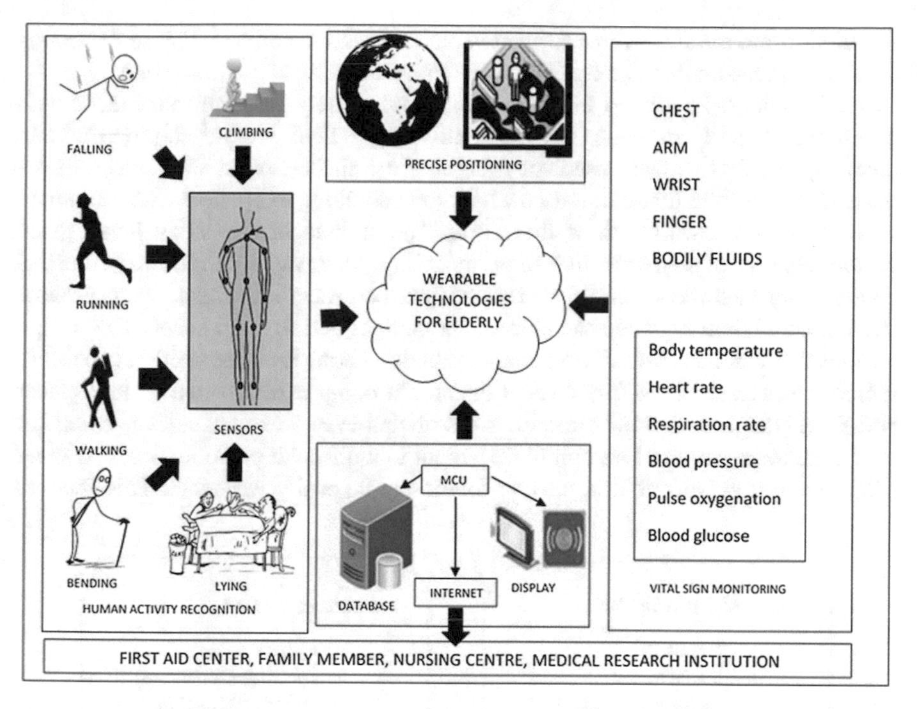

Fig. 7 Types of IoT devices

Smart clothing is a device that helps in capturing information from the body through the sensors connected with the fabric. Smart clothing can capture more information when compared to smart watch and smart phones. There are smart shirts [14] that can capture the heartbeat of a person. There are many similar smart clothes that are designed that could be used for elderly care to monitor physical activity.

Elderly care using IoT is made possible with the help of physical devices positioned for monitoring their activities and health. These devices that are used for monitoring can be categorized as outdoor and indoor positioning systems. Outdoor positioning systems provide services based on locations with nearest accuracy level [20]. Indoor positioning systems are those systems that have the capability to function in real time and thus help in the ambient-assisted living by providing the precise locations of human in the indoor areas [21]. These systems are well suited for detecting and tracking objects. Further, they help in providing support for elderly in their everyday doings.

4.1 Pressure Ulcer Detection in Elderly by Using IoT Devices

From [11] it is clear that friction plays an important role in pressure ulcer formation. Keeping this as a basic cause, bed sheets are designed that could cause reduction in the friction and the shear force formed in patients who are on bed. Figure 8 presents the risk of pressure damage due to microclimate conditions in human body.

Authors in [22] designed a bed sheet that could reduce discomfort for those with pressure ulcer and can reduce the probability of a patient with developing pressure ulcer. Spacer fabrics were used for designing the sheet. Spacer fabrics is a three-dimensional knitted fabric that uses a tuck loop stitching to connect with a filament yarn at the top and bottom of the fabric. The authors in this study investigated various features of the fabric, like air permeability, water vapor permeability, thermal conductivity, absorbency and compression. The bed sheet is designed to ensure low friction coefficient between the skin of the patient and the bed sheet. The design ensures that the skin stays dry by enabling high wicking and evaporation capability which in turn ensures low friction coefficient. The compressibility of a 3D knit spacer bed sheet is high so that the pressure is distributed evenly and enables the caretaker to change the position of an immobile patient to a different position. The bed sheet proposed in this work is designed so that it can be easily washable. This sheet is

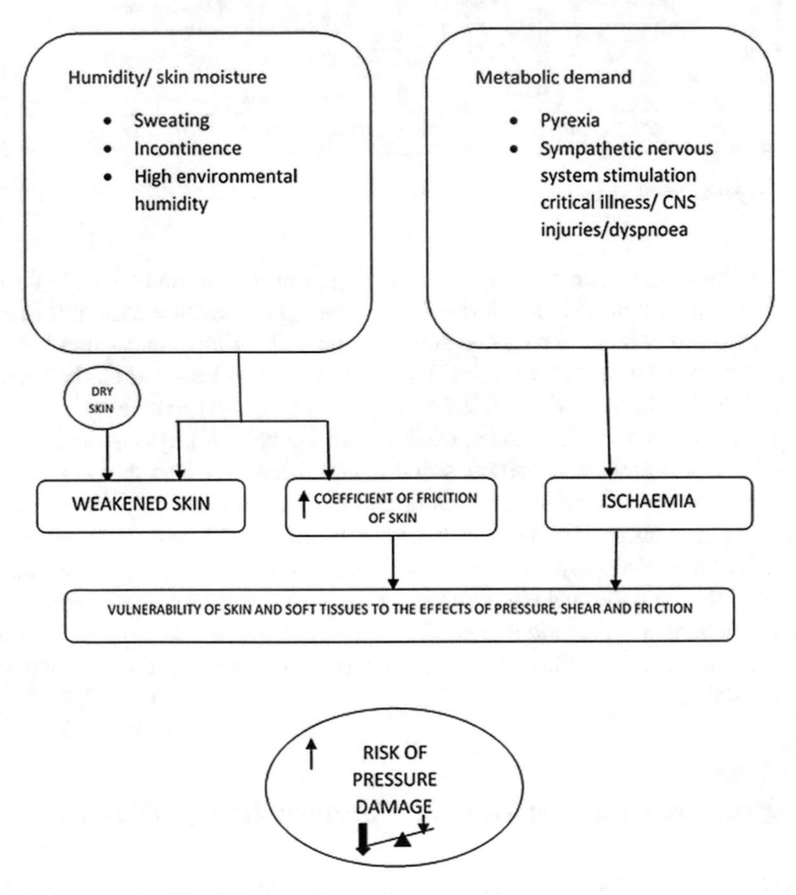

Fig. 8 Risk of pressure damage

also expected to stay longer than a usual bed sheet used in the hospitals. The antimicrobial finishes in the blanket will protect it from pollutants. The anti-creasing finishing used in the sheet will protect the sheet from wrinkling and hence reduces the chance of creating friction points [23].

A pressure-sensitive bed sheet is designed with sensing e-textile layers that help in monitoring pressure ulcer occurrence. The designed sheet involves three different components: an array of pressure sensors, a unit for sampling the data and user interface using a tablet. Sensor array is an e-textile material which has a fiber yarn covered with piezoelectric polymer. The bed sheet has three sheets which are crammed together. The topmost sheet is designed with a normal fabric which has parallel conductive lines 64 in number. The central sheet is the e-textile and the bottommost sheet has 128 conductive lines organized vertically to the upper 64 lines. At each connection of conductive lines, the structure has a pressure-sensitive resistor [24]. Pressure image analysis is carried out to obtain the body part localization. Through continuous monitoring the risk of pressure locations in the body is analyzed to avoid formation of ulcer. This data will be embedded in tablets to perform data analysis so as to track the data and generate alerts [25].

Smart hospital beds are designed that consist of an actuating mechanism that is capable of controlling patient's body without the assistance of a caretaker. When the pressure is exerted at a particular point, the surface of the mattress deforms by distributing force at each contact point. This helps in offloading the pressure with minor repositioning, which in turn decreases the shear on the skin of a patient due to manual turning or repositioning.

Monitor Alert Project (M.A.P) system mat uses a specialized mat that can measure the pressure of contact between the person and the surface. The M.A.P. system of Wellsense, Inc. is an equipment that is designed in such a way that it creates a heat map-like display in real time, which shows the pressure that has high probability of producing ulcers. The disadvantage of the system is that the pressure is measured along the coordinate of the grid rather than the person lying on the mat. Simply indicates that even if the patient is not on the mat and a dummy pressure is applied the system won't be able to differentiate [26].

Dyna-Form Mercury Advance mattresses are tested to be appropriate for patients at very high threat of ulcer development and are very much prone to treatment of the same. Dyna mattress is a fixed mattress that is in combination with the feature of dynamic alternating system. These mattresses can be used within patients home or in a palliative care environment. The major advantage with this mattress is that the parts of the mattress are replaceable. The outer cover of the Dyna mattress is of high-frequency connected, multirigid, vapor-permeable fabric strictly controlling the infection policies so that the patient is safe from causing any kind of infections. This mattress is capable of holding a weight of 254 kg. Studies have proved that the best outcome is when the weight is up to 152 kg [27].

The Softform Premier Active mattress is also used for all those bedridden patients who are at high threat of pressure ulcer development. It comprises a froth mattress with an underlay that dynamically alternates on two-cell 10-min cycle time through the pump. The pump is designed in such a way that it can judge the weight of a patient and accordingly regulate the appropriate amount of air. This helps in controlling the development of pressure ulcer in patients. The weight that this mattress can hold is up to 248 kg.

A system was developed that could be used in home scenarios for monitoring the possibility of pressure ulcer development. The feasibility of the study is conducted with people who are clients of the caregiver company. A pressure ulcer risk screening module is developed that includes a software module developed using android that acquires the pressure ulcer risk of the patient based on the Braden scale of risk assessment. This is integrated with the system for monitoring the pressure ulcer. The system includes three basic modules to detect the motion of the patient using accelerometer and pressure, a module for collection of data and pre-processing the same and a user interface. Authors claim that this system could be mounted on any type of mattresses and it does not have any effect on the sleep comfort of the patient [28].

Figure 9 presents a pressure ulcer risk alert system in which sensor patches are positioned on threat areas on the skin of the patient. These sensors will monitor the pressure, temperature, humidity and motion in communication with the skin. The

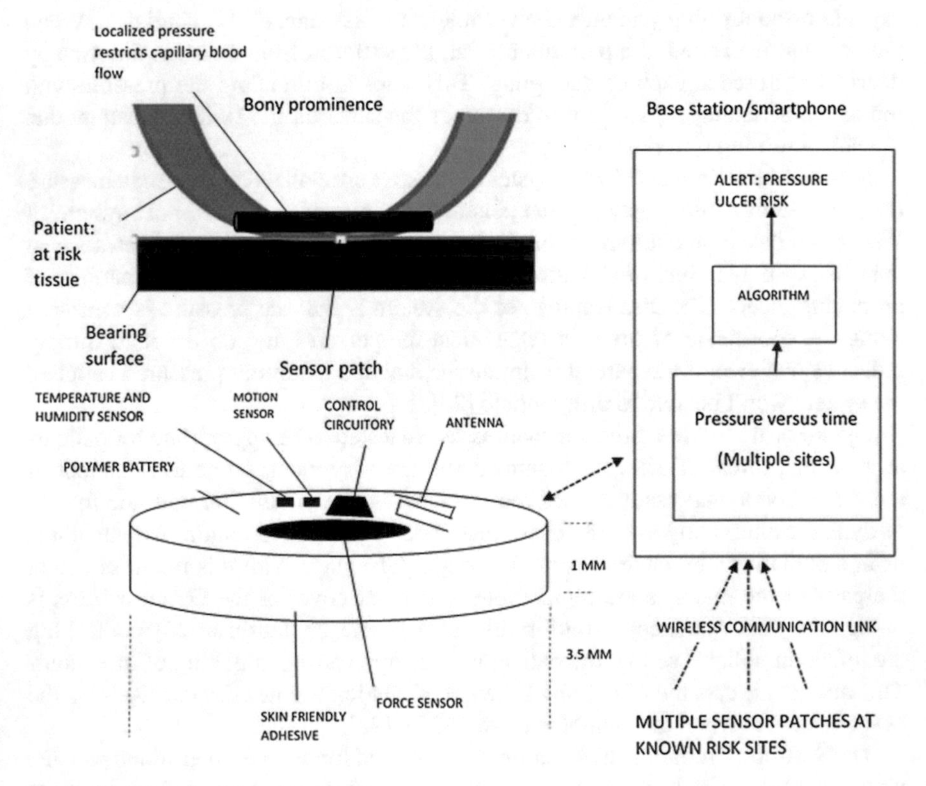

Fig. 9 Pressure ulcer risk alert system

data collected from the sensors are communicated to the base station device or the smart phone [29].

EHealth image system is a pressure preventive sitting mat with components like monitoring sensor, main board, a unit to control the power supply and an electronic switch. The monitoring sensor is used to identify the body position of the patient, the factors like, temperature and humidity and the level of pressure exerted by the patient. With a particularly established EHealth image system for pressure ulcer, all the sensors that are used to collect this information are mounted on the matt. The design uses medical pressure mapping system that can be applied at the interface of the seat/skin. An user interface is designed so that it can display the real-time data from the sensors [30].

Smart bed system is designed to assist the caretakers in nursing of the elderly. Based on the factors, age and body weight, the system can recognize the risk points of the body where ulcers are prone to occur. The smart bed designed in this study is claimed to provide intensity of pressure at risk points or area in the body of a patient. This information helps to determine the posture of the patient, if it is the supine or lateral position. The information regarding the duration of pressure exerted at this particular body position is also captured. These information will help the caretakers in preventing the occurrence of bedsores [31].

The technique designed by Leaf Healthcare is based on an accelerometer-containing electronic sensor. Leaf Healthcare created such a product that could sense the motion and then predict whether or not the patient is at threat of occurrence of pressure ulcer based on the data captured from motion. A motion sensing device claims to increase the accuracy of preventing pressure ulcer when compared to the traditional methods that is followed in hospitals, like turning the patient in a specified interval to avoid the occurrence of pressure ulcer. The main drawback of this device is that it does not measure pressure in the body's at-risk areas, so its predictive capabilities cannot be accurate [26].

Subepidermal moisture (SEM) is a biometric scanner that could be handheld and has various sensors that are incorporated in the device. It helps to detect commencement of pressure ulcers before they actually appear on the skin. This equipment helps in evaluating the subepidermal moisture level, which is a major factor associated with the localized epidemic in the initial inflammatory phase of pressure ulcer. Caretakers or nurses can place it in the body of the patient in the areas that are prone to get ulcers to check if there is tissue damage.

4.2 Wearable Devices

An adhesive patch is developed that adheres to a body area that is prone to the development of pressure ulcer. The idea was that the patch that is designed for detecting the risk of pressure ulcer should stay on the body for at least seven days, be water-resistant and be biocompatible. The material used for the patch was Tegaderm Film dressing by 3 M Co. It remained for an average of 5 days on the participants, was water-resistant after 5 h and caused no skin damage that led the team to select this medical bandage as the final material to be used for detecting the risk of pressure ulcer [26].

The heels of the patient can be easily prone to shear and pressure. Heels are always in contact with bed surface for patients lying down and hence they are more prone to shear. When the patient is lifted out of the bed the patient is more prone to shear if proper handling techniques are not used. Pillow and heel lift boots can be used to reduce the cause of pressure ulcer formation. While using pillows the caregivers need to make sure that the heel does not come in contact with mattress. The caregivers need to make sure to use the heel boot devices very carefully. Straps need to be in place so that it does not come in contact with the skin.

Cervical collars are one more device which surges the risk of increasing pressure ulcer at chin, shoulder and ear. It was found that lengthier period of collar use was connected with amplified risk of developing pressure ulcer in studies of trauma patients with cervical collars. Further than five days, the usage of cervical collars is related with a 38–55% risk of increasing pressure ulcers. Inflexible collars prepared of foam or plastic are related with a greater risk of evolving pressure ulcer than padded collars. When used suitably, padded collars such as the Aspen or Miami cervical collar can stop the progress of pressure ulcer [32].

Intelligent monitoring and caution systems are developed with five functional components: profile of the patient that stores patient data, sensor settings to set up the parameters of the sensor nodes, information management of staff that manages the data of the caretaker, monitoring of patient state that contains dynamic information about the patients state, monitoring pressure contains data monitoring and querying for caretakers to get an update of patients present status. This module also takes care of setting the frequency of data transmission, threshold for the sensors and the threshold for alarms. This system helps to prevent pressure ulcer formation in mobility-impaired people. It also works as a precautionary system. It can monitor the patient while he is in the lying position. Also the data can be continuously monitored, transmitted, processed and recorded. And with all this data, repositioning schedule can also be generated [23].

The wearable sensing system with sensor placed in wearing gowns is an IoT-enabled technique which supports taking care of hospitalized elderly at home and also tele-monitoring them. It is a very useful method which will benefit the elderly patients and their families. Because of such initiative, timely care can be provided in a comfortable environment and also this reduces risk. The sensing system is reliable and robust in monitoring actions through different mobile devices. It manages patient data, alerts nurses and caregivers through web applications [33].

5 Conclusions

There is an immense increase in the number of elderly citizens who are prone to health problems and hence this leads to increase in demand for healthcare services. With advancement in technology, effective support for the elderly in various situations of unpredictable falls; sudden sickness and so on can be provided with continuous monitoring alarm systems. Ambient-assisted living is aimed to support active and healthy aging of the elderly through emerging technology like internet of things (IoT). The concept of AAL is to imbibe the smart technology to assist the elderly or the people with unusual requirements in their day-to-day activities. It helps them to achieve independence or autonomy to a great extent. Since such applications are designed with utmost security concerns, the reliability and acceptability is increasing and resulted in wide usage of AAL applications.

6 Future Scope

With increasing population of elderly and no one to monitor them continuously, there is a need for a system that could help in taking care of the aged. With advancement in technology, there is increase in the development of IoT-integrated devices that help to give a safe and healthy living for elderly. There are many devices that are developed with the objective of assisting the elderly by monitoring their health on a real-time basis. It is very much necessary to encourage people to use AAL systems for a better and safe life. AAL could be extended by establishing a technique that can automatically map the services that are requested. Some of the service mapping tools could be developed that could overcome this challenge of current AAL systems.

References

1. Kudou D, Okamoto A, Murata Y (2018) Internet of Things, 1st edn., Elsevier Ltd., pp 1–380
2. Jing Q, Vasilakos AV, Wan J, Lu J, Qiu D (2014) Security of the Internet of Things: perspectives and challenges. Wirel Networks 20(8):2481–2501
3. Miorandi D, Sicari S, De Pellegrini F, Chlamtac I (2012) Internet of Things: vision, applications and research challenges. Ad Hoc Netw 10(7):1497–1516
4. Roman R, Zhou J, Lopez J (2013) On the features and challenges of security and privacy in distributed Internet of Things. Comput Netw 57(10):2266–2279
5. Gil D, Ferrández A, Mora-Mora H, Peral J (2016) Internet of Things: a review of surveys based on context aware intelligent services. Sensors (Switzerland) 16(7):1–23
6. Sethi P, Sarangi SR (2017) Internet of Things: architecture, issues and applications. Int J Eng Res Appl 07(06):85–88
7. Lin J, Yu W, Zhang N, Yang X, Zhang H, Zhao W (2017) A survey on Internet of Things: architecture, enabling technologies, security and privacy, and applications. IEEE Internet Things J 4(5):1125–1142
8. Gubbi J, Buyya R, Marusic S, Palaniswami M (2013) Internet of Things (IoT): a vision, architectural elements, and future directions. Futur Gener Comput Syst 29(7):1645–1660
9. Ammar M, Russello G, Crispo B (2018) Internet of Things: a survey on the security of IoT frameworks. J Inf Secur Appl 38:8–27
10. Sikder AK, Petracca G, Aksu H, Jaeger T, Uluagac AS (2018) A survey on sensor-based threats to Internet-of-Things (IoT) devices and applications

11. Yacchirema DC, Palau CE, Esteve M (2017) Enable IoT interoperability in ambient assisted living: active and healthy aging scenarios. In: 14th IEEE annual consumer communications & networking conference CCNC, pp 53–58
12. Cedillo P, Sanchez C, Campos K, Bermeo A (2018) A systematic literature review on devices and systems for ambient assisted living: solutions and trends from different user perspectives. In: 5th international conference on eDemocracy & eGovernment. ICEDEG, pp 59–66
13. Spitalewsky K, Rochon J, Ganzinger M, Knaup P (2013) Potential and requirements of IT for ambient assisted living technologies: results of a Delphi study. Methods Inf Med 52(3):231–238
14. Wang Z, Yang Z, Dong T (2017) A review of wearable technologies for elderly care that can accurately track indoor position, recognize physical activities and monitor vital signs in real time. Sensors 17:341
15. Dimitrievski A, Zdravevski E, Lameski P, Trajkovik V (2016) A survey of ambient assisted living systems: challenges and opportunities. In: Proceedings of the 2016 IEEE 12th international conference on intelligent computer communication and processing ICCP, pp 49–53
16. Memon M, Wagner SR, Pedersen CF, Aysha Beevi FH, Hansen FO (2014) Ambient assisted living healthcare frameworks, platforms, standards, and quality attributes. Sensors (Switzerland) 14(3):4312–4341
17. Lloret J, Canovas A, Sendra S, Parra L (2015) Ambient assisted living communications: a smart communication architecture for ambient assisted living. (1):26–33
18. Stefan I, Aldea CL, Nechifor CS (2018) Web platform architecture for ambient assisted living. J Ambient Intell Smart Environ 10(1):35–47
19. Sun H, De Florio V, Gui N, Blondia C (2009) Promises and challenges of ambient assisted living systems. In: ITNG 2009 6th international conference on information technology new generations, pp 1201–1207
20. Dardari D, Closas P, Djuric PM (2015) Indoor tracking: theory, methods, and technologies. IEEE Trans Veh Technol 64(4):1263–1278
21. Gu Y, Lo A, Niemegeers I (2009) A survey of indoor positioning systems for wireless personal networks. IEEE Commun Surv Tutorials 11(1):13–32
22. Gokarneshan N (2018) Role of knit spacer fabrics in treatment of pressure ulcers. Glob J Addict Rehabil Med 5(5):1–5
23. Wang TY, Chen SL, Huang HC, Kuo SH, Shiu YJ (2011) The development of an intelligent monitoring and caution system for pressure ulcer prevention. In: Proceedings of the international conferrence on machine learning and cybernetics, vol 2, pp 566–571
24. Poon CCY, Wong YM, Zhang YT (2006) M-health: the development of cuff-less and wearable blood pressure meters for use in body sensor networks. In: 2006 IEEE/NLM life science systems and applications workshop, pp 1–2
25. Liu JJ, Huang MC, Xu W, Sarrafzadeh M (2014) Bodypart localization for pressure ulcer prevention. In: 2014 36th annual international conference of the ieee engineering in medicine and biology society, pp 766–769
26. Ooyama-searls R, Pachucki B, Parent B (2017) A pressure ulcer patch material study for a wearable sensor
27. Rafter L (2014) Evaluation of patient outcomes: pressure ulcer prevention mattresses. British J Nurs 20(Sup6):S32–S38
28. Hayn D et al (2015) An eHealth system for pressure ulcer risk assessment based on accelerometer and pressure data. J Sensors 2015:1–8
29. Sen D, McNeill J, Mendelson Y, Dunn R, Hickle K (2018) A new vision for preventing pressure ulcers: wearable wireless devices could help solve a common-and serious-problem. IEEE Pulse 9(6):28–31
30. Sung CS, Park JY (2017) A monitoring sensor-based eHealth image system for pressure ulcer prevention. Multimed Tools Appl pp 1–13
31. Hong Y-S (2018) Smart care beds for elderly patients with impaired mobility. Wirel Commun Mob Comput 2018:1–12
32. Karen C (2013) Evidence-based prevention of pressure ulcers. Crit Care Nurse 33(6):57–67

33. Ribon JR, Martin Monroy R, Plinio Puello M (2018) Prevention of pressure ulcers and incontinence-associated dermatitis in home hospitalization of older adults. Indian J Sci Technol 11(1):1–10

Dr. A. Vijayalakshmi works in the Department of Computer Science at CHRIST (Deemed to be University), Bangalore. She completed her Ph.D. in the year 2017 in the field of pattern recognition. Her area of research interests are pattern recognition, internet of things, machine learning and artificial intelligence. She is currently working on a University-funded project in the field of internet of things.

Dr. Deepa V. Jose works in the Department of Computer Science at CHRIST (Deemed to be University), Bangalore. She completed her Ph.D. in the year 2017 in the field of wireless sensor networks. Her area of research interests are internet of things, sensor networks, machine learning and artificial intelligence. She is currently working on a University-funded project in the field of internet of things.

Smart Healthcare Applications and Real-Time Analytics Through Edge Computing

Parul Verma and Shahnaz Fatima

Abstract The healthcare industry is growing with leaps and bounds. These services are getting costlier day by day. As the population is growing and so the number of diseases, there is a need for easy, economical, and reachable healthcare solutions. Technology can help in a great way by just changing the scenario and moving medical regular medical checkups from hospital to your home. Even in the case of chronic diseases, regular remote monitoring of patients can be a great help. IoT has a great impact on healthcare industry and is supporting all sectors of health care. IoT has revolutionized the healthcare systems by connecting medical devices, sensors, equipment to Internet, and collecting invaluable data which is being used for treatment, forecast, study of trends, analytics, and so on. IoT for healthcare systems uses cloud to store and process voluminous data produced by medical devices and sensors. Edge computing has been introduced to reduce overburdening on cloud servers and also facilitates real-time analysis of medical data. The chapter focuses on using edge computing for real-time analysis of healthcare system. The chapter will also discuss challenges of edge computing.

Keywords Healthcare systems · Real-time analytics · Edge computing · Real time · Edge computing use cases · Issue and challenges edge computing

1 Introduction

Health care is huge and dynamic industry which is always ready to adopt revolutionary technologies. Though the industry is changing dynamically, still there are some lacunae due to which the benefits are not reachable to the masses. Collaboration of IoT with healthcare applications is done in order to draw maximum benefits of healthcare applications. IoT-based healthcare services are reducing the cost, enhancing user's experience and hence increasing the quality of life.

Microelectromechanical Systems (MEMS) have been acknowledged to be one of the most sought for technologies for times to come and this MEMS has the potential

P. Verma (✉) · S. Fatima
Amity University, Lucknow, Uttar Pradesh, India
e-mail: pverma1@lko.amity.edu

P. Raj et al. (eds.), *Internet of Things Use Cases for the Healthcare Industry*,
https://doi.org/10.1007/978-3-030-37526-3_11

to transform consumer and industrial products by merging both microelectronics and micromachining technologies. This joint system has been witnessed to initiate and propagate opportunities for implementation of the smart surroundings. It is a great help especially in the field of medical sciences, forensic sciences, applied sciences, and numerous sensors to assess different types of essential symptoms, viz., heartbeat, blood pressure, body temperature, ECG, profile, etc. This is where the emergence and importance of IoT-enabled design of innovative services are found essential for better health care of citizens. The lives of citizens will be dramatically affected by infusion of microelectromechanical system-based devices and technologies [1].

The latest advancements in the design of IoT technologies are stimulating the development of improved version of healthcare systems. With the IoT-enabled range of MEMS sensors and actuators, the observable facts that can be sensed or acted upon with MEMS devices are more of challenge in today's scenario. The system having automatic identification and tracking of individuals and certain specific biomedical machines/devices in healthcare units along with real-time examining of individual's physiological parameters for early or at least timely detection of clinical deterioration are few of the good examples to be mentioned [1].

The health care is a very vast domain and it also includes personal health care, pharmaceutical industry, healthcare insurance, biosensors, ingestible sensors, smart pills and beds, and many other things. The list of IoT applications in health care is endless. Other areas of IoT applications in health care are monitoring, tracking, and maintenance of patient's health status, device's working status, maintenance status of device, and many more.

Most of the organizations look for cloud for data access, analysis, and storage as well. Though there are numerous advantages of using cloud, still it is not a viable solution for storing and analyzing the huge volume of data that is produced by connected medical devices and IoT. Moving all data to a centralized data center is an inefficient way of handling huge volume of data generated by numerous IoT devices. Edge computing provides solution by creating small network of data centers with specific features for data processing. Digital projects that create or require data can be processed much faster when the computing power is close to the device or person generating it. The functioning of edge is quite similar to the traditional data center and it changes the way of processing information and delivery to the end users.

1.1 IoT Application in Healthcare Systems

Application area of IoT is quite diversified. IoT-enabled devices facilitate remote monitoring in the healthcare system. IoT is playing a crucial role in transformation of healthcare industry. IoT has applications in health care that benefit patients, families, physicians, hospitals, and insurance companies.

Following are the various IoT healthcare application areas which can be categorized as follows:

For Patients

Nowadays, it has become a trend of showcasing or having wearable devices driven with the Internet of Things (IoT). However, the fundamental idea is nothing new at all. The latest wearable devices can connect with your existing devices like personal computers, etc. which makes it quite obvious that by getting access to them it can do lot of interesting activities. These devices have gone quite smart and they are helping especially old age people who are living alone or living in some remote areas. The device will not only notify the person itself, besides that the notification will also be to their caretakers may be their family or healthcare centers. Such kind of instant notification will definitely help them in taking crucial decisions related to their health.

For Physicians

Wearable devices used by patients can help the doctors to monitor their patient's health. Doctors can proactively suggest treatment plans for their patients by getting updated information on various parameters through these wearable devices. Identification and persuasion of best possible treatment in record time is one of the major outcomes from IoT-enabled healthcare devices as these devices assist physicians with correct data collection and may assist physicians for suggesting appropriate prescription based on symptoms (data collection).

For Hospitals

IoT can be a big help in hospitals also by facilitating the complete healthcare system in many ways. Doctors or physicians can make use of Real-Time Location Services (RTLS) to locate various IoT-enabled devices in hospitals. While duty shifts, various medical devices kept by earlier staff are difficult to locate, and hence real-time location services can be of real help to them in locating various devices like wheelchairs, nebulizers, pumps, etc.

Doctors can also predict and analyze the arrival of remote patients in Post-anesthesia Care Units (PACU). IoT-enabled healthcare monitoring systems can provide the real-time status of patients to the doctors.

The system of hand hygiene is another very crucial concern to monitor the recklessness caused due to unhygienic touch to patients. As per the records of Center of Disease Control and Prevention in USA, it is about 5% patients who get infections caused by the lack of proper hand hygiene in the hospitals [2].

For Medical Insurance Companies

With reference to processes of health insurance, the recent reports by Growth Enabler refer to a futuristic claim of about 20 billion connected devices by the year 2020. These figures are quite promising and so we can look forward in the direction of digital transformation which will be sensor-powered in many industries including health insurance as well. [3] Insurance companies are now incorporating the monitoring system through various wearable devices and identifying the kind of policy needed by the person.

In current scenario, the whole healthcare system is somewhere revolving around the IoT technology. Be it patient, doctors, hospitals, or medical insurance companies, all are drawing benefits out of this digital innovation.

There are varieties of healthcare system devices available these days like heart rate monitors, electronic wristbands. These devices help physicians and doctors to give more personalized advice to their patients. Patients also interact with the doctors seamlessly and the benefits are increased manifold.

1.2 Devices Being Used in Healthcare Systems

IoT has revolutionized the healthcare system and opened up versatile opportunities. Ordinary medical devices are capable of collecting less valuable data. However, when they are connected to Internet, they collect invaluable data which provides wide insight of patient symptoms, remote monitoring of chronic patients, and they facilitate patients to have control over their lives and treatment. Following devices are popularly being used by patients involved in IoT-based healthcare systems.

Wearables

These devices are getting popular and are first-hand tools to monitor personal health. Wearables are available to keep a track of an individual's health as well as keep alarming them in critical situations as well.

Activity Tracking

The Runtastic Orbit is an activity tracking device which tracks daily movements, sleep, and fitness routine of the end users. Like any other wearable devices, it is also designed for versatile usability. It can be worn on a wrist, belt, or any other location. Orbit features time, alarm, OLED display, and Bluetooth Smart Technology. It is waterproof up to 30 feet.

Weight Loss

Lose It! is one of the weight loss utility. It offers numerous services majorly counting calories, logging meals, sending reminders/reports on weight loss goals, and many more. The real purpose of this wearable device is to motivate people to sustain healthy lifestyle and to lose weight. It is quite compatible with numerous healthcare technologies and fitness devices that include FitBit, Misfit, Google Fit, Strava, and Runkeeper, available a Bluetooth-coupled scale for uploading data to the application.

Consultation with Virtual Doctor

HealthTap is one of its kinds of health and fitness management networks which help patients cum consumers with wide-ranging virtual care from remote.

Hydration Tool

Water balance is a hydration tool introduced in the form of watch. It is quite useful wearable device which helps users to maintain their water level and also help them in improving their hydration habits. Hydration tool identifies the need of the amount of water of an individual depending upon consumers' age, height, weight, and level of burning calories by physical activities. It also keeps needful records of the beverages end user drinks to meet this goal throughout the day [4].

BioSensors

BioSensors are introduced as analytical tools for analyzing the biochemical and biomaterial samples. The biosensors are used for understanding of bio-composition, structure, and functions of the samples by changing a biological response in equivalent electrical signal(s). These analytical devices or tools comprise a biological recognition constituent openly linked to a signal transducer that jointly relates the concentration of an analyte (or group of related analytes) to a well-defined measurable response [5].

Biosensors are quite smart as they record patient's health data in real time and provide updated information to the doctors in order to avoid disease complications. In healthcare systems, biosensor collects various physiological data and then transmits it to the healthcare monitoring systems where the caretakers have a look on the data and reports doctor if any unusual change is found in regular pattern of the data. In this way, biosensors patch up the whole network of healthcare system and are trying to convert it into Medical IoT.

Sensiotec Virtual Medical Assistant

This is the first cardiorespiratory remote patient monitoring system. It is called as Virtual Medical Assistant (VMA). VMA tends to work as a decision support system. It has a potential to identify health crisis at an early stage. The VMA generates continuous cardiorespiratory information, and the data served with such system is having its tremendous usefulness in decision support systems and may also be used fundamentally in recognizing the problems before they take a serious shape.

Freestyle Libre Flash

It is freestyle way of glucose monitoring where you do not have to prick instead of that you can scan. It is a small sensor which automatically measures and stores glucose readings throughout day and night. While doing any activities even if you are swimming or bathing it keeps on monitoring as it is water resistant. It is user-friendly in nature which keeps you updated about the last 8 h glucose status and also shows the direction of high or low glucose level. It provides various types of reports based on various parameters which give detailed and intricate information about the glucose level in your body.

Health Patch

Health patches are a kind of wearable wireless device. It is a waterproof sensor for heart rate monitoring which seems like a Band-Aid which is highly technical. It consists of Bluetooth connectivity, internal memory which can hold data up to a day and a battery that persists for a week and can be easily charged by putting up the strip on an inductive charging pad. It is entirely made up of silicon and has an electronic module with single-lead ECG. It also consists of skin temperature sensor.

2 Challenges of IoT-Based Healthcare Applications

IoT has changed the way healthcare applications were working. Connected devices through healthcare applications allow elderly people to be connected to the healthcare system, people living in remote areas get healthcare advice through medical advisors without visiting their place, and patient's suffering from chronic diseases can be monitored by medical advisors on regular basis. In spite of all these benefits of IoT, there are various challenges also which are given below:

Success Rate of IoT applications

Faster data transmission and convenience of using IoT applications motivate healthcare providers to explore healthcare applications using IoT. As per Cisco research in 2017, it has been revealed that only 26 percent IoT-based projects were successful. The research also revealed the fact that 60 percent of the IoT projects encounter trouble at the stage of proof of concept. However, most of the IoT-based projects utilized external partnership for success. Although Cisco research did not focus on IoT based healthcare applications. Cisco research underlines that organizations should be cautious while planning IoT solutions for their organizations. Organization should focus on prioritizing their business projects and their objectives or needs of patient.

Voluminous data generated by health care

Healthcare initiatives had brought revolution to medical industry. Reducing emergency room waiting times, tracking assets and devices, tracking movement of patients throughout hospitals, and medical device monitoring all such kind of applications generate huge volume of data. The forecast says that by 2025, healthcare sector will only produce major portion of data by IoT devices as compared to any other sector. The flooding data generated by IoT health devices used in healthcare industry could also cause unforeseen problems. Healthcare organizations dealing with that data should be capable enough to handle it properly and also verify its quality.

Vulnerability of IoT devices

The vulnerability of IoT devices increases as its usage. Hackers are using a variety of techniques for data filtration in order to mine valuable data and misuse it. As per the study of Zingbox, it has been observed that hackers could identify the connected medical devices and understand their working by getting into the system. Hackers can break into a healthcare network and can manipulate the readings or data generated by the IoT device, hence affecting patient care. However, serious efforts have been taken by researchers and technology experts by reinforcing security standards and protocols. Organizations should plan in prior and should increase awareness of existing threats of the IoT-based systems and also how to protect their network and devices from these threats.

Obsolete Infrastructure

Even though retrofitting can breathe new life into aging infrastructure, truly taking advantage of IoT is tricky if an infrastructure is outdated. Old infrastructure is a known issue in health care. When hospitals are in dire need of revamped infrastructure, they also have difficulty hiring the staff to make upgrades. Tech talent is in high demand. Prospective candidates may not want to tackle old infrastructure.

3 Cloud Computing/Edge Computing/Fog Computing

IoT devices are flooding the market and our life will seem impossible without IoT devices these days. Sending or receiving data over the internet or the cloud is quite easier now but data processing is quite challenging.

Cloud computing simply means storage of data and access of programs over the Internet instead of accessing it from your own computer. Cloud computing enables organization by providing them computer infrastructure in the form of various resources like virtual machines, storage of data, networking, software, analytics, etc. Cloud may belong to a single organization (private cloud) or it is available to many organizations (public cloud) or it can be a combination of both (hybrid cloud). Cloud provides various services to the client in the form of Software (SaaS), Platform (PaaS), and Infrastructure (IaaS).

Cloud environment has a great impact on the performance of various enterprises. Upgradation of infrastructure is always a big challenge for the enterprises, and hence switching to the cloud-based service helps enterprises to meet the demand instantly. This improvement and flexibility will make a significant improvement in performance of your enterprises. This is one of the reasons for adopting cloud computing which helps in fulfilling the demands of business instantly (Fig. 1).

Fog computing refers to the extension of cloud computing to the edge of the network of enterprise. It is an additional layer of a distributed network and it is closely related

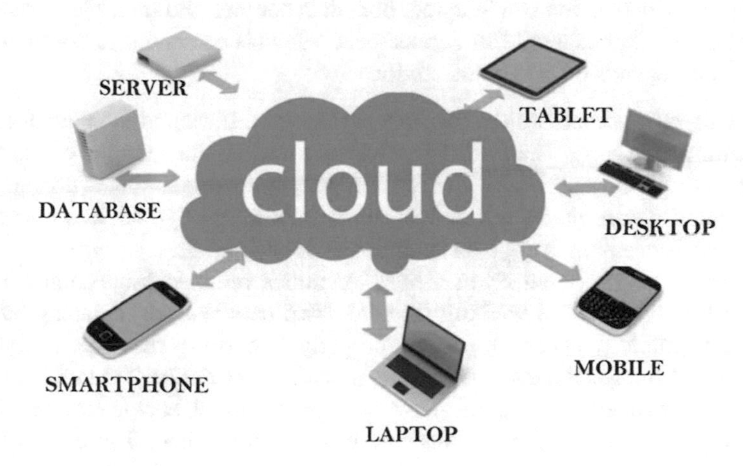

Fig. 1 Cloud computing

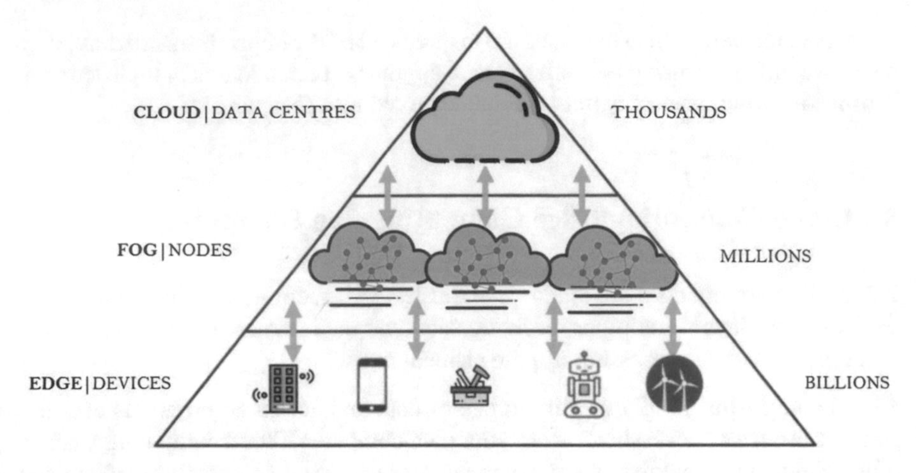

Fig. 2 Fog computing

to cloud computing. Fog network is an extension cloud and hence makes it ideal for IoT and other applications that run on real-time data. Fog networking basically makes use of local resources in spite of accessing remote one and hence decreasing the latency and making it more powerful and efficient (Fig. 2).

It is an improvement over cloud computing by reducing the amount of data to be transported to the cloud for analysis, storage, and processing. Though it makes the things quite efficient, it can also be used for security reasons and it also has low latency in terms of network. It also reduces the amount of data that is sent to the cloud. Mostly fog computing is used for efficient data processing but it can also be used for security and compliance. Low latency of fog computing in terms of network is also one of the reasons for its popularity. It also reduces the amount of data sent over the network, and response time is quite high. Cloud can only integrate multiple data sources, whereas fog can integrate both data sources and multiple devices too. Fog is also popular because of its access speed which is promising in comparison to cloud which depends on VM connectivity.

Edge Computing processes the data where it is created around the network rather than in centralized form. There are dedicated edge devices that are used which enable the entry into the core networks. In edge computing, the processing is done majorly on distributed device nodes referred as smart devices or edge devices opposite to cloud where processing is done on centralized cloud (Fig. 3).

Edge computing is popularly used by autonomous vehicles. Edge computing and its integration with AI are working for automated cars and are replacing humans. However, technology needs to work on properly to perform real-time analytics in order to avoid road accidents. Another great example of the edge technology is the predictive maintenance. The applications of edge computing enable the IoT wireless sensor network to scrutinize the machine health in real time. The data collected through the various edge devices is most of the times sent to the central cloud data center for further analysis.

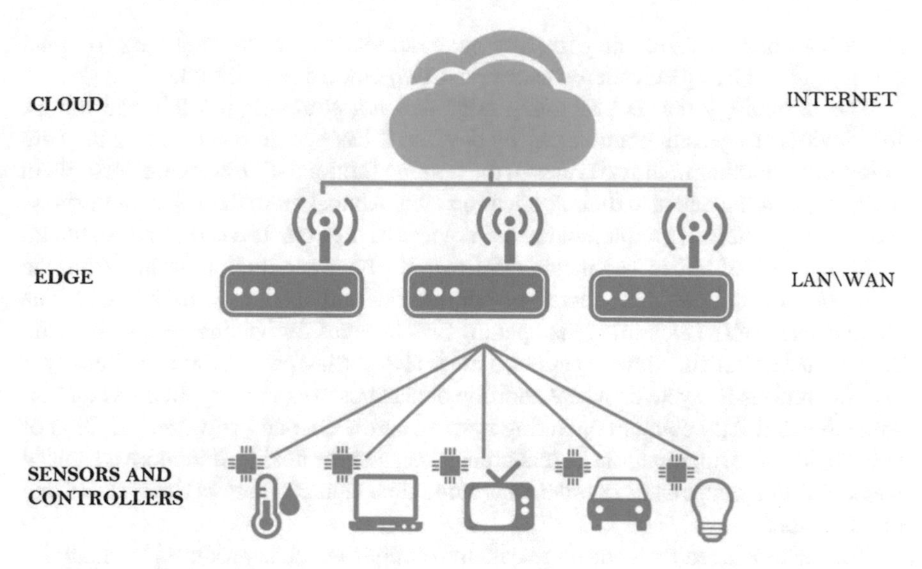

Fig. 3 Edge computing framework

Edge networking offers resource optimization over cloud computing system. All computations are performed at the edge of the network which helps in reducing network traffic, hence decreasing the risk of a data bottleneck.

4 Need for Edge Computing

The virtualization of services is getting popularity with the spread of cloud services everywhere and information technology is undergoing a revolution with the two cutting-edge technologies, edge computing and fog computing. Both the technologies pay emphasis on processing data at the edge of networks and not sending it back and forth to the data center. These technologies play vital role in reducing round trip times, and hence critically increase the performance of various applications.

Cloud is not all a new buzzword in the industry. It has been there for decades. Using cloud simply means storing and accessing data over the Internet instead of your own computer hard drive. Companies these days do not need to develop their own infrastructure and they are exploiting resources like virtual machine, storage, or an application all these as a utility. Cloud computing is providing various services like databases, storage, intelligence, virtual networks, analytics, hybrid cloud intelligence to name a few.

The idea of edge and fog computing is being motivated by introducing improvements upon the model of cloud services currently in use. In 2018 itself, the market of cloud services has been increased by 21%, i.e., which as $145.3 billion in the year 2017. The major cloud market is covered by AWS, Microsoft Azure, and Google cloud but this is not stopping fog and edge computing by standing next to cloud computing and being considered as the next step onward from cloud.

The technology that is promoting edge and fog computing is IoT and things. IoT devices are getting popular day by day and it has been forecasted that they are going to outnumber mobile devices in the coming future. IoT devices are versatile in their shape, sizes, and also their application area. Almost more than 90% of business organizations that have implemented IoT devices have got returns on their investment.

The growth of IoT in healthcare field with the huge production of data from the numerous sensors produces versatile opportunities and challenges in this field. The advancement of the technology is opening new avenues for healthcare systems with the demand of holistic view of patient. This is also putting pressure and challenge for existing healthcare systems where addition or changes in existing systems is cumbersome due to tightly coupled operating system, hardware, and firmware. Addition of new devices and upgradations in technology demand for flexible and more advanced ways of data management in order to provide time valuable data to the systems and organizations.

Technology is ready to converge data into actions which is produced by analytics using AI, machine learning, inference, and deep learning. All these technologies are becoming an integral part of the healthcare systems and are routine for ensuring patient safety and quality of care. Edge computing places the data and the processing capabilities at the edge of the network, which is quite close to the relevant data and its operational or diagnostic module.
Edge computing showcases following benefits of processing data at the edge:

Low latency

The problem of cloud environment is high latency which means that data collected from millions of devices connected in a particular system has to reach the cloud for further processing which is far away from the position data is being generated. Many sensors do not meet the demand of power consumption required for transmission of data to the cloud. Edge computing provides solution to this issue and tries to process the data by sensors or nearly connected device and analyzes it, hence reducing the latency. Even machine-learning algorithms can run directly on edge devices, only interacting with the cloud when needed.

Reliability

Establishing connection with the remote cloud data center can be not unreliable as at remote locations data connectivity is poor or discontinuous. Shifting distributed computing to the edge also ensures reliable processing, in case if one edge device fails, other processing resource will take over.

Scalability

Edge computing expands its capacity with the combination of IoT devices and data centers working at edge. It offers less expensive ways to implement scalability. Adding edge computing devices which are capable of processing does not put an overhead of growth costs as addition of each new device demands for substantial bandwidth at the core of a network.

Cost savings

Transferring data to a cloud needs higher bandwidth. Hence, if all data to be analyzed has to be transferred to cloud, it will be a costly issue. If preliminary analysis of data is performed at edge before sending it to cloud it will save cost and only that data is transferred to the cloud which is required for aggregate analysis.

Security

Data processing at edge or close to IoT device improves security and privacy of data. The data that is transferred to the cloud is prone to be attacked. There are high security concerns as the data transfer relies on the public Internet. Lot of critical information can be intercepted by malicious third parties. An edge computing application can ensure that sensitive data is preprocessed on-site, and only after having passed the data through a first layer of anonymizing aggregation, the application sends the data to the cloud for further analysis.

Versatility

Scalability adds up to the versatility of edge computing. Organizations can promote partnership with local edge data centers, and hence they need not invest in expensive infrastructure. The partnership with these edge data centers allows them to provide efficient services to the end users with low latency. The robustness of edge computing supports IoT devices to gather exceptional amount of data on which certain action can be taken. Edge computing devices are always connected, in spite of waiting for people or device to log in and interact with connected central cloud servers, and it always generates data for future analysis. Huge amount of unstructured data is collected by edge network data centers; either that data is processed locally by edge centers or transferred to the core network servers where robust analytical techniques will analyze it to identify trends and crucial data points. This information can be used by healthcare centers for better decision-making.

5 Edge Computing and Healthcare Systems

Edge computing is drawing attention of companies as it offers basket of benefits and trics to overcome the limitations imposed by cloud-based environment. Though cloud has its own important role, there are numerous possibilities offered by IoT with edge computing. All traditional network architecture used to have data processing center at the heart of it. The devices, systems, and tools forward their data to central hub for storage, processing, and further transmitting to another system, device, or network. The transmission of high volume of data to a centralized location before its analysis and sending it back to the device is not suggested as it is inefficient and leads to bottleneck. Decentralization of data pathways will help in saving time and bandwidth and will result in fast delivery of data. In spite of centralized data centers in edge computing, data centers are shifted to the edge in order to reduce transmission time and processing the data where it has been produced. Data centers added at the edge will give opportunity to doctors and healthcare staff to process their data in the close proximity of the source of data and it can reduce data transmission times also. The basic three benefits of edge computing are easy access to real-time data, security, and data transmission efficiency.

Each data center at edge handles limited amount of data which improves security as volume of vulnerable data at each data center at edge is quite lower. It makes things difficult for cyberattackers as at particular location there is limited volume of data that can be compromised in comparison to centralized data center. Monitoring of security issues is easier as it is all closer to the source and IT staff can react quickly and take serious steps in order to avoid such security breaches. The proactive data security approach is easily implemented in this scenario.

Data access also shows improvement in edge computing as data is quite near to the source. Data can also be accessed even if you are offline as all data is stored near to the source and does not depend on wireless network. Such kind of setup is quite useful in healthcare systems because clinical staff often depends on network channel for easy access of patient information. Since the data transmission distance is reduced due to the closeness of edge data center, the cost of data transmission is also reduced. Not all data generated by the IoT devices have to be transmitted to central cloud as majority of it will be processed by edge data centers, and hence it reduces the cloud storage requirements.

Edge computing can be well exploited in healthcare systems. It can be implemented for closed-loop systems in ICU for the monitoring of seriously ill patients using smart sensors. Clinicians can respond immediately to any adverse situation of patients. In an ICU system, edge computing connects system sensors to localized control system which will handle all processing and communication. "The result of edge computing can be rapid machine-to-machine communication or machine-to-human interaction. This paradigm takes localized processing farther away from the network right down to the sensor by pushing the computing processes even closer to the data sources."

The sensors attached to the system work as a dispatcher. The role of dispatcher is to pass information to another edge device in the close proximity and sometimes even to cloud also. In this way, all edge devices work as a part of the information processing rather than sending all data to a central cloud. In healthcare systems, edge computing distributes workloads on the branch data centers in order to deliver applications and services to remote areas. The effective usage of edge computing in health care can be by bringing services near to the patients by virtualization and helping patients at the remote location in an effective manner.

The edge computing also plays an important role in telemedicine. Doctors in metropolitan areas can treat remote and rural patients reliably. Telemedicine programs can also utilize specialized care especially for patients who travel.

The edge node need not be large enough like cloud and it can be a small entity which basically brings healthcare application and data closer to the patient. Edge devices can have a great impact on telemedicine through patient monitoring.

Wearable devices are, in general, example of edge solution. The purpose of wearable device is to analyze health-related data like blood pressure, heartbeat rate, sleeping patterns, and other activities in order to provide recommendations without connecting to the cloud.

6 Edge Computing General Framework

There are no defined boundaries of edge network; it depends upon a particular application. Edge is basically a logical layer rather than physical. As per the business perspective, location of edge can be defined by the business problems to be handled or key objectives of the business. Basically, edge computing comprises following three layers:

Lowest Layer

It consists of large number of versatile devices ranging from sensors, smartphones, actuators, and wearables. Some of these devices are dynamic in nature like mobile IoT objects while some are static. Voluminous amount of raw data is produced by these devices which are further transmitted to higher layer devices for further processing.

Middle Layer

This layer is actually edge layer. An edge can be a computer or a processor inside an IoT camera, router, local edge, or ISP all can be considered as edge. Edge computing can be defined in terms of relative position of processing power, communication function, and intelligence to the end user. It consists of devices that have computing capability like routers, switches, set-top boxes, etc. The basic role that edge nodes have to perform is to provide services to the end users. These services vary from delivery of service, caching, or may be data storage, especially transient data from cloud to the end users. The basic aim of edge is to divest some tasks from the cloud to the edge. Further edge nodes can provide services to the users in collaboration and cooperation with other edge nodes. For example, Shi et al. [6] introduced a use case of connected health in which hospitals, pharmacies, logistics companies, governments, and insurance companies form a collaborative edge to provide healthcare services.

Highest Layer

This layer is made up of decentralized computing infrastructure which comprises data, computational power, storage space, and various applications which together work in a distributed manner between edge node and centralized data center/cloud. It takes data processing one step further from the preprocessed data from edge nodes. Few tasks are assigned to the edge nodes. In two situations, cloud server requires to provide its services: (i) when edge nodes require coordination among themselves and (ii) when large-scale data analysis is performed; in this case, edge nodes send data to cloud server after preliminary analysis [7].

Edge computing allows data from IoT device to be processed and analyzed at edge local processing and then further transmits it to cloud or corporate data center.

Edge Computing Components

Edge computing setup uses various terms. Following are the terms that are being used with edge computing:

Edge Devices: Any device like sensors, machines, mobiles, or any other device which produces data or collects data.

Edge: The edge does not have standard definition. The boundary of edge varies from application to application, for example, telecommunication filed it can be mobile or may be mobile tower. In the case of automotive edge, it can be a car. Edge can be a machine in a shop floor or a laptop in IT.

Edge gateway: It is a buffer zone where processing is done in between broader fog and edge computing. It basically works as a window between larger environment that exists beyond the boundary of the edge.

Fat client: It is basically an application used for data processing on edge devices in contrast to thin client which simply transfers data.

Edge computing equipment: Various sensors, mobiles, router, and switches can be used as an edge computing equipment simply by connecting them with Internet. A range of computing servers, converged systems, and even storage-based hardware systems like Amazon Web Service's Snowball can be used in edge computing deployments [8].

7 Edge Computing Use Cases

IoT devices are becoming more popular day by day and edge computing has expanded its wings and tries to accommodate every domain. Healthcare industry is also ready to exploit the benefits of edge computing. The healthcare industry is ready to be benefitted by the expanded use of IoT edge devices and other latest advancement in the computing architecture. Edge is considered as a complement to cloud computing rather than as a replacement. Cloud has contributed to several benefits for IT health care but now cloud alone is not considered as the best solution for divesting core applications.

To implement edge computing ecosystem, organizations have to define a use case which describes each and every aspect of an organization which includes IT setup, management, and patient care as well. The healthcare organizations have to perform brainstorming in order to identify which service will have benefit from edge service, like EHR systems, telemedicine, digital imaging to name a few. Organizations have to assess each and every aspect like network bandwidth to handle needs of remote patients and what other devices need to be connected in near future.

Implementing edge computing in the organization is not only the solution. There is a requirement of skilled staff also in order to deploy edge solution. Organizations that attempt to deploy edge network without required expertise will definitely end up in wasting money. Organizations have to decide location, storage system, and amount of data to be processed and people who will access it in order to build secured and compliant edge system. Well-defined and secured edge computing will bestow following benefits:

- Data in a close proximity increases efficiency.
- Integration of IoT data and healthcare systems.
- More precise and in-time data about patient health.
- Telemedicine.
- Real-time monitoring of patients that influences medical devices.
- Health apps and wearables that keep a track of various health metrics.

Edge computing will benefit by reducing transmission costs, improvement in delivery of services, and have a great impact on people lives by managing their health issues. The ultimate result is to make health care available to those people who are in great need of it. It improves patient care and also increases efficiency from business perspective. Following are the use cases that justify the success and usage area of edge computing:

Rural Medicine

Quality health care for the rural areas which are isolated has been a biggest challenge for healthcare industry. Even with the latest innovations in telemedicine, the quality care is not easily reachable to the remote areas in the time of emergency. Traditional healthcare databases are facing challenges and the biggest challenge is connectivity but the edge computing along with the IoT healthcare devices are making it easier in overcoming these difficulties.

Edge computing along with IoT healthcare devices together have the potential to store, process, generate, and analyze critical data of patients without having continuous connection with network infrastructure. Patients using wearable devices can get their diagnosis quite quickly and effectively on-site and gathered information can be fed to the central servers as soon as connection is established. IoT healthcare devices can extend their reach to other existing networks by connecting with an edge data center. By connecting it through edge data center, the medical personnel is ready to access critical patient data in the areas where there is poor connectivity. This particular use case of edge computing has the potential to expand the reachability of healthcare service to a great extent.

Closed-loop system in ICU

Implementation of closed-loop system to monitor patients that are critically ill in an ICU system is also one of the useful use cases of edge computing. The system will respond to the changes in conditions of the patients in ICU.

The implementation of closed-loop ICU can be attained by all the sensors in the system to local control systems which can handle processing and further communication. The edge computing will result in rapid interaction and communication between machines. This system performs localized processing by pushing the computing power close to the source of data. Sensors in the systems work as a dispatcher which transmits information further to another connected edge device or may be to centralized cloud.

Patient's data generated by numerous devices

Patient health-related data is generated by numerous IoT medical devices like wearable devices, glucometer, and other healthcare apps and devices. The data generated by all these devices is being effectively used by healthcare industry experts and creates the potential for improved results. Such data is analyzed by the medical experts to analyze and provide medical help to the patients who are at remote areas.

The huge amount of this PGHD produced by all these devices is putting challenge for the healthcare providers to manage all such unstructured data and also keeping it secure. The data produced by these devices is poorly defined and usually passed to the cloud infrastructure which is not often prepared to analyze it and draw some inferences which can be well utilized by the healthcare providers. By the time data reaches the central servers and is analyzed it may be too late to respond to the critical changes in a patient's condition. The problem can be rectified by keeping the processing of critical data at edge near to the data source. IT architectures gain benefit of collecting data and also performing real-time analytics which can perform to solve or respond to medical emergencies. The medical devices in IoT-based healthcare systems monitor patient's current condition and send alerts the moment anomalies are detected. The system needs to follow rapid response in order to save patient's life.

1. *Improvement in Patient Experience*

IoT medical devices with edge computing are making things easy for patients visiting the hospital. The smart devices are helping patients in finding offices, guiding them through proper notifications. Hence, edge computing with IoT devices has the potential to transform healthcare industry.

Patient health and satisfaction are the ultimate issues of healthcare industry. Edge computing companies play a crucial role in healthcare infrastructure. Numerous healthcare devices are ready to provide their services to patients and are trying to give patients convenient and accommodating results. Many hospitals are ready to offer contents like movies, games, and interactive educational programs by streaming. The data can be decentralized by edge data center and will be made available widely with minimum latency.

2. *Supply Chain System*

IoT edge devices also make a noticeable contribution to the supply chains. The hospitals and healthcare centers in today's era are using numerous edge medical devices along with various hardware components in order to provide best possible care. The hospitals are equipped with various sophisticated medical equipments which are required on daily basis for the lifesaving procedure in hospitals. Keeping these facilities running without hindrance is one of the important aspects of healthcare industry. Disruption to supply chain by any means will break the smooth functioning of healthcare system. The requirement of expensive medical equipment, robotic-assisted tools to the smallest bandage all support the smooth functioning of the systems. Hence, full proof supply chain system should be established.

Healthcare system requires variety of tools, machines, equipment, and medical accessories for their smooth functioning. Any hindrance to the supply of any of these items will create significant effect on the functioning of healthcare systems.

IoT edge devices that are well equipped by sensors have the capacity to manage the inventories in healthcare systems. The whole inventory and supply chain are dependent on the data collected by usage patterns. The predictive analytics can be done to find out about a working status of a particular device and when it will fail. Real-time situation of crucial shipments can be tracked by GPS and sensors. Innovations in supply chain of IoT-based healthcare have given the opportunity to the organizations which are struggling to put a control on the rising cost of supply chain, and hence represent one of the compelling use cases of edge computing.

3. *Cost Driver*

Widespread usage of IoT edge devices is helping healthcare organizations to save up to 25% cost. Few savings come from day-to-day applications of security and surveillance and also from smart building controls but most of the cost saving will come from patient monitoring. IoT medical devices, wearables, implantable sensors, and other IoT services that are based on data analytics are all included as the use case of edge computing which are significantly reducing per patient cost.

Another costly issue involved with IoT-based healthcare systems is interconnectivity among various devices. Healthcare providers are facing issues of incompatible systems and also they have to manage huge recordkeeping which is quite challenging. All this can be handled easily by edge computing devices that communicate quickly and easily across organizational boundaries. The cost of healthcare services is rising day by day. The innovations in healthcare industry with IoT and edge will boost up the efficiency and deliver better value which surely promotes end user to embrace it.

Monitoring of Patients (Critically Ill)

Edge computing gathers the data of patients by monitoring their behavior and watching out for anomalies. For example, epileptic patients in healthcare system's edge computing devices can be utilized to monitor their health condition, an early detection of attack can be notified timely to family members or related people to ensure timely care provided to the patients.

There is software that can create a diary of events and patients' vitals (jerking movements, physical vibrations, whether the body is stable or falling, heart rate, and so on) to determine treatment patterns. These diaries at edge can help in making preemptive analysis for the patient's critical condition.

A. *Response Time*

Huge hospitals have numerous devices connected to the patients; sometimes this number reaches 20 devices per bed. Managing data generated by all those devices is cumbersome job. Transferring this volume of data to a centralized data center for further processing creates a bottleneck and also increases the response time. Edge computing provides solutions in such cases where preliminary analysis and processing of data can be done at the edge and only data that requires supporting data from other devices too will be sent to the centralized cloud data center. This helps in reducing response time and timely decision and care to the patients.

B. *Mobility of Patients*

Hospitals these days have very specific infrastructure, and monitoring of patients is also restricted due to limitations of the infrastructure. The issue is that when the patient leaves the instrumented infrastructure further monitoring of patient's activities has to be ensured by the healthcare systems.

Edge computing is considered as the fruitful resources in such transitional environments and monitoring can be managed effectively. Edge computing along with IoT is considered as the robust solution for both patient and healthcare providers. Following are the different ways of managing these resources with the combination of IoT and edge computing:

On the body: Wearable devices, implants, and peripherals fall into this category. These devices constantly monitor the patient's health patterns and note the abnormalities before sending alerts to the healthcare provider.

At the hospital: The patient will be connected to smart devices and monitors that will continuously monitor the patient's location in real time. The data from all the devices will be networked and analyzed.

At home: There are plenty of home medical devices, activity monitors, and virtual assistants that would aid in monitoring the health condition of the patients, especially elderly patients who live alone.

1. *Identification of Vital Signs in Disasters*

In the case of major disasters, prompt medical help is required in order to save the lives of injured ones in emergency. The basic disaster management in such cases includes wearable biosensors which should be attached to the body of injured person by the medical officer available on-site. The biosensor will provide critical information about the current medical condition of patient and guides in the form of queue of priority action required for patient processing. Very soon the attached sensors start emitting data to the edge devices that are located nearby. These edge devices can perform only basic and lightweight analytics just to determine the current state of injured person and informing the status to the on-site medical officer. On availability of network connection, selected data will be further transferred to the cloud for detailed and complex analysis. This further analysis of data will make more precise predictions for treatment of patients, improving coordination between healthcare centers, time optimization for reaching hospital, and also providing timely information about patient current condition.

2. Identification of Vital Signs in Everyday Life

Biosensors are used to record patient's vital symptoms during everyday life activities. For example, sensors keep on streaming data of electrocardiogram to the nearby edge device which will perform preliminary analysis on the data. In case of any deviation being found from standard data, it will be notified immediately to the emergency services. Filtered and preprocessed data is further sent to the cloud where elaborated analytics on that data is being performed to get better insight about overall health condition of patient that will finally help in precise diagnosis.

3. Activity trackers during cancer treatment

Patients undergoing cancer treatment can make use of wearables and apps to check on the diagnosis and treatment through the data collected on a daily basis. This will also monitor their appetite, lifestyle, activity level, and fatigue level.

4. *Ensuring adherence to treatment plans*

Doctors can now be assured that their patients stick to the treatment plan through devices connected to mobile apps. It will also remind the patients to take their medicines on time.

8 Edge Computing for Real-Time Analysis

It has been notified and justified that there is a need for collaborating cloud with edge computing real-time analysis in order to exploit its maximum benefits. The collaboration also helps in a prompt reaction to the changing state of patient. In cloud computing, the processed data after compilation is sent back to the source of data. Contrast to that edge computing computes and analyzes data near to the data source. In edge analytics, there is a paradigm shift of processing control of all data and applications from cloud to the edge, which is quite near to the source of data. Edge computing glues various technologies together like Cloud, Grid, and IoT. Edge is an additional layer between cloud data center and end user devices. The purpose of this layer is to relocate computational power near to end device. Edge computing can perform real-time analytics which can be applied to all devices, applications, and services.

The most prominent benefit of edge computing is the reduced latency and improvement in quality of service. There are many heavy tasks of big data processing, video processing, and artificial intelligence that require huge computational power. If the computation is required to be done in real time using cloud and Internet, it is simply not preferable. Any real-time system is supposed to react to its environment in the specified time interval.

Real-time computing can be categorized into three types [9].

Hard Real Time: In hard real-time systems, strict real-time clause should be followed. For example, in cars, if airbags deflate after or before the specific time interval it loses its importance and it will be fatal for the consumers [10].

Firm Real Time: It is in between the hard and soft real time. Systems with firm real time can bear some lapses in deadline; however, increase in these lapses will definitely degrade the performance of the system, and hence making system unacceptable [11].

Soft Real Time: The real-time applications which demand for less strict timeline and also have wide deadline interval are called soft real-time applications. For example, voice or video streaming can bear loss of some data packets.

There are systems which produce huge volume of data per second. Since we live in an era where billions of devices are producing data and processing data, there is a need for filtering data at the source itself. In these situations, data can be off-loaded to the edge node for filtering and some preprocessing and perform some real-time analytics. Nowadays, cloud computing and edge are working in tandem to maximize the output of IoT, cloud, and edge computing.

The edge analysis architecture has been utilized by several IoT-based healthcare systems. Lv et al. [7] proposed to analyze physiological data of patients at local end in order to implement authenticity. They mentioned if data will be forwarded to global cloud for analysis it will surely experience some data loss. After local analysis, data is collected and stored to build up an information system for patients.

Bourouis et al. [12] proposed the concept of Intelligent Central Node (ICN) which allows to analyze data on a smartphone. The operating system in a smartphone performs real-time data processing. The role of ICN is to determine whether data needs to be forwarded further to the cloud storage or not using comparison algorithm.

In [13], smartphones perform basic data analysis on the data collected by the sensors. However, in such cases, there is huge risk of data security which can be avoided by getting acknowledgement of user before any critical data processing.

@Home [14] and PhMon [15] are the systems that locally analyze data between its source and control center. Such systems comprise biosensors (wearable) which are connected to a monitoring system through Bluetooth/Zigbee. The monitoring systems work as an efficient alert system and send alarm after processing of data in case it is required. The system presented in [16] carries out some basic analysis on the cell phone by employing wireless sensor networks and some complex detection algorithm.

Kosisochukwu et al. [17] proposed system makes use of edge analysis which is transparent, free, and works for both structured and unstructured data. The proposed platform is used for analysis of raw data produced by various IoT healthcare devices. Their platform also employs KAA platform in the design of an IoT-based healthcare system. Using platform rather than writing algorithms provides a better IoT solution and product for healthcare systems. The proposed system consists of a heart rate sensor which is connected to a mobile application (android based) for remote monitoring of patients. The focus of the platform is to provide easy usage of visualization of data related to patients of different classes.

Few other works of edge computing using real-time analysis are discussed below:

Icare: Real-Time analysis with Edge computing

Icare is the solution for health monitoring of elderly people. It uses the combination of wireless sensor technology along with smartphone, body sensors, and web technology which offers real-time health monitoring. The system will collect physiological data through body sensors and other devices attached. The collected physiological data will be analyzed locally at the edge and it will alarm the emergency healthcare center whenever data collected exceeds the threshold values. The emergency healthcare center will send an ambulance to the current location of the elder person who is in trouble.

Body sensors and other devices will be customized as per the old people's health condition. The data collected will not only be analyzed at the local level, besides that it will be sent to the server in bulk in order to maintain personal health information system. The comparative analysis of history data and current data helps doctors to set the thresholds from remote location and elderly people can be guided accordingly [18].

Serverless Framework for Real-Time Analysis

The purpose of cloud storage and computing is to perform analysis and deriving patterns in a huge amount of data. In the combined architecture of edge and cloud, edge device plays a role of gateway. The edge devices perform preprocessing and also perform filtration of data which is further transmitted to the cloud. The transmitted data at cloud is converted into persistent data and is further available for complicated analysis. The presented framework by researchers establishes the need of combining cloud and edge based analytical technique. The suggested framework will process patient's data at the edge in a real time using low latency algorithms.

The proposed full-stack framework performs uniform real-time data analytics between cloud and edge. The basic role of the cumulative cloud and edge is to facilitate management of the underlying resources in the framework. The cumulative framework also optimizes the placement of various analytics functions in order to support execution of serverless model. This serverless approach combines the benefits of edge like latency, heterogeneous data management along with the computational power of cloud. For example, if in a healthcare system, the patient is visible in some critical position then the particular data is analyzed at the edge in the close proximity where it is generated and some initial results and suggestions are transmitted to the patient. However, further selected data will be forwarded to cloud to perform some powerful analysis and data will be stored for long-term storage.

The serverless framework proposed is capable of managing bottom up approaches of data analytics of varied granularity. This means that the focus of edge is on local analysis that is per edge gateway, whereas cloud supports global views which means analysis of data from varied edge devices that belong to different regions or even domains. Consumption API is used to deliver collected data from the connected devices to the applications. The important fact is that analytics can be performed either on cloud or edge node or may be both and finally delivered to application from any node.

The core concept of the model is a transforming function that encapsulates data analytics logic defined by the user for data processing along the stream. The set of such function is then composed into a topology which facilitates complex data processing applications. The model considered streams as the most important aspect as it is defined throughout all the presented concepts [19].

Real-Time Map-Reduce Framework Using Edge

Kang et al. [20] proposed a framework for soft real-time analysis performed at network edge. The basic feature of framework is (a) transfer of data form adaptive sensor to the edge based on their importance and (b) periodic real-time analytics performed in memory of the edge server handled by real-time scheduling and map-reduce functions originated in functional programming which is not related to a specific implementation [21].

Though the demand for real-time analytics has been increasing drastically, related work is relatively unavailable. There are various advanced data stream management systems, for example, Storm [22], S4 [23], and Spark Streaming [24] that support real-time stream processing but do not consider time deadlines and not ensure timeliness of data processing. Hadoop framework faces the problem of meeting deadlines [25–27] as it is optimized for processing in batches of data in secondary storage space.

To address this issue, the proposed work of a real-time map-reduce framework is suggested as a solution called as Real-Time Map-Reduce framework (RMTR). It provides various unique features (Fig. 4).

Framework offers transfer of periodic data from IoT devices to edge server on the basis of their relative importance mentioned by the sensors/IoT devices.

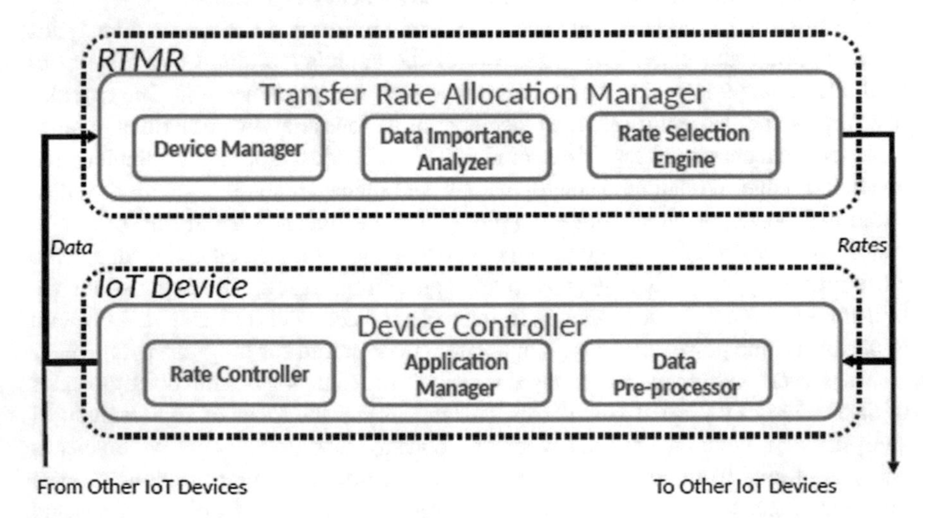

Fig. 4 RMTR framework for real-time analysis (*Source* [20])

Generic transfer adaptation scheme is proposed which supports different parameters of importance of data that depends on a specific real-time analysis application.

Framework provides API for RMTR, which can be used to write serial map() and reduce() functions by application developer for a particular real-time data analytics application and can also specify parameters for timelines and intervals for data analysis task.

Framework provides a test for the earliest deadline first scheduling algorithm in order to check the performance level of computation and data access delay. The framework performs periodic real-time analysis of sensor data.

Framework also supports various efficient mechanisms for in-memory sensor data analysis. These schemes are as follows:

- Sensor data is streamed into main memory directly so that RMTR can fetch information from it on the fly.
- Unlike Hadoop and its variants, intermediate data generated by the map/reduce phase is directly transferred to the next phase without being stored locally in a disk or distributed file system.
- For each input/output and intermediate data memory, reservation is done in prior.
- Wireless transfer of data as per their importance. An RMTR prototype is made which extends Phoenix [28] which is an open-source multicore/multiprocessor map-reduce framework. Phoenix supports RMTR features used for real-time analytics.

Collaborative Framework for Real-Time processing in wireless network

Edge and cloud computing solutions both have their own unique merits and demerits in context of real-time data analytics in wireless IoT networks. The framework combines features of centralized cloud and real-time analysis benefit of edge which is capable of addressing various issues related to wireless network.

Sharma et al. [29] proposed a collaborative edge-cloud framework for wireless IoT networks. In the proposed model, edge gateways are fortified with cache memory which facilitates edge-caching and helps in delivery of local popular contents. The edge nodes may be any device having computational capability along with storage and network connectivity. It may be sensor, router, smartphone, and video camera depending on various application scenarios. IoT networks may be heterogeneous comprising of various unique characteristics.

IoT devices are diversified in nature. They have heterogeneous features of computing capabilities, intelligence, and processing power. There is a need for one monitoring agent that can guide edge nodes to make maximum utilization of available communication and computing resources. The proposed framework in this line works in the same manner and lures benefits of both cloud and edge. The framework uses cloud center as monitoring agent to have effective real-time data processing.

In this framework, information/data is gathered by edge computing from the surrounding radio environment. The role of cloud is to monitor and give suitable instructions to the edge nodes for operations. There are various operations on the edge side like filtering, data compression, power control, and decision-making on the various

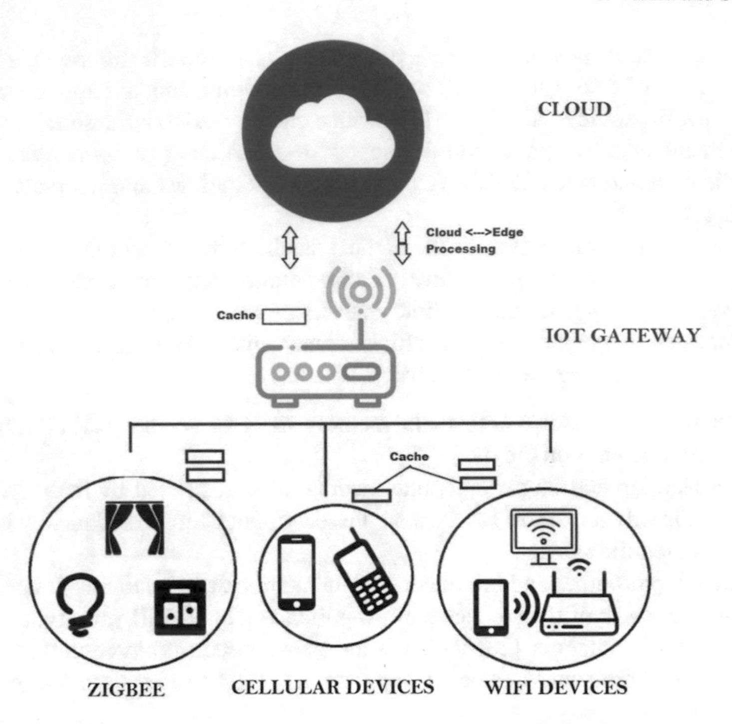

Fig. 5 Collaborative framework for real-time processing in wireless network

types of data which is well supported by cloud center which gives suitable signals (Fig. 5).

Real-Time Analysis of Patients through voice communication

The reachability of technology has now opened doors for early diagnosis of a variety of diseases. Application of voice communication in healthcare application is set to revolutionize health care in many countries. Let us take an example, Person worried for his mother as she has issues related to memory loss and calls to the clinic, nurse at the clinic asks few questions to her and gathers some information for preliminary detection of disease. The analysis has been done on the basis of vocal communication and data collected from her wearable device. The analysis helps the nurse to determine and diagnose Alzheimer's disease to the patient with the high probability. Hence, the preliminary detection helped the patient in taking early medical action for his mother. With the overloaded connected devices available these days, diagnosis by simple voice communications is really ultimate.

Using analytics in voice communications for the diagnosis of early symptoms of any disease is actually quite close to reality. Apple recently released new Apple watch series 4 with a feature of electrocardiogram. The watch is capable of monitoring heartbeat of the person wearing it and will alert them in any undiagnosed condition. This real-time data provided by Apple watch helps in diagnosis of certain health conditions. It alerts the users to consult their health provides detecting any significant reaction or change in standard health data.

Role of Analyst in detecting medical fraud

Healthcare industry is dealing with numerous frauds. In 2017, US faced $1.3 billion of false billings as per the records of Inspector General of the U.S. Department of Health & Human Services. Real-time analysis can play a vital role in detection of these medical frauds.

Analytics at the medical call center using voice analytics can deal with this issue. The tone of patient's voice can be detected and the person at call center can pinpoint it. The person attending the call could alert the concerned person to investigate the case to the deeper level. The role of analytics is to identify medical fraud in order to warn organizations at the preliminary stage of appointment scheduling.

The real-time analytics with edge computing has the great potential in order to meet varied challenges of healthcare industry. The efforts are made to propel health care to next generation and deploy real-time analytics for early medical diagnosis and fraud detection.

9 Challenges for IoT-based Edge computing

The future of edge computing seems bright and promising. But there are always some loopholes of every technology. Security, performance level, managing so many devices all these issues are quite challenging.

9.1 Security

The edge devices are quite vulnerable and lot of security measures is needed to be implemented for its secure implementation. Security is one of the complicated issues while implementing the edge computing environment. The security issue of edge computing has different reviews. Few people mention that security in edge computing is better as compared to cloud as data need not to travel over a network and is closer to the place of generation. Opposite to it, few believe that edge devices are quite vulnerable. Hence, security issue should be vital while deployment of edge. Security also makes deployment of edge complicated. Displacing important device toward the edge makes them vulnerable.

Following measures can be taken in order to implement secure edge computing framework:

Secure Data Collection: The first and foremost step of data processing is to collect data from various sources. The quality and integrity of data affect the data analysis accuracy. Hence, there is a need of secure data collection methods. Following strategies can be followed for secure data collection:

Authentication of the User

A foolproof user authentication mechanism is required in case of outsourcing data analytics which is a crucial requirement for the reliability of data source. The authentication mechanism will validate the user identity and guarantees that the user accessing the cloud server and the edge node is legitimate [30]. There are some common authentication ways that can be utilized for authentication of users. **Password-based authentication method**: This is the most basic one where every user while registering sends their user ID and password. Every time the user accesses the network its identity will be authenticated by the remote server. Smart Card-Based Authentication Method: It is a non-reproducible card and while registration it is being issued and authenticity of the user is verified by its details. Dynamic Password: It allows user to change their passwords dynamically number of times. Biometric Authentication: In this, users' unique credentials are stored for authentication purpose while registration.

Data Processing in a Secure Manner

The data is being outsourced to cloud or edge node for analysis. Once the data moves out of the users' end, the owner of the data loses the control. The personal data on the healthcare system can be revealed or shared by attackers. Following methods are used to secure data processing. **Encryption**: Encryption of all data that is being outsourced to edge through end user device. **Differential Privacy**: It is one of the privacy-preserving techniques which is used to guarantee privacy for users by adding a random noise to user data [31]. **Pseudonym**: This technique allows the users to request for services offered by edge or cloud using pseudonym. Users do not reveal their identity on cloud. Hence, their personal data cannot be related to them and if accessed by intruders it will not harm them personally [32].

Secure Data Storage

Due to cost of data storage, some results of data processing are stored on edge nodes or cloud. These results can be tampered or misused by the attackers. If we keep all processed data in encrypted form, it will hinder further processing. Hence, other mechanisms are used to handle this issue.

Access Control

This mechanism allows only authenticated user to access processed data results. There are various access control mechanisms. **Role-Based Access Control**: In this mechanism, the access policies are related to different roles and these roles are assigned to the users to authorize them for particular roles [33]. **Attribute-Based Access Control**: It is a cryptographic technique where secret key of the owner and ciphertext relies on attributes of recipients. This technique offers fine-grained access control by providing ability to data owner to set its own access policy in order to prevent private data of data owner. The recipients can only encrypt data when their attributes match to the specific access policy.

Searchable Encryption

It is being proposed by Song et al. [34] which is capable of performing data encryption along with keyword search over ciphertext. It is one of the promising solutions for the security of the outsourced data on edge/cloud which is kept in encrypted manner. The data need not be decrypted for searching purpose. There are two categories of searchable encryption, symmetric and asymmetric.

9.2 Performance and Deployment of Edge

Performance of the device is another one challenge and deployment of edge computing is also a complicated process. Engineers and founders quote that the life cycle of deployment of edge computing has many iterations and experiments before landing up to the feasible solution. Going through much iteration, many projects did not work out because of the complex production. There are many profiling tools available for developers but they are quite limited in guiding how to optimize the entire hardware and software layers.

9.3 Defining Use Case

Use case definition is another bottleneck for edge computing projects. There are idea and concept but sometimes unavailability of clear definition of use case becomes a barrier. The reason is not properly defined requirements of patients or end users and improper alignment of requirements with management. It is not mandatory that an edge expert can only define use case for its deployment. The basic requirement is to align infrastructure and business requirements to ensure that your use case or plan for the project can take off.

9.4 Less Expertise

There is a serious lack of expertise when we are deploying edge solutions. Even if a health care or any other business organization has well-defined use case, lack of expertise puts a hindrance on successful implementation of edge solutions. The reason behind all these complications is that edge is quite different from typical data center. The deployment needs to consider various parameters like space, power, connectivity, management, density to name a few. To manage all these parameters, we require skilled person for planning and implementation.

9.5 *Data Management*

This is also a major concern while deploying edge solutions. Data is the most crucial aspect of any edge computing solutions. The requirements and management of data need to be crystal clear. There are various issues regarding data management in edge like which data has to be processed where and is data transient or it will be stored. The integrated solution for edge has to define solutions for these aspects. Security of data is also one of the crucial issues that should be taken care while deployment of edge solutions.

10 Conclusion

IoT-based healthcare systems are in use over the last decade. These healthcare systems are quite complex to be managed effectively. With the growing technology, various solutions have been given time in order to handle IoT-based healthcare systems effectively. Latest transformation of healthcare system is making use of effective edge computing. Edge computing provides analysis and processing closer to the source of data. Hence, it improves security, latency, and real-time analysis to add on to the performance of the IoT-based healthcare systems. Edge computing is considered as an efficient way to solve the issue of moving all data to a central cloud. It forces to create small data centers near to point of data source. It is true that there are benefits of using edge in IoT-based healthcare systems but there are some challenges of planning, creating, deploying, and maintenance of edge-based healthcare systems.

References

1. Sivagami S, Revathy D, Smart healthcare system implemented using IoT. Int J Contemp Res Comput Sci Technol (IJCRCST) 2(3):641–646
2. https://www.cabotsolutions.com/2016/02/applications-iot-healthcare-industry
3. https://www.elinext.com/industries/healthcare/trends/how-iot-disrupts-health-insurance
4. https://www.ansys.com/en-in/Campaigns/internet-of-things/wearables-and-medical-devices
5. http://nanohub.org/resources/2261/download/nanobiotechnology_and_biosensors.pdf
6. Shi W, Cao J, Zhang Q, Li Y, Xu L (2016) Edge computing: vision and challenges. IEEE Internet Things J 3(5):637–646
7. Lv Z, Xia F, Wu G, Yao L, Chen Z (2010) iCare: a mobile health monitoring system for the elderly. In: Green computing and communications (GreenCom), IEEE/ACM international conference on cyber, physical, social computing (CPSCom), Hangzhou, China, pp 699–705
8. https://www.networkworld.com/article/3224893/what-is-edge-computing-and-how-it-s-changing-the-network.html
9. Gezer V, Um J, Ruskowski M, An introduction to edge computing and a real time server architecture. https://www.networkworld.com/article/3224893/what-is-edge-computing-and-how-it-s-changing-the-network.html
10. Olderog E, Dierks H (2008) Real-time systems: formal specification and automatic verification. Cambridge University Press

11. Kaldewey T, Lin C, Brandt S (2006) Firm real-time processing in an integrated real-time system. University of York, Department of Computer Science - Report, vol 398, p 5
12. Bourouis A, Feham M, Bouchachia A (2011) Ubiquitous mobile health monitoring system for elderly (UMHMSE). Int J Comput Sci Inf Technol 3(3):74–82
13. Morón MJ et al (2007) A smart phone-based personal area network for remote monitoring of bio-signals. In: 4th international workshop on wearable and implantable body sensor networks, vol 13, Spain, pp 116–121
14. Sachpazidis I (2002) @Home: a modular telemedicine system. In: Proceedings of 2nd workshop mobile computing in medicine, Heidelberg, Germany
15. Kunze C, Grossmann U, Stork W, Müller-Glaser KD (2002) Application of ubiquitous computing in personal health monitoring systems. In: Proceedings of 36th annual meeting German society for biomedical engineering, pp 360–362
16. Wan-Young C, Chiew-Lian Y, Kwang-Sig S, Risto M (2007) A cell phone based health monitoring system with self analysis processor using wireless sensor network technology. In: 29th annual international conference of the IEEE engineering in medicine and biology society
17. Madukwe KJ, Ezika IJF, Iloanusi ON (2017) Leveraging edge analysis for internet of things based healthcare solutions. In: IEEE 3rd international conference on electro-technology for national development
18. Lv Z, Xia F, Wu G, Yao L, Chen Z, iCare: a mobile health monitoring system for the elderly
19. Nastic S, Rausch T, Scekic O, Dustdar S (2017) A serverless real-time data analytics platform for edge computing. IEEE Internet Comput 21(4)
20. Kang KD, Chen L, Yi H, Wang B, Sha M (2017) Real-time information derivation from big sensor data via edge computing. Big Data Cogn Comput, MDPI
21. Bird R, Wadler P (1998) Introduction to functional programming, 2nd edn. Prentice Hall, Upper Saddle River, NJ, USA
22. Apache Storm. https://storm.apache.org/
23. S4: Distributed Stream Computing Platform. http://incubator.apache.org/s4/
24. Spark Streaming. https://spark.apache.org/streaming/
25. Basu A (2017) Q learning based workflow scheduling in hadoop. Int J Appl Eng Res 12:3311–3317
26. Phan LTX, Zhang Z, Zheng Q, Loo BT, Lee I (2011) An empirical analysis of scheduling techniques for real-time cloud-based data processing. In: Proceedings of the international workshop on service-oriented computing and applications, Irvine, CA, USA
27. Kc K, Anyanwu K (2010) Scheduling hadoop jobs to meet deadlines. In: Proceedings of the international conference on cloud computing technology and science, Washington, DC, USA
28. Phoenix. https://github.com/kozyraki/phoenix
29. Sharma SK, Wang X, Live data analytics with collaborative edge and cloud processing in wireless IoT networks. In: IEEE access, special section on future networks: architectures, protocols, and applications
30. Alizadeh M, Abolfazli S, Zamani M, Baharun S, Sakurai K (2016) Authentication in mobile cloud computing: a survey. J Netw Comput Appl 61:59–80
31. Dwork C, Roth A (2014) The algorithmic foundations of differential privacy. Found Trends Theor Comput Sci 9(3–4):211–407
32. Lysyanskaya A, Rivest RL, Sahai A, Wolf S (1999) Pseudonym systems. In: Proceedings of international workshop on selected areas in cryptography, pp 184–199
33. Zhou L, Varadharajan V, Hitchens M (2013) Achieving secure role based access control on encrypted data in cloud storage. IEEE Trans Inf Forensics Secur 8(12):1947–1960
34. Song DX, Wagner D, Perrig A (2000) Practical techniques for searches on encrypted data. In: Proceedings of IEEE symposium on security privacy, pp 44–55

Parul Verma is working as a Faculty at Amity Institute of Information Technology, Amity University, Uttar Pradesh, Lucknow. Her research interests are Natural Language Processing, Web Mining, Deep Mining, Semantic Web, Edge, and IoT. She has published and presented almost 30 papers in Scopus and other indexed national and international journals and conferences. She has been actively involved in research being a supervisor to research scholars and postgraduate students. She has been nominated as a member of Technical Program Committee and Organizing Committee of many International Conferences. She is also a member of many International and National bodies like ACM (Association for Computing Machinery), IAENG (International Association of Engineers), IACSIT (International Association of Computer Science and Information Technology), Internet Society, and CSI (Computer Society of India).

Shahnaz Fatima is MCA and Ph.d. She has completed her Ph.D. from Integral University. Her research area is human–computer interaction. Currently, she is working as an Assistant Professor at Amity University. She has published many of the valuable research papers in various national and international conferences and journals. She has been nominated as a member of Technical Program Committee and Organizing Committee of many International Conferences. She has been actively involved in research being a supervisor to research scholars and postgraduate students. She is the member of International Association of Computer Science and Information Technology (IACSIT) and other similar organizations.

Clinical Data Analysis Using IoT Data Analytics Platforms

R. Sujatha, S. Nathiya and Jyotir Moy Chatterjee

Abstract Public aid knowledge management needs actions, definitions, and laws so as to produce enhancements over public health treatment and designing. These enhancements have often supported a collection of data and indicators, and the health administrators must own admittance to machines that offer elasticity to manage the efficient analysis. Several technologies will cut back overall prices concerning the interference about the administration of persistent diseases. The clinical study intends to discover novel and better ways to recognize, diagnose, check, or manage a distinct disordered manner. With the IT support supervision of chronic pathogenesis, home rehabilitation, patient direction, and coordination of clinical pathways including multiple actors' makes it potential and IT adoption permits innovating or re-engineering lending divisions to market the commercial property of lending assistance and enhance their feature. Healthcare assistance supports the continual therapy, observance of victims at intervals the unit, and offers around the timekeeper help and makes sure that the encircling setting does not hinder their treatment and observance. Recently, an IoT (Internet of Things) possesses interesting in the eyes of creators of care systems. World Health Organization is integrating numerous medical practices with IoT technologies to supply top-quality cheap care services to patients. Additionally, few IoT gadgets communicate with cellular gadgets through wireless device-to-device communication networks for the transmission of knowledge, which may be obtained via the apps for data retrieval, creating choices or information warehouse for eventual way.

Keywords Health care · Big data analytics · Distributed analytics · Edge intelligence · Hospital management

R. Sujatha (✉) · S. Nathiya
School of Information Technology & Engineering, Vellore Institute of Technology, Vellore, India
e-mail: r.sujatha@vit.ac.in

S. Nathiya
e-mail: nathiya.s@vit.ac.in

J. M. Chatterjee
Lord Buddha Education Foundation, Kathmandu, Nepal
e-mail: jyotirchatterjee@gmail.com

P. Raj et al. (eds.), *Internet of Things Use Cases for the Healthcare Industry*,
https://doi.org/10.1007/978-3-030-37526-3_12

1 Introduction

1.1 Clinical Data

In hospital and healthcare environment, information about patient acts as a vital ingredient in taking decision. Visit of each time and tests taken needs to be in cumulative manner to help in the process of diagnosis. Irrespective of the past, present, or future, this is going to be inevitable in clinical perspective. Papers and filing of the same in the name of physical charts were maintained for the past so many years. Invention of digitalization and Internet utilization made the drastic change in this field in the name of Electronic Health Record (EHR). In this process, electronic information pertaining to patient is stored and retrieved based on the requirement.

To discuss, in precise, clinical data holds collection of data gathered by observing a sick person's health condition over time span. Normally, a datum comprises of the patient, the attribute, value of the attribute, and observation time. The data pops from disease, follow-up of the same, screening data and examination data. Based on the nature of data it is classified into various types, namely, narrative documented by clinician, numerical reading like blood pressure, lab values, coded data gathered from terminals, textual data in the form of text, recorded signals like EEG, ECG, and pictures like radiographs, and so on. Uses of clinical data are manifold in nature by acting as source of historical record, future health could be diagnosed, aids in clinical research, helps in coding and billing purpose, communication, and provide glimpse of preventive measures in times of spread of epidemic disease when considered in cumulative manner.

National committee on vital and health statistics has been established in the last decade and acts as the statuary body in handling the rules governing to health data of US citizens. Ultimate aim of the committee is to handle the data in meticulous manner to get great insights. They have illustrated the data stewardship for individual personal health information in tactical manner as mentioned below.

Data sources—hospital, payer, public health, person/patient, ambulatory centers, prescriptions, and labs.

Data users	Data uses
Hospital	Discharge summary, quality reporting, operational assessment
Physicians	Office visits, quality reporting
Person/Patient	Personal health record
Labs	Test results
Public health	Communicable disease reporting
Payer	Benefit checking claims quality audits
Researchers	Research studies

2 IoT World

The IoT denotes a setup of physical devices and alternative things, implanted with natural philosophy, software, sensors, and network property that allows those objects to gather and reciprocate knowledge. By 2020, four-hundredth of IoT-related technology based on health-related issue is quite possible of creating $117 billion business. The confluence of drugs and knowledge technologies, like medical information science, can improve health care as we all acknowledge it, curb prices, decreasing incompetence, and protecting lives [1].

2.1 Medical IoT (mIoT)

Wearable and portable apps these days sponsor fitness, health training, symptom pursuit, including cooperative illness administration and care coordination. All these principles of analytics will increase the relevance of information interpretations, degrading the number of times that finish user's pay to piece along with knowledge outputs. Insights obtained from massive information outline can stimulate the digital separation of the attention world, marketing methods, and period decision-making. A brand-new class of "personalized preventative health coaches" (Digital Health Advisers) can rise. These employees can maintain their abilities, and therefore the capacity to evaluate and perceive strength and welfare data. They are going to facilitate their shoppers to avoid chronic and diet-related sickness, improve cognitive features perform, deliver the goods, enhanced subjective strength, and deliver the goods obtained lifestyles overall. Several technologies will cut back overall prices for the interference or administration of persistent diseases. Certain embody materials that perpetually control health indicators, tools that auto-administer treatments, or a device that tracks the period health information once a patient self-manage a medical aid. As a result of the need for expanded admittance to fast web and smartphones, several victims have begun to utilize cellular applications (apps) to achieve varied health desire. These methods and movable apps square measure currently more and more related and are used with telemedicine and telehealth through the medical IoT (mIoT). mIoT may be an important section of the digital conversion of concern because it permits distinct market patterns to develop and allows modifications in business methods, productivity enhancements, price containment, and increased client practices [2].

2.2 *Linked Medical Data*

The clinical analysis intends towards finding new and more reliable systems to learn, diagnose, monitor, or handle a definite neurotic method, e.g., complaints or unfavorable situations. It includes three chief sections:

(i) The patient-centric examination which suggests individual subjects;
(ii) The hygienics and social researches which explore the distribution of infection and the agents that harm circumstance; and
(iii) The results and health assistance investigation which tries to recognize the best persuasive and adequate mediations, procedures, and services.

Linked Medical Data Access Control (LiMDAC) methodology which capitalizes on linked information methodologies to facilitate measuring access to preventive information among classified origins having distinct access limitations. Linked data is a method for obtaining and attaching information using free network standards. The Linked Data publishing method normally starts with actual, organized information in different organizations (CSV, social information, XML, and so forth), which are changed over to RDF. The distribution depends on a Linked information model that can be delivered either by formulating an unmistakable nearby pattern (in RDF Schema, OWL, and so forth), or by reusing existing, broad lexicons, (for example, FOAF, Dublin Core, and SKOS). From that point, URIs are relegated to the things in the dataset on the occasion level and between connections are set up with various datasets. There are commonly several models of areas that can be built up used to relate URI anonyms and other space explicit RDF bonds. The impact of announcing restorative information as Linked Data coordinates obviously in the event that we reuse generally utilized philosophy or connected datasets [3].

2.2.1 LiMDAC

LiMDAC principles are to empower controlling access to restorative information. Aside from the LiMDAC measures, the structure contains an authorization mechanism module and an authorization interface module. The authorization interface lies between data clients and suppliers. It empowers data customers to (i) create client structures dependent on the LiMDAC client profile model and (ii) mission for shared restorative data. The data shopper characterizes the extent of getting therapeutic data being either persistent arranged examination or epidemiological study. The exploration principles depend on the components of the data cubes that are saved in the conveyed RDF data stores. Following each mission principles, there is a range for choosing its incentive from a drop-down rundown of conceivable keys. Moreover, the authorization interface makes an interpretation of data purchasers' investigation into SPARQL inquiries and moves them over the authorization mechanism. At first, the authorization mechanism recovers the entrance strategies from conveyed data suppliers. From that point, the authorization mechanism checks whether the profile of the data purchaser coordinates the client profile characterized by each entrance strategy. On account of progress, the authorization mechanism makes and sends SPARQL questions to disseminated data suppliers. The inquiries scan for data that match both the data customer's inquiry and the fulfilled access approaches. On account of accomplishment, they came about datasets are come back to the data customer by means of the authorization interface. The impact of this technique is except if (i) (for patient-arranged investigation purposes) the quantity of exploited people coordinating explicit examples, alongside the name of the data supplier issuing certain data or (ii) (for epidemiological examinations sees) the few connected data cubes [3].

3 Electronic Health Record Data (EHR)

Healthcare analytics influences clinical and managerial knowledge in EHRs and data regarding clinical observe patterns and pointers, to maintain metric-driven feature enhancement. Objects combine characteristic incapability in healthcare delivery and deviations from the following criteria: characteristic possibilities for increasing aids assumed to boost the degree of responsibility, economical targeting of inadequate supplies, and also examination of risk-adjusted performance to count establishments. Procedures embrace retrospectively characteristic groups with large or below risk-adjusted metric records that describe patterns of top-quality concern and measures for development, severally. Subject features, or phenotypes, with sturdy similarities with effects of care, might facilitate to make a case for such records. Phenotypes obtained from EHR information additionally could also obtain organized as variables within prophetical figures that prospectively cipher including gift patient-specific prospects through clinical call comfort. Certain analytic strategies need to experience EHR implementations. EHRs with the desired extent of information more and more square measure obtainable at giant hospital systems. Establishments might create certain data obtainable throughout a clinical information repository, some computer database maintained by AN EHR's transactional systems which promote economic population questions. Federal storehouses of body and general clinical information give establishments with admittance to comparative information, e.g., UHC's CDB. Certain native and general datasets along describe an expensive potential supply of data for analytics; however, others gift abundant trials in their practice. Examinations, co-morbidities, and schemes usually square measure described indirectly as request principles. Clinical information like lab takes a look at results and medical histories could also be marked as native rules or in the document, and those they might need abundant clinical circumstances to perform. Attempts square measure afoot to form in public obtainable institutions of phenotypes outlined in the duration of patterns in systems and distinct information like eMERGE. eMERGE's phenotypes are in public obtainable in a record kind. Accessories for transposing these phenotypes into questions of native information repositories and national storehouses may create data-driven quality gain higher generally sensible [4].

4 Analytic Information Warehouse

Analytic Information Warehouse (AIW) is to deal with the requirement of EHR. This maintains defining phenotypes through a database-agnostic practice as teams about body systems, classes of digital take a look at outcomes and important symbols, also incidence, consecutive, and different temporary designs in coded and separate information. The capacity permits defining phenotypes like Victims with replicated high-pressure level studies that have diagnosed hypertension and continue signifying handled with a water pill in the duration of those information. The AIW obtains information and determined variables denoting phenotypes of concern into delimited records appropriate for applied math analysis and mining with customary tools. I2b2 (Informatics for integration Biology and therefore the Bedside) may be a generally utilized clinical analysis information repository operation. The AIW's growth becomes initiated and managed by an operational scheme through our establishment to grasp the elements of clinic readmissions regionally and across the nation [5].

The AIW may be a care analytics sandbox. Its code well reaches a temporal concept method, PROTEMPA, to maintain information retrieval and make up discovery in performance analytics, a capacity that was not antecedently approved by PROTEMPA's architecture. Fields of expansion embody versatile configuration to provide immediate admittance by the code to enterprise information repositories; a configurable tool to remodeling information from its supply mode illustration toward a typical information design; guide for stipulating considerations in terms of knowledge as diagrammatical in the traditional pattern to permit theirs reprocess over datasets; guide for investing connections within information parts within the standard form in concept estimate; economical process of enormous databases that manage cradle of, however, considerations were calculated and the AIW will estimate to tens of immeasurable conflicts, corresponding to a various classes of measure increases in advanced statistics as analyzed with PROTEMPA, and configurable maintenance for commerce treated information and located phenotypes into existing review, mining, and question tools. The most participation of the practice is this software's widespread design and free supply implementation. Whereas quality development analytics has been the driving clinical drawback for AIW development, AIW is additionally extended during a kind of comparative effectiveness and different in-progress studies that use EHR information. The AIW code involves abundant extensions of PROTEMPA as corresponded therewith represented in AN earlier notification. Certain expansions maintain the info amount, information and makeup representation and distribution, and product form desires of clinical analytics. The AIW design defines cooperation implementing online database access (data source), descriptions of data also concepts (knowledge source), and implementations of algorithms that cipher groups of your time-series data (algorithm source). The work fiduciary part achieves processing flows via organizing notes to the assistance suppliers to recover data and abstraction outlines, and cipher recurrence, and regular and different temporary designs. Expansions being associated with PROTEMPA embody the following:

(1) A data supply service provider which enables defining nontemporal, additionally, to temporary concepts during temporal abstraction metaphysics;
(2) A data source service supplier which executes the VDM capability and produces including performs SQL applicable for databases of interest;
(3) Re-architected information supply and work fiduciary parts that flow information from supply orders within temporary concept process, thus permitting tens of immeasurable polyclinic encounters to be treated expeditiously on customary server hardware configurations and while not this requirement for on-disk caching; and
(4) A plug-and-play method within the work fiduciary referred to as the Yield Handler for performing and configuring; however, PROTEMPA products calculated periods and data [5].

The AIW permits feature development knowledge to leverage phenotypes represented in EHR knowledge as classes of principles and ideas and as frequency, consecutive, and different temporary attachments. It promotes the process and measurement of different knowledge experts through skills to justify phenotypes in database-agnostic form and rework reclaimed knowledge toward that type. These characteristics provide a large-scale measurement of readmitted subjects on our establishment with these during a general dataset. The AIW's temporal abstraction capacity contributes vital and required versatility in defining phenotypes in quality improvement. Its data mapping ability might eventually offer a method for cross-institutional clinical constitution reprocess. The provision of software which permits easy reading of constitution repositories might considerably boost the appliance of EHR data in related and clinical effectiveness [5].

5 Data Warehousing

Public aid knowledge management needs actions, definitions, and laws to produce enhancements to public health treatment and designing. These enhancements have often supported a collection of data and indicators, and the health administrators must own access to tools that offer versatility to handle the efficient study. The info Warehouse (DW) is a vital tool for such circumstances, as a result of its outlined as comprehensive information designed to help on the higher cognitive process in business management. DW holds the features of being integrated, subject-oriented, nonvolatile, and time-variant. Knowledge reposting could be a wide setting targeted in an exceeding DW. Its implementation needs the mixing of knowledge returning from many inward and outward sources (legacy and internal transactional environments), to larger functional information. This setting affords a complete read of the whole system by the way to traditional and authentic knowledge to promote the decision-making, with the most limited potential overload on the transactional practices.

Typical knowledge reposting design includes a mix of components that creates an upscale setting for the data warehouse, namely, operational supply systems, knowledge frame-block, data presentation area, and data access tools. The primary component of the info reposting design is that the operational source systems that embrace varied heterogeneous knowledge experts with completely various formations and compositions, such as relative and non-relational databases, flat files, spreadsheets, etc. The next component is the knowledge field that includes some knowledge preprocessing tasks, like as services of cleanup, connecting, regulating, and knowledge storing, and therefore the sorting and consecutive process. The third component is the performance space whereby the info is organized in data markets (a subset of a DW) supported one business process; furthermore, the info markets are settled in an exceedingly regulated thanks to being additionally integrated. The last component represents the info access devices, which include circumstantial question tools, article writers, analytic applications, information processing, and others. Among the primary, second, and third components, there is the Extract, Transact, and Load (ETL) method. Essence entails that knowledge is obtained by varied information sources and derived to different integrated information for additional preparation. Remodel entails correcting knowledge inconsistencies, cleansing and mixing knowledge returning from various origins, and reducing data repetitions. The load is the transportation of the ready knowledge to the DW repository. Other necessary component of an information reposting setting is that ODS (Operational Data Store) that is AN extension of the DW design and it includes operational data that are integrated from bequest data experts' systems [6].

6 Clinical Data Warehousing

Clinical data warehouses signify typically headed to combination and investigation of coded information. Designed on high of EHRs, Clinical Data Warehouses (CDWs) modify assortment and subsequent practice of tending information for several functions as well as analysis. CDWs are used for several kinds of statements comprising all the areas of medication: Phenome-wide summary, record mining, epidemiologic police investigation, pharmacovigilance, etc. CDWs are typically won't leverage structured information (for example, asking principles, procedures, laboratory outcomes, and treatments). However, despite vital purpose approaching the regularity of knowledge assortment, an oversized portion of the medicinal information remains implanted in free-text clinical narrative [7].

7 Process Analytics Techniques

Most recent subjects and healthcare practices are frequently increased in Electronic Healthcare Records (EHR) generating an enormous quantity of information. Further, especially, Process Analytics (PA) procedures could help us using certain penetrations because of the active outlook others contribute to the captured entity. The benefits of PA can perform to the healthcare conditions and more particularly the diabetes domain. Type 2 diabetes mellitus (T2DM) is a growing and highly existing disorder in our community. Furthermore, it suggests extra requests both from a cultural and informatics perspective.

PA can address important penetrations into patients' concern courses though the existing challenges in the healthcare field bring with its difficulties. Hence, the analysis displays a procedure comprising of six stages toward applying PA on human services data. This system plans to control clients through the different difficulties experienced while applying PA to EHRs. Besides, the various advances must be considered as an iterative method of progress toward well-supported outcomes. As such, explicitly consider the need for iterative utilization as a deficiency of earlier studies [4].

Log preparation: This stage includes the collection of event data from various data experts into a single event record. The aggregation of EHRs brings along its challenge. Although PA procedures can help to identify and determine data feature issues.

Log inspection: In this phase, it relates to the initial search of the data utilizing statistics and easy PA techniques. The purpose of this level is to fully experience the dataset and its constraints and possibilities. General abnormalities can previously be found. As such, one can examine which medicinal sources provided the numerous preventive aids and whereby numerous medical services the common subject accepted. This previously presents an abundance of knowledge for health coverage and preventive situations. A common idea in PA is the method plan which reflects the patient's care course. This could be connected to event incidence, i.e., how frequently a victim suffered a cooperation at most concise earlier and certain regularity, i.e., how regularly service is supported in certain courses.

Abstraction and selection: This phase is a necessary measure for unorganized methods. Abstraction eliminates unnecessary features and supports to concentrate on the numerous vital features of the method. An identity solution is to combine practiced information. Based on custom and communication with a medicinal specialist, we obtained information on the divisions about attention and their classification principles. Hence, we substituted the exercises with this abstraction. Keep in mind, in any case, that one can no longer dispread ways between exercises inside these classifications. Another arrangement dynamic practices consequently. The structure thought methodology bunches the tasks that normally perform all in all. The client can figure out how to digest these examples into an alternate exercise in the occasion log. This technique can likewise be connected iteratively when the first occasion log is utilized as data for the module. Another procedure is movement grouping mining. This method distinguishes exercises that consistently occur in arrangement and that offer a few qualities, for example, indistinguishable therapeutic specialist co-ops. Both computerized deliberation techniques were chosen as a result of their appropriateness on human service datasets, and be a reason for their inside on the dynamical highlights of the dataset. Separation systems are exciting to concentrate on a subpart of the occasion log which frequently prompts progressively organized outcomes. Occasion logs were separated per subgroup for specific classifications, for example, training to contrast patients that match a few rules and sufferers who do not, or, for example, "ophthalmology" to coordinate on this period of the diabetes procedure.

Clustering: This stage manages dependable tracks into discrete parts with their qualities. A sub-log is made by bunching the follows in gatherings that have fundamentally the same as qualities. Patients are hence bunched not (just) founded on the patient data however on the attributes of their consideration ventures. There are two significant grouping strategies from an expert less point of view, specifically follow bunching and succession bunching. Follow bunching groups care adventures dependent on follow profiles. A follow profile contains certain qualities of the follow that one finds significant, for example, exercises, a specific arrangement of activities, preventive specialist organizations, and so forth. ActiTrac has actualized this technique. ActiTrac is especially valuable because it explicitly recognizes health projects, because of its visualization attributes, and because of its assuring outcomes in former benchmark research. Sequence clustering directs totally on the series of actions in shades and designs more easy patterns than trace clustering. Clustering not only allows discovering numerous comprehensible models but also allows identifying or confirming subgroups based upon their performance.

Process mining: When the event log is isolated and collected, the genuine procedure mining can start. The strategies are the specked graph examination and the fluffy excavator from a procedure point of view, and the job chain of command module and the informal community digger from a hierarchical perspective. The specked diagram can incorporate a prepared perception of the scope (a category) of cases. This technique was expressly picked for its optical and reasonable outcome which, additionally, improves collaboration with human service specialists. This may be utilized for verifying agreement with preventive guidelines or to the optimization of sources and methods.

Validation: Hence, the outcomes must be granted to the healthcare situation and approved by experts. Furthermore, private communication with authorities during the performance of the early levels is meant to manage the examination (as illustrated in Fig. 1).

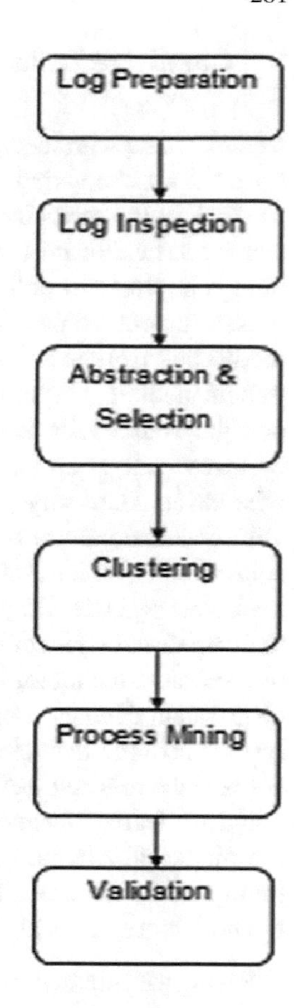

Fig. 1 Process analytics techniques

8 Mobile Health Care (M Health Care)

Phone and tablet area units help doctors to solve issues quicker with less stress. Physicians will use mobile devices to record patient history with borderline errors. These devices offer higher access to the latest drug info, and therefore facilitate to create higher choices. The mobile health care (mhealthcare) appeals with the IoT area unit allowing the assorted dimensionalities and therefore the online assistance. These applications should afford brand unique principles to the many folks for obtaining profit above the health advice often for being a healthy life. Once the initiation of IoT technology and therefore the connected tools that area unit employed in the medical field reinforced the assorted options of those aid online requests. The massive amount of huge knowledge is formed by IoT gadgets in aid atmosphere. Cloud computing technology is employed to manage the massive amount of information and also additionally offers the convenience of usage. During this state of affairs, a cloud primarily based utilization area unit is taking part in a significant role during this quick environment. These preventive treatments also have used the cloud computing for secured storage and convenience [8].

9 Cognitive Data Transmission Method (CDTM)

Medical trade with medicinal knowledge is growing day by day. It is simple to diagnose and handle varied forms of conditions efficiently. It is a chance for improving the QoS in the medicinal analysis. Cognitive feature technology could be a higher answer in healthcare trade to open the medicinal benefits. Cognitive feature technology implements policies for medical examiners to mix different patient data into massive extent medicinal big data, wherever this serves to diagnose and determine the medication from the obtainable related medicinal reports. Varied analysis purposes, patient medicinal reports, success stories of medication ways, and literature are the possible sources for medicinal examiners and doctors to try effectively diagnosing and treatment, if and as long as, it is simple to locate the present medicinal data, whereas standard ways cannot scale the medicinal data of a brand unique outpatient with crucial conditions. Varied styles of medical information from totally different sources will give innovative and fascinating data to decide, to permit, and to assist the medicinal practice. Cognitive feature technology performs the corrective examiners to grasp varied styles of medicinal data connected to the patient's fitness status. Cognitive feature technology obtains the medicinal information victimization healthcare observation devices, converts into helpful data and then transfers to medicinal analysts, where the medicinal examiners will get the patient information, analyze, and counsel the relevant treatment supported the patient's fitness status. In this manner, cognitive feature technology serves to enhance the clinical call method wherever the medicinal examiners will connect with the present reports and counsel higher therapy [9]. Numerous benefits are obtained from cognitive feature technology in the healthcare trade, as follows:

- Rising the interaction between the consultant and outpatient,
- Economical administration of medicinal information frequency and content authority,
- Integration of the structured and unstructured information, and
- Grants information access.

10 Digital Health Ecosystem

Modern courses in aid assistance offering support-integrated and patient-centric attention afforded by multidisciplinary groups and various supplying perspectives on the time of sickness. Before position, the victim during attention suggests that additionally to target interference and well-being, and to serve to the physical, mental, and non-secular wants of the national. The existent tending practices do not seem to be appropriate to fulfill these requests as a result of their homeward-bound to acute sickness care, emphasize low conflicts of victims with their caregivers wherever the tending experts square measures the most leads, promotes designation and treatment of modern signs, and typically maintains the caregiver's exercise in isolation. Tending methods square measure, however, for the most part paper-based mostly, ignore data tools which will promote evidence-based most excellent methods, and performance while not analytics to restrict and quantify the problem they supply. Medicinal choices square measure created in keeping with absolute standards located within the physician's logic and data instead of express criteria that square measure external data which will be reviewed, estimated, and refreshed. To meet such a demand, the change of the fitness standard a scientific selection of tending Data Technologies (IT) is taken into account necessity, not solely a chance. With the IT support authority of enduring diagnostics, home recovery, patient direction, and coordination of clinical pathways with various actors' makes it potential and IT support allows innovating or re-engineering tending areas to market the commercial property of tending services and improve their condition. The tending it is additionally the instruments which will remodel tending to resist the unsustainable price drop. For this, applications, methods, and workflows will enhance quality, protection, access, and value potency square measure required. Fostering Electronic Health Record (EHR) methods have existed among the earliest analysis issues of the eHealth strand. The constant assurance has begun to repay as numerous eHealth solutions square measure being adopted on AN increasing scale [10].

11 IoT-Based Healthcare Devices and Technologies

Healthcare assistance promotes the continual practice, observance of patients at intervals the unit, offers around the clock help, and makes sure that the encircling setting does not hinder their treatment and observance. Implants area unit devices are designed for a few specialized care services provided by medical specialty. These embrace aids granted to watch or handle internal body organs. Mobile care assistance talks to help that ought to not be affected even though the patient's area unit toward the progress and so needs design and technologies which will assist a patient's quality. Remedy suggests to, however, the particular doses of medicine provided to victim's area unit established or controlled with the help of technology. This may be a specialized technology-based medicine invented to handle sure illnesses and disorders. Surgical health services peoples, who need a read of the inner organ to control on a victim to revise any exception or make a certain process. To attain certain objects, the care division has been utilizing numerous kinds of hardware, software, and networking technologies in their Information and Communication Technology (ICT) framework. Most recent IoT becomes attracting the eye of creators of care practices. World Health Organization is integrated with numerous medicinal practices and IoT technologies to provide top-caliber cheap care assistance to subjects [11].

- Mobile Device

Mobile devices (e.g., smartphones) and tablets became the foremost widespread handheld computing systems. They are currently omnipresent and possess filtered each facet of life. Once connected with cellular package applications (apps) which are produced for numerous user desires, mobile devices will reduce personal communication and contributes numerous sorts of settings. Additionally, fascinating IoT tools interact mainly with cellular gadgets through broadcast device-to-device communication networks for the transfer of knowledge, which may be located via the apps for data accumulation, creating choices or information storage for ultimate access.

- Wearable Device

Wearable gadgets are tiny, on-body gadgets worn by individuals. They are perpetually attached, hands-free, less distractive, and have various information access interfaces. These tools embody hand-worn terminals, body-mounted cameras, or increased reality headsets. The wearable innovation is supplemented by cell phone innovation (cell phones) and mobile package applications (apps). The program of a wearable is an application that is accessible on a cell phone or an individual system. Hence, cell phones are expected to hold out the task of the procedure and sending the data delivered by a wearable gadget to the cloud for capacity.

- Body Area Network (BAN)

A BAN might be a healthcare custom-made communication correspondence network that advances the perception of the health remaining of somebody wherever, whenever. Sensors with remote correspondence ability are inserted in the internal or potentially outer pieces of a patients' body. The detecting component data got is then forwarded over a low control remote system to the worthy server inside a door gadget. For the IoT-based medicinal services applications, the Wireless BAN (WBAN) is acquiring quality in light of the fact that the range additionally sorts of wearable gadgets still develop and become less expensive. To understand certain reasons, the medicinal services division has been using various sorts of equipment, programming, and organizing advances in their ICT frameworks.

12 Healthcare Monitoring System

Healthcare observation is usually rising because of completely different IoT capabilities and instrumentality that should track a patient's health parameters unendingly. Because of the vital nature of healthcare systems, several healthcare devices square measure developed using numerous ideas and procedures like distant monitoring/diagnostics and air ambulances that are launched in several countries to contend among the quick-growing requirements of health care throughout difficulties and promote sufferers' recoveries. The description of the transmission protocol and practice design describes attention-grabbing and difficult assignments during the aspect healthcare observation ought to be continuous to trace the patient's body parameters and supply a standardized and substantial knowledge to the experts or the preventive unit for designation. These approaches specifically are going to be of a nice facility to patients and old users once assistance is required just in case of medical emergencies. Healthcare observation ought to be continuous to trace the patient's body parameters and supply a standardized and substantial knowledge to the doctors or the preventive unit for designation [12].

13 Smartification of IoT

The IoT is an associate in nursing scheme which comprises gadgets implemented with sensors, computing, associate in nursing networking methodologies cooperating to make an independent setting within which sensible assistance area unit is produced to boost the standard of individual life. The current administration field wherever the conception of IoT is presently being examined and used combines voltage conservation and management, transportation, health, logistics, urban living, and education [13]. In IoT, smartification implies to nearly each gadget (home appliances to wearable devices) within the scheme. IoT smartification discusses a fascinating level of intelligence to a policy providing assistance among the scheme. Hence, guaranteeing ability and QoS is of dominant influence within the performance of any sensible service [14].

14 Secure Health Using IoT

Commonly for home primarily based health care, the organization embraces information, imaging, sensing, and personal laptop cooperation technologies mobilized at identification, practice, and observance subjects while not perturbing the standard of mode. It may be able to attain the event of an occasional price preventive sensing, information, and analytics device that is period observance net allotted subjects' physical fitness. IoT network can give fresh and period selection of the subject, clinics, guardian, and experts except this the acquired information transmission from supply purpose to address for the aim of primitive observance there would be like of the design of an occasional price secured principles for web-based observance. The further observance is formed attainable by mistreatment numerous medical specialty designs, and they exist and broadcast information through Bluetooth/ZigBee to a system which controls devices (PC, iTV). The handled data is also kept on the device or transmitted to a center that has an entire observance, for each fitness specialist and subjects. Introduction to the medical center may be approved through the web and through mobile devices or computers. The IoT and RFID additionally execute an important part in object detection and private description that might be using classified person, whereas remote observance once a variety of individual data have determined which can be used for distinctive identity of every patient and their individual information are going to be stored [15].

15 Healthcare Information Systems

Healthcare info systems analysis (often named as health info technology or HIT research) in info Systems (IS), and therefore the IS discipline to expand its "contextual envelope" by grasp the fitness care division as a sociably necessary and in theory fascinating circumstances to improve and clarify info systems approach similarly on offer contextually relevant penetrations on healthcare info methods extension and management. This ascent in HIT analysis may be attributed in massive half to socioeconomic and technological advancements at intervals in the healthcare division that have contributed further possibilities and demand for HIT analysis. In most social prosperity, healthcare defrayment proceeds to develop speedily as a community period and measures chronic illnesses further. HITs, which embrace software system and support utilized in the clinical observe of drugs similarly as technologies to collect, distribute, and examine fitness info, are touted as important elements to scale back healthcare prices and conjointly to boost healthcare status, admittance, and fitness concerns [16].

16 Long Short-Term Memory and DeepCare

Personalized prognostic medication requires the modeling of subject unhealthiness and application manners that essentially have large temporary dependencies. Aid views keep in automated restorative reports are episodic and variable in time. DeepCare is the associate end-to-end deep dynamic neural network which shows medicinal reports, reserves earlier unwellness history, suggests common unwellness states, and divines expected medicinal consequences. At the info level, DeepCare expresses care events as vectors and registers stable fitness status trajectories by the vision of ancient documents, engineered on Long Short-Term Immediate Memory (LSTM); DeepCare introduces ways to achieve on an occasional basis regular effects by lenitive forgetting and compression of memory. DeepCare additionally expressly models medical gadgets which modify the course of unwellness and form future medical risk. DeepCare associates end-to-end deep dynamic memory neural network which discusses the four aforesaid challenges. DeepCare is made on Long Short-Term Memory (LSTM), a repeated neural network furnished with memory cells to save activities [17]. About each time step, the LSTM states associated information, updates the memory cell, and associated returns an output. Memory is managed over an overlook portal that moderates the passing of memory from just one occasion level to a different and is renewed by attending different data at any time level. The product is set by the memory associated tempered by an output gate. In DeepCare, the LSTM displays the unwellness mechanical phenomenon and aid rules of a patient encapsulated in an exceedingly time-stamped series of admittances. The information to the LSTM is data derived from admittances. The outputs express unwellness events at the point of admittance [18]. To review, through offering DeepCare, there are four modeling supplements:

(i) Managing large dependences in health care;
(ii) Presenting a unique illustration of variable-size disclosure as mounted size continuous vectors;
(iii) Molding indirect reporting and strange timing; and
(iv) Capturing contradictory communications among sickness including interventions.

17 Clinical Pathways

A complete simulation of patient responsibility implemented in the aid units needs analysis of this method from various positions of reading. The method includes multiple activities, several sorts of projects, completely distinctive actors with specific tasks, experience level, information, etc. Further, the various fields and phases of the aid method are thought-about (departments' source capacity, hospital accounting systems, patients' practices throughout the care method, and lots of others). It becomes far more necessary as patient care (including unwellness progress and medication) prolongs on the far side of the clinic visit [19]. Operating with such approaches typically needs a practice of automated or semiautomatic methods to investigate numerous information sources, together with medical records, exploitation machine learning, data processing, method mining procedures, communication with victims, and alternative strategies. The list of issues includes the absence of flexibility, completeness, and accuracy of corrective information to be examined, low coverage of unique problems with Clinical Pathways (CP), weak rationalization, and huge change in core preventive information. To beat these problems, a composite strategy with a mix of techniques from information, method, and text mining is projected to support computer-aided simulation [20].

18 Online Health-Oriented Chat Logs

Easy and Internet-based friendly communications like online healthcare-oriented discussion associations offer a handy way for victims and other peoples involved concerning tendency to speak and partition data. The chat logs of a web healthcare-oriented chat cluster will doubtless be accustomed to obtain potential issues, to promote cooperation, and to suggest relevant aid data to users. Online healthcare-oriented discussion groups typically turn out an oversized quantity of chat logs, which could include necessary data that is instantly or lengthily associated with potential issue analysis and preventive assistance performance. As a result of potential issues in aid, chat logs are significantly connected among the public health considerations of patients, aid experts, and customers, and agency ordinarily utilizes friendly communications to begin discussions among one another; the matter of identifying these potential issues signifies an encouraging and fascinating analysis subject within the area of health data processing [21].

19 Wearable IoT Data Stream

Among the IoT, available devices (or articles) like sensible sensors and different environmental materials that area unit ideally negatively viewed as processors will act with few social interferences. This has provided an increase to the distinct application within the administration and associating private information with doctors wherever sensors and smartwatches will circulate particular vitals, a region referred to as wearable IoT. This can be ordinarily observed in fitness and health watching applications. But, in wearable IoT, for example, users of World Health Organization area unit running their vital organ to backend services (e.g., fitness info systems within the cloud) or across various private agents (e.g., streaming within sensors and smartphones for health tracking) is not solely in danger from hackers. Still, there are units of rising care system problems with the correct management of the various information streams and that constitutes the requirement to supply analysis solutions on the way to dependably discover, record, and balance the patients to their scheme in shared designs [22].

20 Big Data Analytics with Application to Health Care

With the advanced ordered endorsement of EHRs by the US Department of Health and Human Services (HHS), tending professionals have gotten access to luxuriant volume of knowledge which may give additional insights and higher takeaways that were not attainable before. EHRs do not seem to be the sole ample and wealthy supply of care information, for example, broadcast forms observance tools and activity-friendly communication origins additionally give additional possibilities and will be dangerous game changers. Various information analytics computer code merchants are producing devices that are related to those origins and are specifically tailored to care. Several enterprises are driving the flow of massive information because the current period of data-driven deciding is unveiling. The sector of massive information analytics is obtaining quick traction in business, domain, and also administration; the care field is not any different. During this chapter, huge information analytics are employed to care information that is gathered from various experts to realize feature penetrations and comprehend the most excellent systems of the sector (handling distinct care-specific huge information devices). Health consultants perpetually advocate nearer immersion in one's fitness and additional commitment to precautionary care [23].

21 Big Data and Analytics in Mobile Healthcare Market

With the recent mandated adoption of electronic health record EHRs by the HHS, tending professionals have gotten access to luxuriant amounts of knowledge that may give additional insights and higher takeaways that were not attainable before. EHRs do not seem to be the sole ample and wealthy supply of care information, for example, wireless health observance devices and activity social media sources additionally give additional opportunities and will be serious game changers. Multiple information analytics computer code vendors are building tools that are connected to those sources and are specifically tailored to care. Several industries are riding the wave of massive information because the new era of data-driven deciding is unveiling. The sector of massive information analytics is gaining quick traction in business, domain, and also the government; the care arena is not any totally different. During this paper, huge information analytics are applied to care information that is collected from multiple sources to realize quality insights and apprehend best practices of the sector (using new care-specific huge information tools). Health consultants perpetually advocate nearer immersion in one's health and additional engagement with preventive care [24].

22 Big Data in Health Care

Big Data Analytics (BDA) are making gigantic effects in various fields, together with retail, account informal communities, and so forth. In consideration division, BDA has shown unmistakable advantages on up consideration power. BDA will recognize people's consideration conditions, set up dangers for genuine medical problems, supply customized care administrations, and so forth; moreover, BDA conjointly has possibilities to decrease care cost by trademark care assets squander, giving closer perception and expanding care intensity. Inside the strategy for BDA execution in consideration segment, wearable gadgets territory unit demonstrated to be a much better data supply looking on its regular advantages in consideration and its quality. The consideration wearable gadgets will gather and redesign constant timeframe care data and uncover concealed checking and tangible alternatives. As of now, wearable gadgets territory unit is widely utilized in consideration field. The wellness screens as Fitbit, Jawbone, Garmin, and Suunto, zone unit intended for the clients to watch day-by-day care conditions. Furthermore, some consideration wearable gadget provider's territory unit is making endeavors on exploring new gadgets with restorative capacities. For instance, Apple has an enthusiasm for blood perception through skin and medicinal sensor-loaded gadgets that expect to explore aldohexose levels [25].

23 Big Data Privacy in Health Care

The present pattern toward digitizing medicinal services work processes and moving to electronic patient records has seen a change in outlook inside the social insurance business. The measure of clinical information that square measure offered electronically will be then drastically swelled as far as quality, assorted variety, and practicality, following what is called immense learning. Driven by important necessities and along these lines the possibility to improve care spare lives and lower costs, enormous learning holds the guarantee. To hinder ruptures of delicate information and elective types of security occurrences, a proactive and preventive methodology and measures ought to be taken by every medicinal services association focusing on future security and protection wants. Driven by vital necessities and in this manner the possibility to upgrade care, spare lives and lower costs, tremendous information hold the guarantee of supporting a decent shift of uncommon chances and use cases, together with these key models: clinical call support, protection, wiped outness police examination, populace well-being the board, unfavorable occasions recognition, and treatment improvement for infections moving various organ systems [26].

24 Challenges of mIoT

The mIoT is patching up consideration administrations as people have begun exploitation of IoT to deal with their well-being needs. For instance, people will utilize IoT gadgets to advise those with respect to arrangements, changes in power per unit region, calories consumed, and substantially more. One among the best components of the IoTs inside the consideration business is that the remote well-being watching framework, where patients will be observed and recommended from wherever. Continuous area administrations zone unit is another real approach IoT offers. By exploitation of the administration, specialists will basically follow gadget areas, which straightforwardly diminish overabundance time spent. Cell phone utilization is expanding apace, and people have begun utilizing versatile applications for basically everything. When it includes the consideration business, portable applications will improve correspondences among patients and specialists over a verified association. The essential obligation of Digital Health Advisors and likewise the clinicians will be to figure cooperatively once the association is moving toward IoT-empowered foundation. Right training and input zone unit are essential for higher arrangement.

The standard technique for recording a patient's subtleties, i.e., a stack of paper holding tight the patient's bed, is not intending to work anymore, since such records region unit exclusively available to a confined few and can be lost or complicated. This can be an application with any place on-field portable/tablet innovation may work, since they give bother free record the executives on the applications inside the two gadgets. Well-being learning data will be offered in definitely a spigot when information is recorded electronically, when security and protection issues region unit is met [2].

25 Conclusions

Along with the support of vastly complicated procedure, the medical field has grown up exponentially with good quality in the numerous accomplishment time of handling and makes a diagnosis. Healthcare inspection is typically expanding because of totally unlike IoT capability and instrumentality that must follow a patient‘s health parameters continuously. Because of the crucial nature of healthcare systems, healthcare approach square measure is developed using various thoughts and techniques like distant monitor/diagnostics and air ambulances that are launched in several countries so as to compete with the rapid mounting demands of health care throughout emergencies and speediness aware of patient's recoveries. The identification of the communication procedure and structure plan represents really mesmerizing and complex responsibilities during this perception healthcare inspection necessity to be constant so as to trace the patient's body parameters and deliver consistent and trustworthy information to the health center or the medicinal panel for description. The software system and communications utilized in the medical survey of drugs, likewise as technologies to accumulate, collectively investigated physical condition info, are touted as vital essentials to balance back healthcare prices and conjointly to improve healthcare feature, right to use, and health outcomes.

References

1. Dimitrov DV (2016) medical internet of things and big data in healthcare. Healthc Inform Res 22(3):156
2. Sodhro AH, Pirbhulal S, Sangaiah AK (2018) Convergence of IoT and product lifecycle management in medical health care. Future Gener Comput Syst 86:380–391
3. Kamateri E, Kalampokis E, Tambouris E, Tarabanis K (2014) The linked medical data access control framework. J Biomed Inform 50:213–225
4. Lismont J, Janssens A-S, Odnoletkova I, Broucke S, Caron F, Vanthienen J (2016) A guide for the application of analytics on healthcare processes: a dynamic view on patient pathways. Comput Biol Med 77:125–134
5. Post AR, Kurc T, Cholleti S, Gao J, Lin X, Bornstein W, Cantrell D, Levine D, Hohmann S, Saltz JH (2013) The Analytic Information Warehouse (AIW): a platform for analytics using electronic health record data. J Biomed Inform 46:410–424
6. Oliva SZ, Felipe JC (2018) Optimizing public healthcare management through a data warehousing analytical framework. IFAC PapersOnLine 51(27):407–412

7. Garcelona N, Neurazb A, Salomona R, Faoura H, Benoita V, Delapalmea A, Munnicha A, Burgun A, Rance B (2018) A clinician friendly data warehouse oriented toward narrative reports: Dr. Warehouse. J Biomed Inform 80:52–63
8. Kumar PM, Lokesh S, Varatharajan R, Babu GC, Parthasarathy P (2018) Cloud and IoT based disease prediction and diagnosis system for healthcare using Fuzzy neural classifier. Futur Gener Comput Syst 86:527–534
9. Arun Kumar M, Vimala R, Aravind Britto KR (2019) A cognitive technology based healthcare monitoring system and medical data transmission. Measurement 146:322–332
10. Serbanati LD, Ricci FL, Mercurio G, Vasilateanu A (2011) Steps towards a digital health ecosystem. J Biomed Inform 44:621–636
11. Zeadally S, Bello O (2019) Harnessing the power of Internet of Things based connectivity to improve healthcare. Internet of Things 1–14
12. Jayaratne M, Nallaperuma D, De Silva D, Alahakoon D, Devitt B, Webster KE, Chilamkurti N (2019) A data integration platform for patient-centered e-healthcare and clinical decision support. Futur Gener Comput Syst 92:996–1008
13. Sakra S, Elgammal A (2016) Towards a comprehensive data analytics framework for smart healthcare services. Big Data Res 4:44–58
14. Bello O, Zeadally S (2019) Toward efficient smartification of the Internet of Things (IoT) services. Futur Gener Comput Syst 92:663–673
15. Zanjala SV, Talmaleb GR (2016) Medicine reminder and monitoring system for secure health using IOT. Procedia Comput Sci 78:471–476
16. Davidsona E, Bairdb A, Princec K (2018) Opening the envelope of health care information systems research. Inf Organ 28:140–151
17. Pham T, Tran T, Phung D, Venkatesh S (2017) Predicting healthcare trajectories from medical records: a deep learning approach. J Biomed Inform 69:218–229
18. El Zouka HA, Hosni MM (2014) Secure IoT communications for smart healthcare monitoring system. Research Article
19. Almeida A, Mulero R, Rametta P, Urosevic V, Andric M, Patrono L (2019) A critical analysis of an IoT aware AAL system for elderly monitoring. Futur Gener Comput Syst 97:598–619
20. Kovalchuka SV, Funknera AA, Metskera OG, Yakovleva AN (2018) Simulation of patient flow in multiple healthcare units using process and data mining techniques for model identification. J Biomed Inform 82:128–142
21. Wang T, Huang Z, Gan C (2016) On mining latent topics from healthcare chat logs. J Biomed Inform 61:247–259
22. Lomotey RK, Pry J, Sriramoju S (2017) Wearable IoT data stream traceability in a distributed health information system. Pervasive Mob Comput 40:692–707
23. Batarseh FA, Latif EA (2016) Assessing the quality of service using big data analytics with application to healthcare. Big Data Res 4:13–24
24. Wua J, Li H, Liu L, Zheng H (2017) Adoption of big data and analytics in mobile healthcare market: an economic perspective. Electron Commer Res Appl 22:24–41
25. Wang Y, Kung LA, Wang WYC, Cegielskid CG (2018) An integrated big data analytics-enabled transformation model: application to health care. Inf Manag 55:64–79
26. Abouelmehdi K, Beni-Hssane A, Khaloufi H, Saadi M (2017) Big Data security and privacy in healthcare: a review. Procedia Comput Sci 113:73–80

R. Sujatha completed the Ph.D. degree in Vellore Institute of Technology in 2017 in the area of data mining. She received her M.E. degree in computer science from Anna University in 2009 with university ninth rank and has done Master of Financial Management from Pondicherry University in 2005. She received her B.E. degree in computer science from Madras University in 2001. She has 15 years of teaching experience and has been serving as an Associate Professor in School of Information Technology and Engineering in Vellore Institute of Technology, Vellore. She has organized and attended a number of workshops and faculty development programs. She actively involves in growth of institute by contributing to various committees in both academic and administrative levels. She gives technical talks in colleges for symposium and various sessions. She acts as advisory, editorial member, and technical committee member in conferences conducted in other educational institutions and in-house too. She has published a book titled software project management for the college students. She has also published research articles and papers in reputed journals. She used to guide projects for undergraduate and postgraduate students. She currently guides doctoral students and is interested to explore different places and visit the same to know about the culture and people of various areas. She is interested in learning upcoming things and gets herself acquainted with student's level. Her areas of research interest include Data mining, Machine learning, Image processing, and Management of Information systems.

S. Nathiya is a first year Ph.D. student and Teacher cum Research Assistant in the School of Information Technology and Engineering in Vellore Institute of Technology, Vellore. She received her M.E. degree in Computer Science and Engineering from Kingston Engineering College, Vellore in 2015 and Master of Science Degree in Software Engineering from Sathyabama University, Chennai in 2013 with university third rank. Her doctoral research investigates the Deep Learning approaches.

Jyotir Moy Chatterjee is currently working as an Assistant Professor (IT) at Lord Buddha Education Foundation (Asia Pacific University of Technology & Innovation), Kathmandu, Nepal. Prior to this he worked as an Assistant Professor (CSE) at GD Rungta College of Engineering & Technology (CSVTU), Bhilai, India. He has completed M. Tech in Computer Science and Engineering from Kalinga Institute of Industrial Technology, Bhubaneswar, India and B. Tech in Computer Science and Engineering from Dr. MGR Educational and Research Institute, Chennai, India. He has more than 36 international publications, 2 authored books, 2 edited books, and 2 book chapters in his account. His research interests include the Cloud Computing, Big Data, Privacy Preservation, Data Mining, Internet of Things, Machine Learning, and Blockchain Technology. He is a member of various professional societies and international conferences.

Index

P. Raj et al. (eds.), *Internet of Things Use Cases for the Healthcare Industry*,
https://doi.org/10.1007/978-3-030-37526-3

P

R

S

Printed in the United States
by Baker & Taylor Publisher Services